The Influence of Antibiotics on the Host-Parasite Relationship III

Edited by
G. Gillissen, W. Opferkuch, G. Peters,
and G. Pulverer

With 84 Figures and 100 Tables

Springer-Verlag
Berlin Heidelberg New York
London Paris Tokyo

Professor Dr. Dr. GÜNTHER GILLISSEN
Institut für Medizinische Mikrobiologie
der Medizinischen Fakultät der RWTH Aachen
Pauwelsstrasse, D-5100 Aachen

Professor Dr. WOLFGANG OPFERKUCH
Abteilung für Theoretische und Klinische Medizin
Lehrstuhl für Medizinische Mikrobiologie
Ruhr-Universität Bochum, Universitätsstrasse 150
D-4630 Bochum

Professor Dr. GEORG PETERS
Professor Dr. Dr. h.c. GERHARD PULVERER
Hygiene-Institut der Universität zu Köln
Goldenfelsstrasse 19–21, D-5000 Köln 41

ISBN-13: 978-3-642-73655-1 e-ISBN-13: 978-3-642-73653-7
DOI: 10.1007/978-3-642-73653-7

Library of Congress Cataloging in Publication Data. The Influence of antibiotics on the host-parasite relationship III / edited by G. Gillissen ... [et al.]. p. cm. Papers from proceedings of a conference. Includes bibliographies and index.
1. Host-bacteria relationships – Effect of drug on – Congresses. 2. Antibiotics – Side effects – Congresses. 3. Bacterial diseases–Chemotherapy – Complications and sequelae – Congresses. I. Gillissen, G. [DNLM: 1. Antibiotics-immunology – congresses. 2. Antibiotics-pharmacology – congresses. 3. Bacteria – physiology – congresses. 4. Host-Parasite Relations – congresses. QV 350 I43] QR201.B34I755 1989 615'.329–dc19 DNLM/DLC for Library of Congress 89-4293 CIP

Softcover reprint of the hardcover 1st edition 1989

2127/3130-543210 – Printed on acid-free paper

Preface

When comparing the number of contributions for the proceedings of the third symposium on *The Influence of Antibiotics on the Host–Parasite Relationship* with those of its two predecessors, one becomes aware of the progress that has been made in this field. It is obvious that the design of experiments has substantially refined and therefore the clinical relevance of the results has gained in significance.

The editors of this volume would like to thank all the colleagues who contributed to this book. It is hoped that interest in this field will develop further and that it will finally yield results which one day may be the basis for an improvement of antibiotic therapy.

Bochum WOLFGANG OPFERKUCH

Contents

List of Contributors

Adams, M. K., Lubbock, Texas, USA

Afnan, M., Hamilton, Ontario, Canada

Amaral, L., Bronx, New York, USA

Andres, B., Bochum, Federal Republic of Germany

Babin-Chevaye, C., Paris, France

Bersani, C., Pavia, Italy

Beuth, J., Cologne, Federal Republic of Germany

Blümel, P., Berlin, Federal Republic of Germany

Brasseur, R., Brussels, Belgium

Breuer-Werle, M., Aachen, Federal Republic of Germany

Brown, M. R. W., Birmingham, United Kingdom

Bryskier, A., CHG d'Argenteuil, France

Büscher, K.-H., Darmstadt, Federal Republic of Germany

Chaperon, E. A., Omaha, Nebraska, USA

Ciborowski, P., Warsaw, Poland

Cullen, R. T., Edinburgh, United Kingdom

Domingue, P. A. G., Calgary, Alberta, Canada

Dougherty, S. H., El Paso, Texas, USA

Easmon, C. S. F., London, United Kingdom

Ehlers, S., Berlin, Federal Republic of Germany

Escande, M. C., Paris, France

Fietta, A., Pavia, Italy

Filipp, G., Homburg, Federal Republic of Germany

Forsgren, A., Malmö, Sweden

Friedman, H., Tampa, Florida, USA

Gemmell, C. G:, Glasgow, United Kingdom

Gialdroni-Grassi, G., Pavia, Italy

Giesbrecht, P., Berlin, Federal Republic of Germany

Gillissen, G., Aachen, Federal Republic of Germany

Gmeiner, J., Darmstadt, Federal Republic of Germany

Grassi, F. M., Pavia, Italy

Greening, A., Edinburgh, United Kingdom

Hahn, H., Berlin, Federal Republic of Germany

Hakim, J., Paris, France

Hand, D. L., Atlanta, Georgia, USA

Hand, W. L., Atlanta, Georgia, USA

Haranaka, K., Tokyo, Japan

Haranaka, R., Tokyo, Japan

Hauss, K., Aachen, Federal Republic of Germany

Heim, O., Homburg, , Federal Republic of Germany

Hentges, D. J., Lubbock, Texas, USA

Hessen, M. T., Philadelphia, Pennsylvania, USA

Horn, W., Giessen, Federal Republic of Germany

Hübscher, U., Zürich, Switzerland

Husson, M., Brussels, Belgium

Huynh, U. D., Zürich, Switzerland

Jantzen, R., Giessen, Federal Republic of Germany

Jeljaszewicz, J., Warsaw, Poland

King-Thompson, N. L., Atlanta, Georgia, USA

Klein, T. W., Tampa, Florida, USA

Ko, H. L., Cologne, Federal Republic of Germany

Kroll, H.-P., Wuppertal, Federal Republic of Germany

Labro, M. T., Paris, France

Lagrange, P. H., Paris, France

Lahav, M., Jerusalem, Israel

Levison, M. E., Philadelphia, Pennsylvania, USA

Leying, H., Bochum, Federal Republic of Germany

Lingaas, E., Oslo, Norway

Lorian, V., Bronx, New York, USA
Lücke, J., Heppenheim, Federal Republic of Germany
Mandell, G. L., Charlottesville, Virginia, USA
Mandell, L. A., Hamilton, Ontario, Canada
Marsh, W. W., Lubbock, Texas, USA
Melzer, B., Aachen, Federal Republic of Germany
Midtvedt, T., Stockholm, Sweden
Neftel, K. A., Zürich, Switzerland
Ohshima, Y., Cologne, Federal Republic of Germany
Opferkuch, W., Bochum, , Federal Republic of Germany
Ostendorp, H., Aachen, Federal Republic of Germany
Overbeek, B. P., Utrecht, The Netherlands
Patselas, T. N., Norfolk, Virginia, USA
Peters, G., Cologne, , Federal Republic of Germany
Pfeiffer, R., Cologne, Federal Republic of Germany
Pitsakis, P. G., Philadelphia, Pennsylvania, USA
Poyart-Salmeron, C., Paris, France
Pulverer, G., Cologne, Federal Republic of Germany
Pusztai-Markos, S., Aachen, Federal Republic of Germany
Quie, P. G., Minneapolis, Minnesota, USA
Raeburn, J. A., Edinburgh, United Kingdom
Remington, J. S., Palo Alto, California, USA
Roszkowski, K., Warsaw, Poland
Roszkowski, W., Warsaw, Poland
Ruysschaert, J. M., Brussels, Belgium
Sakurai, A., Tokyo, Japan
Santagada, T., Pavia, Italy
Satomi, N., Tokyo, Japan
Schell-Frederick, E., Cologne, Federal Republic of Germany
Schultze, P., Homburg, Federal Republic of Germany
Schumacher-Perdreau, F., Cologne, Federal Republic of Germany
Schwarz, G., Bochum, Federal Republic of Germany

Schwarzinger, E., Vienna, Austria

Steinberg, T. H., Atlanta, Georgia, USA

Stonnington, A. C., Omaha, Nebraska, USA

Suerbaum, S., Bochum, Federal Republic of Germany

Sullivan, G. W., Charlottesville, Virginia, USA

Sutherland, R., Edinburgh, United Kingdom

Szentivanyi, A., Tampa, Florida, USA

Szentivanyi, J., Tampa, Florida, USA

Thal, W. R., Lubbock, Texas, USA

Van der Auwera, P., Brussels, Belgium

Verhoef, J., Utrecht, The Netherlands

Warren, G., Philadelphia, Pennsylvania, USA

Wecke, J., Berlin, Federal Republic of Germany

Wendt, S., Bochum, Federal Republic of Germany

Wesokowska, B., Warsaw, Poland

Yassin, A., Cologne, Federal Republic of Germany

List of Sponsors

Deutsche Gesellschaft für Hygiene und Mikrobiologie

Paul-Ehrlich-Gesellschaft

Bayer (Leverkusen)

Beecham-Wülfing (Neuß)

Boehringer Mannheim (Mannheim)

Cyanamid-Lederle (Wolfratshausen)

Deutsche Abbott (Wiesbaden)

Eli Lilly (Bad Homburg v. d. H.)

Grünenthal (Stolberg)

v. Heyden (München)

Hoechst (Frankfurt)

Hoffmann La Roche (Grenzach-Wyhlen)

Johnson & Johnson (Düsseldorf)

Kölner Brauereiverband (Köln)

Madaus (Köln)

Merck (Darmstadt)

MSD Sharp + Dohme (München)

Pfizer (Karlsruhe)

Procter & Gamble (Bad Schwalbach/Taunus)

Takeda-Pharma (Stolberg)

Upjohn (Heppenheim)

Opening Remarks

P. G. Quie

I am honored to have this opportunity to welcome all of you to this Third Symposium on "Influence of Antibiotics on the Host-Parasite Relationship" and to participate for these next 3 days in this exciting program. I had the privilege of participating in the planning of this symposium while I was in Cologne last year.

A remarkably stimulating program has been developed which includes discussion of a great variety of microorganisms and examines many aspects of the complex inflammatory and immune response influenced by antimicrobial agents. I am proud I had a little part in the birth of this program.

I note that some of the presentations today directly respond to the admonition of G. B. Shaw to "stimulate the phagocyte," although some indirectly. The influence of subinhibitory concentrations of antibiotics on the capacity of phagocytes to kill bacteria has important clinical implications. This phenomenon appears to be related to the sometimes paradoxical good clinical response of patients to an antimicrobial agent when in vitro sensitivity tests suggest the antibiotic would not be effective. The susceptibility of several bacterial species to the bactericidal actions of phagocytic cells appears to be greatly enhanced by levels of antibiotics which are *not* effective against these organisms in vitro [1]. Demonstration of synergy between antibiotics and the phagocytic system is important, practical information.

Other positive effects of antibiotics on bacteria in addition to inhibition or killing are those described in the last symposium about antibiotics potentiating release of antigens from gram-negative bacteria, resulting in an amplified antibody response and bacterial protoplast formation with increased susceptibility to serum bactericidal factors.

Another major topic of this symposium is the influence of antibiotics on the surface structures of bacteria and relationship of these changes to adherence of bacteria to host surfaces. Since attachment is a necessary first step in colonization and persistence of bacteria, influence of antibiotics on lectins and other adhesins is especially important. The many actions of penicillin on streptococci, for example, include loss of surface lipoteichoic acid, a primary streptococcal adhesion. A similar loss of adherence of *E. coli* has also been demonstrated using subinhibitory concentrations of antibiotics. Lectin-related adherence of these organisms is compromised by antibiotics [2]. The successful prevention of recurrences of rheu-

University of Minnesota, Department of Pediatrics, Medical School, Box 483, Mayo Memorial Building, Minneapolis, MN 55455, USA

The Influence of Antibiotics on the Host-Parasite Relationship III
Edited by G. Gillissen, W. Opferkuch, G. Peters, and G. Pulverer

matic fever with exquisitely low doses of penicillin and clearing of urinary tract infection with single-dose antibiotic therapy may be related to effect of antibiotics on adherence of bacteria to mucosal surfaces.

We are experiencing an increase in rheumatic fever in the United States now which is an interesting phenomenon since even after 40 years of use there is no epidemiologic evidence of increased resistance of group A streptococci to penicillin. A streptococcal type M-18 has been associated with several of the cases of rheumatic fever in the United States and an interesting characteristic of this strain is that it grows as a "matted" or mucoid colony form.

A colleague of Jan Verhoef, Frank Visseren, is in our laboratory at Minnesota this summer and is conducting a series of experiments examining the mucoid group A streptococcal strains that have been associated with rheumatic fever. These strains are nearly totally resistant to phagocytosis, in contrast to strains of a similar M type which are not mucoid. There is less attachment to phagocytic cells. As you may know, uptake of surface-attached group A streptococci is quite efficient in the absence of opsonin. Uptake of mucoid streptococci does not occur and the most important host defense system is circumvented.

It is interesting that Isaac Ginsburg reported a few years ago that subinhibitory concentrations of penicillin result in increased hyaluronic acid capsular production by group A streptococci. Is it possible that group A streptococcal persistence is increased because of the survival advantage of mucoid strains with hyaluronic acid capsules? Have these strains increased because of the widespread use of penicillin?

Jack Remington and William Hauser reviewed the direct effect of antibiotics on the immune system 7 years ago and concluded that in most cases clinical correlations could not be made between direct effect of antibiotics on the immune system and susceptibility to infection [3]. More carefully controlled studies in humans are needed to define the clinical significance of antibiotic-mediated immunomodulation.

It will be interesting to learn at this meeting how much progress has been made in correlating in vitro observations on direct effect of antibiotics on isolated parts of the immune system with clinical response to therapy. The symposium program includes discussion of several clinical conditions including cystic fibrosis, malignancy, and primary immunodeficiency in which the patients' very life depends on antimicrobial agents. The welfare of these patients is the goal of the research all of us are involved with, and knowledge of the role of antibiotics on bacterial attachment mechanisms to surfaces and interactions with the phagocytic system and effect on specific adaptive immunity are profoundly important. The very duration of life for these patients depends on this knowledge. Since immunodeficiency accompanies the aging process, this knowledge has a direct personal interest for each of us as well. I am looking forward with great anticipation to the next 3 days.

References

1. Gemmell CG (1984) Potentiation of phagocytosis of pathogenic bacteria by exposure to low concentration of antibiotics. J Antimicrob Chemother 13:407
2. Hauser WE, Remington JS (1982) Effect of antibiotics on the humoral and cell-mediated immune responses. In: LD Sabath (ed) Action of antibiotics in patients. Hans Huber, Stuttgart, pp 127–147
3. Eisenstein BI, Ofek I, Beachey EH (1981) Loss of lectin-like activity in aberrant type I fimbriae of *Escherichia coli*. Infect Immun 31:792–797

Interactions Between Antibiotics, Phagocytes, and Bacteria *

W. L. HAND, N. L. KING-THOMPSON, T. H. STEINBERG, and D. L. HAND

Antibiotics have biological effects other than direct antimicrobial activity (i.e., other than growth inhibition or killing of organisms). We have been especially interested in the ability of antimicrobial agents to interact with phagocytes and to influence the fate of bacteria ingested by these cells. A major reason for this interest is that survival, and even multiplication, of pathogenic organisms after ingestion by phagocytes may lead to chronic or progressive disease [1, 2]. Bacteria which fully exhibit this capability include *Mycobacterium tuberculosis* and *Legionella pneumophila.* To a lesser extent many bacteria, including *Salmonella* and *Staphylococcus aureus,* can manifest intraphagocytic survival. The efficacy of an antibiotic in therapy of infections, especially those due to facultative intracellular organisms, will depend upon both the extracellular drug-bacterial interaction and the capacity of the antibiotic to penetrate phagocytes and influence the functions of host cells and organisms. Thus, it is important to study the interactions between antibiotics, phagocytes, and bacteria in detail. In an effort to define certain of these interactions we have studied: the uptake of antimicrobial agents by various phagocytic cells, the mechanisms of this entry process for specific antibiotics, the effects of certain factors (phagocytosis, smoking) on drug uptake, the influence of antibiotics on survival of intraphagocytic bacteria, and the consequences of exposure to antibiotics on phagocyte oxidative metabolism.

Materials and Methods

Collection of Phagocytic Cells

Rabbit alveolar macrophages (AMs) were collected from the lower respiratory tract of normal New Zealand rabbits as previously described [3]. Human AMs from cigarette smokers (healthy or with pulmonary disease) and from healthy nonsmokers were obtained by bronchoalveolar lavage during fiberoptic bronchoscopy [4, 5]. Human polymporphonuclear leukoytes (PMNs) and monocytes were isolated from peripheral blood by dextran sedimentation and Hypaque-Ficoll density gradient centrifugation [6, 7]. Separation of monocytes from lym-

* Veterans Administeration Medical Center (Atlanta), Decatur, and the Department of Medicine, Emory University School of Medicine, 69 Butler St., S.E., Atlanta, GA 30303, USA.
This work was supported by the Medical Research Service of the Veterans Administration

The Influence of Antibiotics on the Host-Parasite Relationship III
Edited by G. Gillissen, W. Opferkuch, G. Peters, and G. Pulverer

phocytes was accomplished by centrifugation on Nycodenz monocytes (Nyegaard, Oslo) [8]. Total and differential cell counts, as well as viability assays, were performed as previously described [6, 9].

Antibiotic Uptake by Phagocytes

The following radiolabeled antibiotics were used in our studies: [^{14}C]rifampin; clindamycin-[^{3}H]HCl; lincomycin-[^{3}H]HCl; chloramphenicol [dichenoactyl-1-2 ^{14}C]; tetracycline [7-^{3}H(N)]; benzyl [^{14}C]penicillin potassium; cephalexin [^{14}C]; cefazolin [^{14}C]; cefamandole [^{14}C]nafate; [thiazolyl-2-^{14}C]cefotaxime; [ring-2-^{14}C]imipenem; [^{14}C]erythromycin; [^{14}C]erythromycin propionate; [^{14}C]roxithromycin (RU 965); [G-^{3}H]isoniazid; [G-^{3}H]gentamicin sulfate; [^{14}C]ethambutol dihydrochloride; [^{14}C]metronidazole; and [^{3}H]trimethoprim. These preparations were provided by pharmaceutical companies or purchased from commercial sources.

Phagocytes were suspended in tissue culture medium 199 (TC 199) at a concentration of 1×10^{7} cells/ml (5×10^{6} cells/ml for human AMs). The cells were incubated with clinically appropriate concentrations of radiolabeled antibiotics ($\sim 2.5 \times 10^{-5}$ *M*). At intervals, 0.2-ml aliquots of the incubation mixture were removed, and the phagocytic cells with their associated antibiotic were separated from the extracellular antibiotic solution by velocity-gradient centrifugation [Beckman Microfuge B] in a microcentrifuge tube [3–6, 10, 11]. Cellular uptake of antibiotics was determined by centrifugation of phagocytes through a water-impermeable silicone oil barrier into formic acid, which dissolves the cells. The contents of the tubes were then frozen, and the frozen layers were separated by slicing the tubes with a razor. The radioactive content of the lower layer, containing the radiolabeled antibiotic which was taken up by the cells, and the upper layer, containing the antibiotic which was still in solution, was determined in a liquid scintillation counter. Antibiotic uptake was expressed as the ratio of the cellular concentration of antibiotic to the extracellular concentration (C/E). A ratio of >1 indicates a selective concentration of antibiotic within the phagocyte. A value of less than 1 implies poor penetration of antibiotic into the cell.

Characterization of Antibiotic Uptake and Membrane Transport

First, we examined the environmental and metabolic requirements of the uptake process for those antibiotics which enter phagocytes readily. Thus, the influences of cell viability, environmental temperature, pH, and metabolic inhibitors on antibiotic accumulation by macrophages and PMNs were examined [3, 4, 6, 10, 12].

Kinetic analysis of antibiotic uptake during the initial exposure of phagocytes to the drug was performed. Cells were exposed to a wide range of radiolabeled antibiotic concentrations for 45 s. Velocity of transport was determined for each concentration, and a double-reciprocal (Lineweaver-Burk) plot of uptake velocity versus drug concentration data was constructed. This allowed calculation of the maximal velocity (rate) of uptake (V_{max}) and the apparent binding affinity (K_m) for these transport systems [6, 10, 12].

Phagocytes have specific carrier-mediated membrane transport systems for hexoses, amino acids, and nucleosides. Therefore, we examined the possibility that one or more of these systems might transport the tested antibiotics into PMNs and macrophages [10–12]. Potential inhibitors (L-amino acids, D-glucose, nucleosides) were preincubated with phagocytes for 20 min prior to determination of radiolabeled antibiotic uptake.

Next, we evaluated the influence of phagocytosis and other membrane stimulation on antibiotic accumulation by phagocytes [11–14]. PMNs (1×10^7 cells/ml) were incubated with ingestible particles (opsonized zymosan or *S. aureus*) or with a soluble membrane-perturbating agent FMLP (n-formyl-methionyl-leucyl-phenylalanine), Con A (Concanavalin A), or PMA (phorbol-12-myristate-13-acetate) for 30 min at 37 °C, washed and resuspended in TC 199, after which antibiotic uptake was determined.

Antibiotics and Intraphagocytic Bactericidal Activity

The influence of antibiotics on survival of intraphagocytic *S. aureus* was determined by means of a modified phagocytic-bactericidal assay [13–15]. In these experiments the antimicrobial agent was added after the ingestion of antibiotic-sensitive, radiolabeled *S. aureus*. PMNs (5×10^6 cells) were incubated with 2×10^7 to 3×10^7 radiolabeled *S. aureus*. After the phagocytosis period (60 min), radioactive and bacterial counts were determined on leukocyte pellets from some tubes. After washing, the remaining leukocytes were suspended in fresh media, in the presence or absence of antibiotics, and incubated for an additional period. At 1 and 3 h samples were removed for quantitation of viable intracellular (and any extracellular) bacteria.

Effects of Nucleosides and Antibiotics on Oxidative Metabolism of PMN

We examined the consequences of phagocyte exposure to antimicrobial agents on oxidative killing mechanisms in these cells [16]. Superoxide generation by human PMNs was determined as superoxide dismutase (SOD)-inhibitable reduction of ferricytochrome C [17–19]. PMNs (2×10^6 cells/3 ml) in Hank's balanced salt solution (HBSS) containing 100 μM ferricytochrome C were preincubated with or without antibiotics or nucleosides. Cytochalasin B and the stimulating agent (zymosan, *S. aureus*, FMLP, PMA, or Con A) or control media were added, followed by additional incubation and determination of optical density (OD) at 550 nm. Duplicate samples contained SOD. Hydrogen peroxide release was measured by the extinction of scopoletin fluorescence during its oxidation by horseradish peroxidase [20, 21]. Nucleosides or antibiotics were added to half of the tubes in each assay system. Baseline recordings in the spectrofluorometer (excitation wavelength 350 nm and emission wavelength 460 nm) were made for several minutes before addition of stimulating agents.

Results

Antibiotic Uptake by Phagocytes

Antibiotics varied greatly in their abilities to enter phagocytic cells. However, the relative entries of drug groups into the various phagocytes were similar even though the absolute values differed between phagocytes [3–6, 12]. Beta-lactam antibiotics (penicillin G, cephalosporins) and gentamicin were taken up poorly by all phagocytic cells (Table 1). Thus, the cellular levels of these drugs were lower than the extracellular concentrations ($C/E<1$). Metronidazole and isoniazid achieved cellular levels which were equal to or somewhat less than the extracellular levels. More lipid-soluble antibiotics, such as rifampin and chloramphenicol, entered cells to a greater degree than the agents already mentioned. These drugs were concentrated severalfold by phagocytes ($C/E=2$–5). Tetracycline, which is also rather lipid soluble, reached cellular levels equal to or greater than the extracellular concentration. In comparison with the other antibiotics tested, ethambutol, two erythromycin preparations, clindamycin, trimethoprim, and roxithromycin (RU 965) were avidly concentrated by all of the phagocytic cells ($C/E=5$–49) [3–6, 12].

Clindamycin uptake was especially rapid and was maximal in 15–30 min (Fig. 1) [3–6, 10, 11]. Roxithromycin was also taken up rapidly by human PMNs and monocytes (the only cells evaluated thus far) and was concentrated to a greater degree by these phagocytes than any of the other antibiotics we have studied [12].

Table 1. Uptake of antibiotics by normal phagocytes (C/E). [3–6, 12]

Ratio of cellular to extracellular concentration				
Antibiotic	Rabbit	Human phagocytes		
	AMs	AMs	PMNs	Monocytes
Penicillin	0.07	0.9	0.4	0.8
Cefamandole	0,4	0.8	< 0.01	1
Cefazolin	0.08	–	< 0.01	–
Cefotaxime	–	–	0.1	–
Gentamicin	0.6	1	0.3	1
Isoniazid	0.9	1	1	–
Metronidazole	–	–	1	–
Tetracycline	0.9	4	–	–
Rifampin	2	5	2	–
Chloramphenicol	2	2	3	3
Ethambutol	7	4	5	–
Trimethoprim	–	–	8	4
Erythromycin	21	18	13	–
Erythromycin propionate	32	16	10	5
Clindamycin	49	24	11	8
Roxithromycin	–	–	34	15

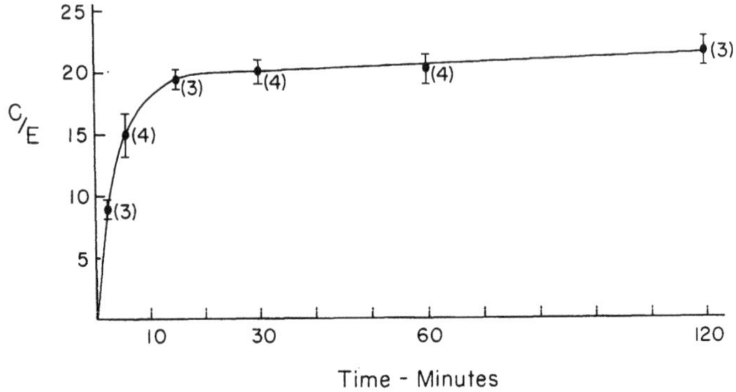

Fig. 1. Uptake of clindamycin (*C/E*) by human alveolar macrophages from healthy nonsmokers. Results are presented as the mean ± SEM values and numbers of observations at each time point

Table 2. Antibiotic uptake (C/E) by human AMs from smokers and nonsmokers. [4, 5]

Antibiotic	Nonsmokers	Smokers
Penicillin G	0.8	0.5
Gentamicin	1.0	1.2
Isoniazid	1.0	1.4
Lincomycin	2.9	3.5
Chloramphenicol	2.0	3.9
Rifampin	5.2	9.8
Ethambutol	4.3	5.4
Erythromycin propionate	15.9	28.1
Clindamycin	23.5	56.1

It is of interest that human alveolar macrophages from cigarette smokers, most of whom had pulmonary disease, accumulated certain antibiotics more readily than did macrophages from nonsmokers [4, 5]. Thus, rifampin, erythromycin, and clindamycin attained significantly higher levels in smoker's alveolar macrophages (Table 2).

Characterization of Antibiotic Uptake and Membrane Transport

We evaluated the environmental and metabolic requirements of the uptake process for erythromycin, clindamycin, and roxithromycin, those antibiotics which are most efficiently concentrated by phagocytes. Cellular uptake of these drugs was dependent upon cell viability and a physiological environmental temperature (Table 3) [3, 4, 6, 10, 12]. Unlike these antibiotics, trimethoprim entered PMNs more readily at 25 °C than at 37 °C [12]. Next, inhibitors of cellular metabolism were examined for their effect on antibiotic accumulation. It is of note that in each type of phagocytic cell the inhibitors of the predominant energy source depressed

Table 3. Influences of cell viability and environmental temperature on entry of clindamycin, erythromycin propionate, roxithromycin, and trimethoprim into human PMNs. [6, 12]

Experimental group (incubation temperature)[a]	C/E			
	Clindamycin	Erythromycin propionate	Roxithromycin	Trimethoprim
Viable cells (37 °C)	10.5	6.8	31.4	8.2
Viable cells (25 °C)	7.2	3.5	23.6	12.8
Viable cells (4 °C)	0.6	0.5	0.9	6.0
Dead cells (37 °C)	2.5	2.6	6.4	1.9

[a] Incubations were for 60 min.

antibiotic uptake. Thus, sodium cyanide and 2,4 dinitrophenol, inhibitors of mitochondrial oxidative respiration, depressed clindamycin and erythromycin uptake in rabbit and human alveolar macrophages [3, 4, 10]. In contrast potassium fluoride, which inhibits glycolysis, decreased clindamycin entry into human PMNs [6, 11]. In a somewhat different fashion, both cyanide and fluoride modestly decreased roxithromycin entry into phagocytes [12].

Kinetic analyses of clindamycin (rabbit AMs, human PMNs) and roxithromycin (human PMNs) uptake were performed [6, 10, 12]. Uptake of both drugs displayed saturation kinetics, characteristic of carrier-mediated systems. The system transporting clindamycin has a high binding constant ($K_m = 2$ mM in PMNs), i.e., a low binding affinity, and a high rate of uptake ($V_{max} = 5$ nmol/45 s per 10^6 PMNs) for the drug [6]. Comparable values for roxithromycin uptake in PMNs were $K_m = 238$ μM and $V_{max} = 1.43$ nmol/min per 10^6 cells [12].

Since macrophages and PMNs have specific carrier-mediated systems for hexoses, amino acids, and nucleosides, we evaluated the possibility that clindamycin and macrolide antibiotics (erythromycin, roxithromycin) might enter phagocytes by one or more of these systems [10–12). Clindamycin transport was not altered in the presence of hexoses or amino acids, but was inhibited by nucleosides (e.g., adenosine) in a manner typical of competitive inhibition. Conversely, clindamycin inhibits nucleoside transport in a competitive fashion [10, 11]. Thus, clindamycin is transported into macrophages and PMNs by the cell membrane nucleoside system. In spite of considerable effort, we still do not have a clear idea of how the macrolide antibiotics (erythromycin, roxithromycin), which are actively accumulated by phagocytes, actually enter these cells. We do know that entry of erythromycin and roxithromycin into PMNs was greater in studies performed in HBSS as compared with TC 199. This observation suggested that components of the complex tissue culture medium inhibited entry of the macrolides. No single component of TC 199 completely reproduced the inhibitory effect of the complete medium ([12]; W.L. Hand and N.L. King-Thompson, unpublished observations).

The consequences of ingesting microbial particles or exposure to PMA on clindamycin uptake by PMNs were striking [11, 13, 14]. After ingestion of opsonized zymosan particles or *S. aureus*, cells concentrated clindamycin to a much

Table 4. Effect of *S. aureus* or zymosan ingestion on antibiotic uptake (C/E) by human PMNs. [11–14]

Antibiotic	PMNs (control)	PMNs + *S. aureus*	PMNs + zymosan
Clindamycin	11	19	30
Erythromycin	12	11	–
Erythromycin propionate	15	–	11
Roxithromycin	34	22	28
Rifampin	4	5	6
Gentamicin	0.7	0.5	–
Penicillin	0.5	0.3	0.6

greater degree, reaching C/E values of 30 and 19 respectively [11]. PMA also stimulated clindamycin uptake by PMNs. Since clindamycin uptake by phagocytes is mediated by the nucleoside transport system, we studied adenosine uptake after phagocytosis. Adenosine uptake reached a C/E of 2 in control PMNs, but this increased to a C/E of 6 after zymosan ingestion and a C/E of 4 after phagocytosis of *S. aureus*. The presence of clindamycin inhibited the phagocytosis-enhanced uptake of adenosine [11].

These experiments documented that clindamycin uptake (mediated by the nucleoside transport system) as well as nucleoside transport per se were augmented by phagocytosis in PMNs. However, phagocytosis and other membrane perturbation does not stimulate antibiotic uptake by PMNs in a nonspecific fashion. Rifampin uptake ($C/E = 4$ in controls) increased slightly after ingestion of zymosan or *S. aureus* ($C/E = 5$–6) [13, 14]. In contrast, entry of macrolide antibiotics into PMNs was slightly decreased after phagocytosis [11–13]. For example, after ingestion of *S. aureus*, C/E values for roxithromycin decreased from 34 to 22 [12]. The entries of penicillin G and gentamicin into PMNs were unaffected by particle ingestion (Table 4) [11, 13].

Antibiotics and Intraphagocytic Bactericidal Activity

The obvious next step was to examine the consequences of antibiotic uptake by phagocytes on subsequent intracellular bactericidal activity. These studies to date have been performed in human PMNs [13, 14], and to a limited extent in rabbit alveolar macrophages (W. L. Hand and N. L. King-Thompson, unpublished observations), and we will summarize them briefly. For experiments in PMNs we used five antibiotics which differ markedly in their ability to enter phagocytes [13]. These antibiotics were clindamycin, erythromycin, rifampin, gentamicin, and penicillin G. PMNs were incubated in the presence or absence of antibiotics after ingestion of *S. aureus*. The most striking aspect of the study was the discrepancy between antibiotic entry into phagocytes and the effect of this drug uptake on intraphagocytic bactericidal activity. Of particular interest was the finding that clindamycin, which is markedly concentrated by phagocytes, had little influence on intracellular survival of organisms ingested by human PMNs and rabbit AMs (Table 5, Fig. 2) [13, 14].

Table 5. Effect of antibiotics on the survival of *S. aureus* ingested by human PMNs. [13]

Experimental group	Number of viable *S. aureus*		
	Start (0 time)	1 h	3 h
Bacteria only	$1.2 \pm 0.2 \times 10^6$	$1.5 \pm 0.2 \times 10^6$	$4.4 \pm 1.0 \times 10^7$
PMN control	$1.4 \pm 0.2 \times 10^6$	$8.1 \pm 1.1 \times 10^5$	$5.7 \pm 0.8 \times 10^5$
PMNs + antibiotic	$1.4 \pm 0.2 \times 10^6$		
Clindamycin		$5.2 \pm 1.1 \times 10^5$ $P=0.09$	$3.4 \pm 0.7 \times 10^5$ $P=0.07$
Erythromycin		$5.9 \pm 0.9 \times 10^5$ $P=0.17$	$5.2 \pm 2.1 \times 10^5$ $P=0.81$
Rifampin		$3.3 \pm 0.7 \times 10^5$ $P=0.02$	$2.3 \pm 0.5 \times 10^5$ $P=0.03$
Penicillin		$7.3 \pm 1.2 \times 10^5$ $P=0.70$	$6.0 \pm 1.3 \times 10^5$ $P=0.85$
Gentamicin		$1.8 \pm 0.3 \times 10^5$ $P=0.0008$	$7.0 \pm 0.1 \times 10^4$ $P=0.0002$

P values reflect differences between control (PMNs only) and experimental (PMNs+antibiotic) groups.

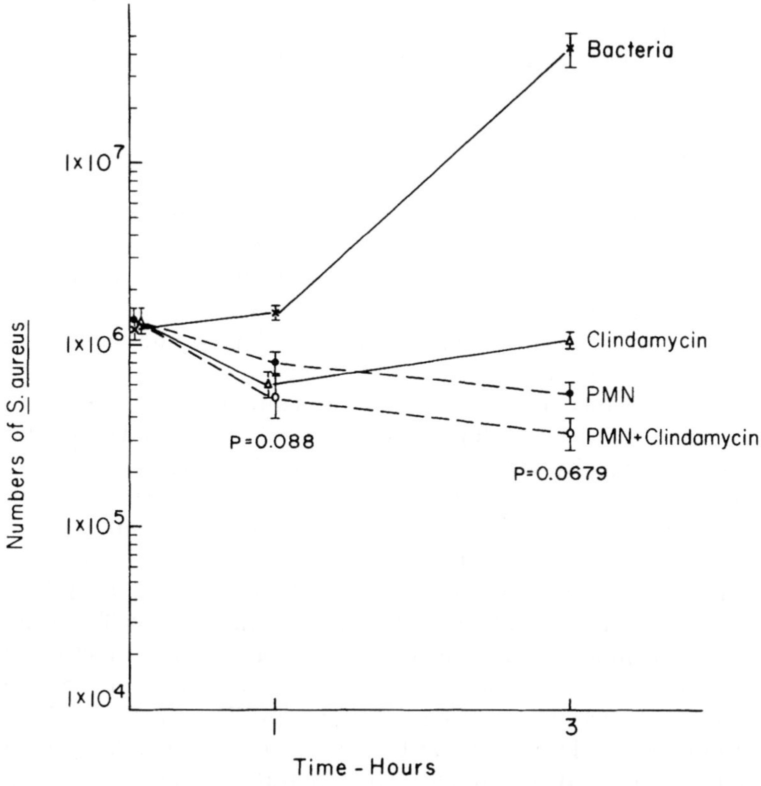

Fig. 2. Influence of clindamycin on the viability of *S. aureus* ingested by PMNs or in the absence of phagocytes. Results are expressed as the mean ± SEM of observations at each time point. *P* values reflect differences between control (PMNs only) and experimental (PMNs+antibiotic) groups

Effects of Nucleosides and Antibiotics on Oxidative Metabolism of PMNs

Human PMNs incubated in the presence or absence of nucleosides or antibiotics were exposed to substances which stimulate oxidative respiratory burst activity and degranulation [16]. Adenosine, certain other nucleosides, and clindamycin inhibited superoxide and H_2O_2 generation, but not degranulation, by PMNs stimulated by microbial particles, FMLP, or Con A. Neither nucleosides nor clindamycin decreased the oxidative respiratory burst stimulated by PMA, which, in contrast to other activators of the respiratory burst in PMNs, bypasses receptor-related mechanisms of activation and directly stimulates protein kinase C. The accumulated evidence strongly suggests that inhibition of the oxidative respiratory burst by both nucleosides and clindamycin may be mediated via the binding of cell membrane nucleoside receptors.

Unlike clindamycin, other antibiotics, including erythromycin, chloramphenicol, lincomycin, gentamicin, and penicillin G, had little effect on stimulated superoxide production in PMNs [16]. Very recently we have documented that two other antibiotics – roxithromycin and trimethoprim – inhibit oxidative metabolism in PMNs. These two antibiotics, as well as clindamycin, also block stimulated superoxide production in human peripheral blood monocytes (W. L. Hand and D. L. Hand, unpublished observations).

Discussion

An ideal antibiotic would not only be active against extracellular bacteria but would enter phagocytic cells and eradicate the surviving intracellular organisms. Unfortunately, intraphagocytic organisms are protected from the action of certain antimicrobial agents (e.g., [22–27]). With these points in mind, we have attempted to establish those characteristics of drugs and cells that determine the interactions between antibiotics and phagocytes.

It is obvious that entry of antibiotics into phagocytic cells is a prerequisite for activity against intracellular organisms. Thus, we studied the uptake of antimicrobial agents by several populations of phagocytic cells – rabbit AMs, human AMs from smokers and nonsmokers, and human peripheral blood PMNs and monocytes [3–6, 12]. Relative entries of drug groups into the various phagocytes were similar, although absolute values differed considerably. Beta-lactam antibiotics and gentamicin entered phagocytes poorly. Lipid-soluble drugs such as rifampin and chloramphenicol were concentrated severalfold (due to simple solubility partition) by all phagocytes. Ethambutol and trimethoprim were concentrated four- to eightfold by phagocytic cells but the entry mechanisms for these drugs are unclear and apparently complex. The most remarkable feature of the antibiotic uptake studies was the striking entry of clindamycin and three macrolide antibiotics (two erythromycin preparations and roxithromycin) into all types of phagocytic cells. These antibiotics reached cellular concentrations which were from 5–50 times the extracellular levels. Uptake of these drugs was found to require active, energy-dependent transport [3, 4, 6, 10, 12]. In the case of clindamycin, the mechanism for the avid concentration by phagocytes was identified as the cell membrane nucleoside transport system [10, 11]. As yet we have been unable to identify the means by which macrolides enter phagocytic cells [12].

It is of interest that human alveolar macrophages from cigarette smokers, most of whom had pulmonary disease, accumulated certain antibiotics more efficiently than did macrophages from nonsmokers [4, 5]. Thus, rifampin, erythromycin, and clindamycin attained significantly higher levels in smokers' alveolar macrophages. It is probable that cigarette smoking per se causes these changes, since the known structural and functional alterations observed in alveolar macrophages from healthy smokers could account for the augmented accumulation of specific antibiotics. Thus, the increased lipid content of smokers' macrophages may enhance uptake of rifampin (a lipid-soluble drug) by these cells. Stimulated metabolic pathways and altered membrane function in smokers' AMs might account for the increased uptake of erythromycin and clindamycin, antibiotics which enter phagocytes by active cell membrane transport systems.

Since a number of pathogens may persist within phagocytes, we felt it was important to evaluate the entry of antibiotics into these cells under conditions which mimic in vivo infection. Ingestion of microbial particles stimulated the entry of clindamycin (and rifampin slightly) but not of other antibiotics, into PMNs [11, 13, 14]. Indeed, erythromycin and roxithromycin uptake by PMNs was decreased after phagocytosis, but cellular levels of these drugs remained quite high [11–13].

Obviously, the next step was to examine the consequences of antibiotic uptake by phagocytes on intracellular bactericidal activity. The most striking finding in that study was the discrepancy between this antibiotic entry into phagocytes and the subsequent effect of drug uptake on intraphagocytic bactericidal activity. For our purposes it is especially noteworthy that clindamycin, which is avidly concentrated by all of the phagocytic cells, had little influence on the intracellular survival of sensitive *S. aureus* ingested by rabbit AMs and human PMNs [13, 14].

There are a number of possible explanations for this phenomenon. The intrinsic antibacterial properties of an antibiotic are probably crucial in determining the intraphagocytic activity of the drug. In the case of clindamycin, an important factor might be the native inability of this bacteriostatic antibiotic to kill the organism. However, the intracellular clindamycin concentration in both AMs and PMNs exceeded the MBC (minimum bactericidal concentration) for the test strain of *S. aureus*. Therefore, the possibility that clindamycin might adversely influence phagocyte antibacterial function was considered. A theoretical basis for an inhibitory effect of clindamycin on phagocyte antimicrobial function does exist. As we have shown, clindamycin enters phagocytes by means of the cell membrane nucleoside transport system. Since nucleosides (especially adenosine) may play a role in regulating the generation of superoxide by activated human PMNs, via binding of membrane nucleoside receptors [28, 29], we thought it possible that clindamycin might influence oxidative metabolism in a similar manner. Such inhibition of oxidative antibacterial function might, at least in part, account for the failure of clindamycin to kill intraphagocytic bacteria. Human PMNs incubated in the presence or absence of nucleosides or antibiotics were exposed to substances which stimulate oxidative respiratory burst activity and degranulation. Adenosine, certain other nucleosides, and clindamycin inhibited superoxide and H_2O_2 generation, but not degranulation, by PMNs stimulated by microbial particles, FMLP, or Con A. Neither nucleosides nor clindamycin decreased the oxidative respiratory burst stimulated by PMA which, in contrast to other activators of the respiratory burst in PMNs, bypasses receptor-related mechanisms of activation and directly stimulates protein kinase C [30]. The accumulated evidence strongly suggests that inhibition of the oxidative respiratory burst by both nucleosides and clindamycin may be mediated via the binding of cell membrane nucleoside receptors.

Unlike clindamycin, other antibiotics, including lincomycin, erythromycin, chloramphenicol, gentamicin, and penicillin G, had little effect on stimulated superoxide production in PMNs. In current ongoing studies we have documented that two of the most recent antibiotics we have studied – roxithromycin and trimethoprim – inhibit oxidative metabolism in PMNs. These two antibiotics, as well as clindamycin, also block stimulated superoxide production in human peripheral blood monocytes (W. L. Hand and D. L. Hand, unpublished observations). It seems unlikely that roxithromycin and trimethoprim influence oxidative respiratory burst activity via cell membrane nucleoside receptors, the postulated mechanism for clindamycin inhibition. We are currently investigating other possible mechanisms of action for these antibiotics. Whatever the mechanism, the possibility that this inhibition of oxidative antimicrobial function might interfere with the ability of phagocytes to kill ingested organisms is of concern. We are now investigating the consequences of antibiotic-mediated alteration of phagocyte activity in respect to antimicrobial function.

Antibiotic entry into phagocytes is only one of the factors which determine a drug's activity against intracellular organisms. Intraphagocytic antibiotic function is undoubtedly determined by multiple factors. Such factors might include: (1) specific location and local concentration of the drug, (2) the agent's intrinsic antibacterial properties (mechanism of action, type of activity), (3) influence of the intracellular environment on biological activity of the antibiotic and susceptibility of the organism, and (4) the drug's effect on phagocyte cellular function (e.g., cell movement, microbicidal systems, phagocytosis). Many of these factors are difficult to evaluate, and our own studies to date have not addressed each of these points directly.

In conclusion, it is apparent that the interactions of antibiotics with organisms and phagocytes are interesting, important, and complex. Much work remains if we are to understand these relationships clearly.

Summary

Antibiotic efficacy in therapy of infections due to facultative intracellular bacteria will depend in part on the ability of the drugs to enter and influence the functions of host cells and organisms. To better define these interactions we studied the uptake of radiolabeled antibiotics by rabbit and human alveolar macrophages (AMs), human polymorphonuclear leukocytes (PMNs), and human monocytes. Penicillin G, cephalosporins, metronidazole, and gentamicin were taken up poorly by phagocytes. Lipid-soluble antibiotics, such as rifampin and chloramphenicol, were concentrated severalfold by phagocytes. Clindamycin, two erythromycin preparations, and roxithromycin were markedly concentrated (10- to 50-fold) by phagocytes. Uptake of these drugs was shown to be by active cell membrane transport systems. Human alveolar macrophages from cigarette smokers accumulated certain antibiotics (rifampin, erythromycin, and clindamycin) more efficiently than did macrophages from nonsmokers. Ingestion of microbial particles markedly stimulated the entry of clindamycin, but not other antibiotics, into PMNs. A striking finding was the discrepancy between antibiotic entry into phagocytes and the subsequent effect of this drug uptake on intraphagocytic bactericidal activity. Clindamycin, which is avidly concentrated by PMNs, had little influence on the intracellular survival of sensitive *S. aureus*. Therefore, we considered the possibility that clindamycin, which enters phagocytes by the cell membrane nucleoside transport system, might inhibit PMN oxidative antibacterial function in a manner similar to that demonstrated for nucleosides. Indeed, clindamycin, as well as roxithromycin and certain nucleosides, did inhibit superoxide and H_2O_2 production by stimulated PMNs. A number of other antibiotics had no effect on the oxidative respiratory burst. The potential biological significance of this antibiotic-mediated alteration of phagocyte oxidative activity requires elucidation.

Acknowledgment. We thank Brenda Bagwell for preparation of the manuscript.

References

1. Horwitz MA (1982) Phagocytosis of microorganisms. Rev Infect Dis 4:104–123
2. WHO Scientific Group (1973) Cell-mediated immunity and resistance to infection. Int Arch Allergy Appl Immunol 44:589–648
3. Johnson JD, Hand WL, Francis JB, King-Thompson NL, Corwin RW (1980) Antibiotic uptake by alveolar macrophages. J Lab Clin Med 95:429–439
4. Hand WL, Corwin RW, Steinberg TH, Grossman GD (1984) Uptake of antibiotics by human alveolar macrophages. Am Rev Respir Dis 129:933–937
5. Hand WL, Boozer RM, King-Thompson NL (1985) Antibiotic uptake by alveolar macrophages of smokers. Antimicrob Agents Chemother 27:42–45
6. Prokesch RC, Hand WL (1982) Antibiotic entry into human polymorphonuclear leukocytes. Antimicrob Agents Chemother 21:373–380
7. Boyum A (1976) Isolation of lymphocytes, granulocytes and macrophages. Scand J Immunol Suppl 5:9–15
8. Boyum A (1984) Separation of lymphocytes, granulocytes, and monocytes from human blood using iodinated density gradient media. Methods Enzymol 108:88–102
9. Cantey JR, Hand WL (1974) Cell-mediated immunity after bacterial infection of the lower respiratory tract. J Clin Invest 54:1125–1134
10. Hand WL, King-Thompson NL (1982) Membrane transport of clindamycin in alveolar macrophages. Antimicrob Agents Chemother 21:241–247
11. Steinberg TH, Hand WL (1984) Effects of phagocytosis on antibiotic and nuceloside uptake by human polymorphonuclear leukocytes. J Infect Dis 149:397–403
12. Hand WL, King-Thompson NL, Holman JW (1987) Entry of roxithromycin (RU 965), imipenem, cefotaxime, trimethoprim, and metronidazole into human polymorphonuclear leukocytes. Antimicrob Agents Chemother 31:1553–1557
13. Hand WL, King-Thompson NL (1986) Contrasts between phagocyte antibiotic uptake and subsequent intracellular bactericidal activity. Antimicrob Agents Chemother 29:135–140

14. Steinberg TH, Hand WL (1987) Effect of phagocyte membrane stimulation on antibiotic uptake and intracellular bactericidal activity. Antimicrob Agents Chemother 31:660–662
15. Hand WL, King-Thompson NL, Johnson JD (1984) Influence of bacterial-antibiotic interactions on subsequent antimicrobial activity of alveolar macrophages. J Infect Dis 149:271–276
16. Hand WL, Hand DL, King-Thompson NL Inhibition of oxidative metabolism in human polymorphonuclear leukocytes by clindamycin and nucleosides. (manuscript submitted)
17. Hand WL, King-Thompson NL (1983) Effect of erythrocyte ingestion on macrophage antibacterial function. Infect Immun 40:917–923
18. Johnston RB Jr, Keele BB, Misra HP, Lehmeyer JE, Webb LS, Baehner RL, Rajagopalan KV (1975) The role of superoxide anion generation in phagocytic bactericidal activity. J Clin Invest 55:1357–1372
19. Crapo JD, McCord JE, Fridovich I (1978) Preparation and assay of superoxide dismutase. Methods Enzymol 53:382–393
20. Root RK, Metcalf J, Oshino N, Chance B (1975) H_2O_2 release from human granulocytes during phagocytosis. I. Documentation, quantitation, and some regulating factors. J Clin Invest 55:945–955
21. Root RK, Metcalf JA (1977) H_2O_2 release from human granulocytes during phagocytosis. Relationship to superoxide anion formation and cellular catabolism of H_2O_2: studies with normal and cytochalasin β-treated cells. J Clin Invest 60:1266–1279
22. Holmes B, Quie PG, Windhorst DB, Pollara B, Good RA (1966) Protection of phagocytized bacteria from the killing action of antibiotics. Nature 210:1131–1132
23. Mandell GL, Vest TK (1973) Killing of intraleukocytic *Staphylococcus aureus* by rifampin: in-vitro and in-vivo studies. J Infect Dis 125:486–490
24. Solberg CO (1972) Protection of phagocytized bacteria against antibiotics. Acta Med Scand 191:383–387
25. Vandaux P, Waldvogel FA (1979) Gentamicin antibacterial activity in the presence of human polymorphonuclear leukocytes. Antimicrob Agents Chemother 16:743–749
26. Jacobs RF, Wilson CB, Laxton JG, Haas JE, Smith AL (1982) Cellular uptake and intracellular activity of antibiotics against *Haemophilus influenzae* type b. J Infect Dis 145:152–159
27. Easmon CSF, Crane JP (1984) Cellular uptake of clindamycin and lincomycin. Br J Exp Pathol 65:725–730
28. Cronstein BN, Kramer SB, Weissman G, Hirschhorn R (1983) Adenosine: a physiological modulator of superoxide anion generation by human neutrophils. J Exp Med 158:1160–1177
29. Cronstein BN, Rosenstein ED, Kramer SB, Weissmann G, Hirschhorn R (1985) Adenosine: a physiologic modulator of superoxide anion generation by human neutrophils. Adenosine acts via an A_2 receptor on human neutrophils. J Immunol 135:1366–1371
30. Castagna M, Takai Y, Kaibuchi K, Sano K, Kikkawa U, Nishizuka Y (1982) Direct activation of calcium-activated phospholipid-dependent protein kinase by tumor-promoting phorbol esters. J Biol Chem 257:7847–7851

Influence of Antibiotics on the Cell Surface of *Escherichia coli*

H. Leying [1], S. Suerbaum [1], H.-P. Kroll [2], J. Gmeiner [3], and W. Opferkuch [1]

Introduction

Many studies have shown that various host-parasite interaction processes like adherence, phagocytosis, serum resistance, or immune response to outer membrane (OM) components can be altered by preincubation of bacteria in sub-minimal inhibitory concentrations (sub-MICs) of antibiotics [6, 18, 24, 26, 27, 29, 30]. Though all these effects appear to be cell surface mediated, only few authors have investigated the influence of antibiotics on cell surface properties. James [12] reported that mecillinam selectively increased the formation of certain OM proteins. Kadurugamuwa et al. [13, 14] and Taylor et al. [30] observed an influence of antibiotics on the production of capsular polysaccharides in *Escherichia coli* and *Klebsiella pneumoniae*.

In this study we performed a quantitative analysis of the cell envelope of *E. coli* after preincubation in sub-MICs of different β-lactam derivatives and one quinolone. We measured the amounts of phosphlipids (PLs), lipopolysaccharides (LPSs), and protein and investigated the influence of antibiotics on qualitative OM properties, such as OM protein pattern, LPS chain length, and fatty acid substitution of PLs. Furthermore we determined the amounts of diaminopimelic acid (DAP) in the OM preparations as a marker of their content of peptidoglycan.

Finally, we examined whether the antibiotics had an effect on the production of capsular K1 polysaccharide, a further component of the cell envelope closely associated with bacterial virulence [1, 7, 11, 25].

Materials and Methods

Bacteria. *Escherichia coli* WF 96 (serotype 07 : K1 : H6) and BK 136 (02 : K1) were used for the experiments. Bacteria were grown in Mueller-Hinton broth (E. Merck AG, Darmstadt, FRG) with or without antibiotics and with agitation.

[1] Abteilung für Medizinische Mikrobiologie und Immunologie, Ruhr-Universität Bochum, 4630 Bochum, Federal Republic of Germany
[2] Pharma-Forschungszentrum, Bayer AG, Institut für Chemotherapie, 5600 Wuppertal 1, Federal Republic of Germany
[3] Institut für Mikrobiologie, Technische Hochschule Darmstadt, 6100 Darmstadt, Federal Republic of Germany

The Influence of Antibiotics on the Host-Parasite Relationship III
Edited by G. Gillissen, W. Opferkuch, G. Peters, and G. Pulverer

Antibiotics. The following antibiotics were used: ciprofloxacin (Bayer AG, Leverkusen, FRG), cephaloridine (Glaxo, Greenford, UK), imipenem (Merck, Sharp & Dohme, Rahway, NJ, United States), and moxalactam (Eli Lilly & Co., Indianapolis, IN, United States).

Minimal Inhibitory Concentration Determination. The MIC determination was performed by microtiter plate assay DIN 58940. The following MIC values (in micrograms per milliliter) were determined: (1) WF 96: ciprofloxacin – 0.063, cephaloridine – 8, imipenem – 0.25, moxalactam – 0.25; (2) BK 136: ciprofloxacin – 0.0078, cephaloridine – 4, imipenem – 0.25, moxalactam – 0.25.

Preparation of OM Vesicles. Membranes were prepared by the method of Kroll et al. [17] with the modifications described previously [18].

Extraction of Lipopolysaccharide and Phospholipids. LPS was extracted by the phenol/water method of Westphal and Jann [32]. PLs were extracted by the method of Folch et al. [5].

Analytical Methods. 2-Keto-3-deoxyoctulosonic acid (KDO) was determined by the method of Karkhansis et al. [16]. PLs were assessed by phosphate determination according to the method of Lowry et al. [20]. Protein was measured by the method of Markwell et al. [22]. All determinations were performed at least three times. Standard deviations were always smaller than 10% of the mean value. The amino acid analysis was performed as previously described [8]. Discontinuous sodium dodecyl sulfate-polyacrylamide slab gel electrophoresis (SDS-PAGE) was performed as described by Lugtenberg et al. [21] with 11% acrylamide in the separating gel. Protein (60 μg) and LPS corresponding to 0.5 μg KDO were applied to each slot of the gel. LPS gels were stained by the method of Karch et al. [15], and protein gels were stained with Coomassie brilliant blue R-250 (LKB, Rockville, United States).

Fatty Acid Analyses. Fatty acids in PL were transesterified and converted into methyl esters as described by Gmeiner and Martin [9], method B.

Gas Liquid Chromatography. For gas liquid chromatography of fatty acid methyl esters a Varian model 3700 equipped with flame ionization detector was used. Samples were analyzed on a Fused Silica capillary column, FS-FFAP-LB-0.25 (Macherey-Nagel, Düren, FRG). The column temperature was 140°–200 °C, the injector temperature 220 °C, and the detector temperature 250 °C. Nitrogen served as carrier gas (30 ml/min). The methyl ester peaks were identified by comparison of their retention time with methyl ester standards.

Determination of Capsular K1 Polysaccharide. K1 polysaccharide was quantitated by rocket immunoelectrophoresis according to the method of Weeke [31]. The equine *Meningococcus* B antiserum that was used for the determination was a gift from John B. Robbins.

Table 1. Composition of the OM of *E. coli* strain WF 96 after treatment with sub-MICs of different antibiotics

	Phospholipids (nmol PL-P/ μmol AA)	Lipopolysaccharide (nmol KDO/ μmol AA)	Peptidoglycan (nmol DAP/ μmol AA)
Control	61.0	14.5	1.66
$^1/_8$ MIC cephaloridine	63.6	15.0	2.71
$^1/_8$ MIC ciprofloxacin	52.1	17.3	2.11
$^1/_8$ MIC imipenem	45.3	15.4	1.89
$^1/_{12}$ MIC moxalactam	51.5	14.9	2.03

PL-P, phospholipidphosphate; KDO, 2-keto-3-deoxyoctonate; DAP, diaminopimelic acid; AA, amino acids.

Results

Quantitative Analyses of OM Preparations

The values obtained for the amounts of PL-phosphate, KDO, and DAP are shown in Table 1. OMs were prepared from late-logarithmic phase bacteria grown in the presence of subinhibitory concentrations of antibiotics or without antibiotics. Ciprofloxacin, imipenem, and moxalactam induced a significant reduction of the PL/amino acid ratio. This reduction was dependent on the concentration of the antibiotic. Cephaloridine had no significant effect on the PL content.

The content of KDO as a marker of LPS was significantly increased only in the OM preparations from ciprofloxacin-treated bacteria. The amount of DAP was determined as a marker of their content of peptidoglycan. DAP was increased in all OM preparations from antibiotic-treated bacteria, indicating that the degree of linkage between OM and peptidoglycan via lipoprotein was increased, or that antibiotics altered the digestibility of peptidoglycan by lysozyme.

Fatty Acid Analysis of OM Phospholipids

Fatty acids of OM phospholipids were analyzed by gas chromatography, and amounts of palmitic acid ($C_{16:0}$), palmitoleic acid ($C_{16:1}$), stearic acid ($C_{18:0}$), and vaccinic acid ($C_{18:1}$) were calculated as percentages of total fatty acids. Values are given in Table 2, together with a calculated ratio of unsaturated/saturated fatty acids. All preparations from antibiotic-treated bacteria had an increased relative amount of unsaturated fatty acids.

Qualitative Analyses of OM Components

Outer membrane proteins and LPS were analyzed by SDS-PAGE. The OM proteins of cells grown in subinhibitory concentrations of the antibiotics used did not

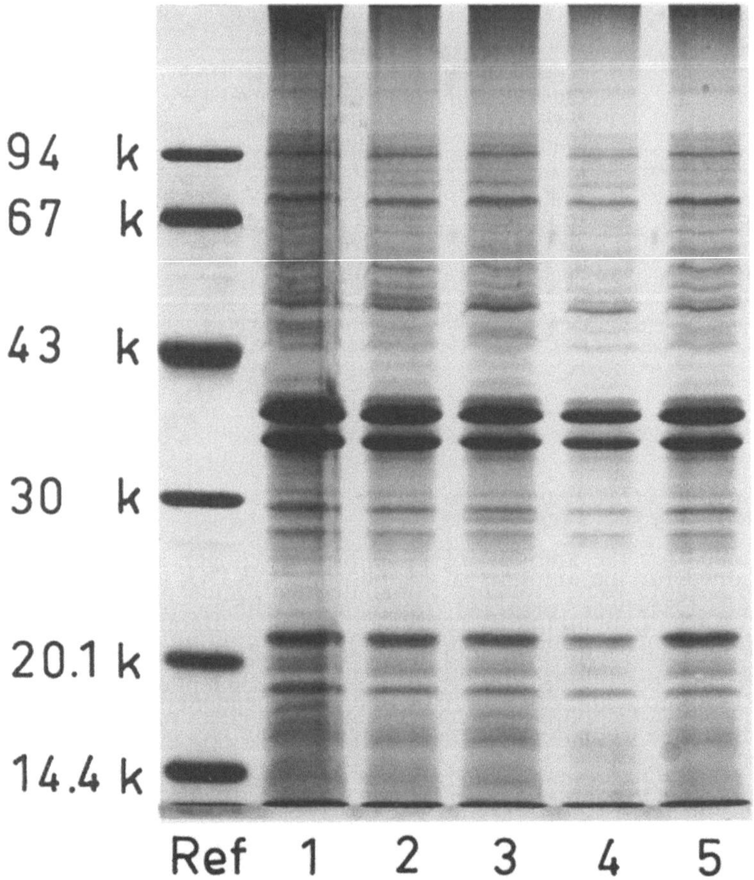

Fig. 1. SDS-Page of OM proteins of *E. coli* WF 96 grown in the absence of drug (*lane 1*) and in the presence of one-fourth the MIC of cephaloridine (*lane 2*), ciprofloxaxin (*lane 3*), imipenem (*lane 4*), and moxalactam (*lane 5*). *Ref*, reference proteins

Table 2. Fatty acid analyses of phospholipids in OMs of antibiotic-treated bacteria and the untreated control

	% Fatty acid/total fatty acids				Unsaturated/Saturated
	$C_{16:0}$	$C_{16:1}$	$C_{18:0}$	$C_{18:1}$	
Control	49.7	16.9	8.7	24.4	0.71
1/4 MIC cephaloridine	49.7	21.9	4.9	23.0	0.82
1/4 MIC ciprofloxacin	48.1	22.3	2.6	26.6	0.96
1/8 MIC imipenem	43.8	22.3	4.8	29.1	1.06

$C_{16:0}$, palmitic acid; $C_{16:1}$, palmitoleic acid; $C_{18:0}$, stearic acid; $C_{18:1}$, vaccinic acid.

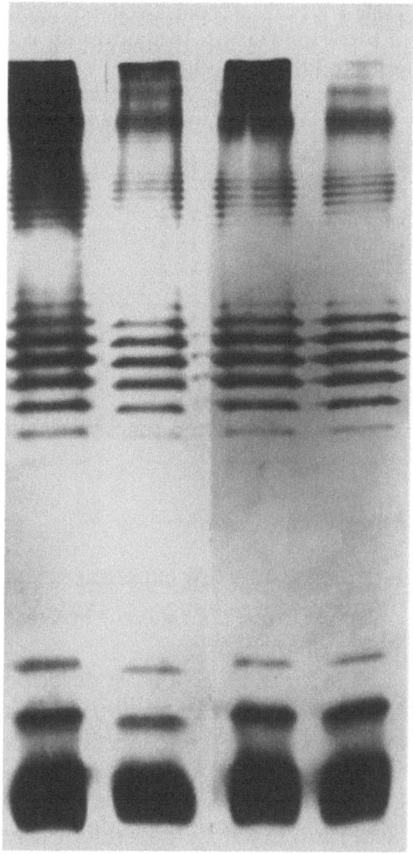

1 2 3 4

Fig. 2. SDS-Page of LPS of *E. coli* WF 96 grown in the absence of drug (*lane 1*) and in the presence of one-fourth the MIC of ciprofloxacin (*lane 2*), imipenem (*lane 3*), and moxalactam (*lane 4*)

exhibit any differences from those of control cells (Fig. 1). In addition to this, no significant alterations of the LPS patterns after antibiotic treatment were observed (Fig. 2). This means that none of the antibiotics tested had any influence on the degree of polymerization of the 0 side chain. The PL of antibiotic-treated and untreated bacteria showed identical migration properties in thin-layer chromatography.

Influence of Antibiotics on K1 Production

When the amount of K1 in whole early stationary phase cells of *E. coli* BK 136 grown in the presence and absence of ½ the MIC of antibiotics was determined, we found a reduction of K1 production under the influence of imipenem, cepha-

Table 3. K1 capsular polysaccharide content of *E. coli* BK 136 after treatment with ½ the MIC of different antibiotics

	µg K1/mg cell protein
Control	18.4
Cephaloridine	7.5
Ciprofloxacin	13.4
Imipenem	12.4
Moxalactam	17.7

loridine, and ciprofloxacin (Table 3). The most effective antibiotic was cephaloridine, which reduced the amount of K1 by more than 50%.

Discussion

Up to now only few experiments have been conducted to demonstrate qualitative or quantitative changes of the OM after growth of bacteria in the presence of sub-MICs of antibiotics.

Taylor et al. [30] have described an influence of mecillinam on the length of 0-side chains in LPS from *E. coli* O7:K1, James [12] found that mecillinam selectively increased the formation of certain OM proteins. In this study we could not detect qualitative changes in the main OM constituents, OM proteins, and LPS.

In contrast to this, we found that the antibiotics tested reduced the PL/amino acid ratio in a dose-dependent way by up to 26%, which is likely to be associated with an impaired fluidity of the membrane. Our findings are consistent with those reported by Dougherty and Saukkonen [3], who described a reduction of lipid content of the cell envelope after treating *E. coli* with nalidixic acid. They are also consistent with our finding [19] that antibiotics inhibit PL translocation into the OM. Whether this is the only mechanism leading to the reduction of PL, or if there is also an increased secretion of lipids into the medium after prolonged incubation times as described by Horne et al. [10] for different streptococci, remains to be investigated.

The observed increase of the relative amount of unsaturated fatty acids in PL of antibiotic-treated bacteria might be a reaction to the reduction of total OM phospholipids in order to maintain membrane fluidity. This is consistent with data published by Marr and Ingraham [23], who observed an increase of the relative amount of unsaturated fatty acids after growing bacteria at lower temperatures, which also reduces membrane fluidity.

Our procedure for preparation of OM is likely to leave small peptidoglycan fragments bound to the OM via lipoprotein. The amount of these fragments can be assessed by determination of DAP. We found that all antibiotics tested increased the amount of DAP bound to the OM in a dose-dependent way. These data are quite consistent with the findings of Braun and Wolff [2] and Essig et al. [4], who described that mecillinam and, less effectively, nalidixic acid and penicillin G increased the degree of linkage between peptidoglycan layer and OM. Another explanation for the increased DAP content of OM material from antibiotic-treated bacteria could be an alteration in digestibility of peptidoglycan by lysozyme.

When we investigated the influence of subinhibitory concentrations of antibiotics on the amount of capsular K1 polysaccharide produced by early stationary phase cells of *E. coli*, we found that imipenem, moxalactam, and ciprofloxacin dose-dependently inhibited K1 production. Similar results were published by Taylor et al. [30], who found a reduction of the extractable amount of K1 after treating *E. coli* with mecillinam, and also by Kadurugamuwa et al. [13], who reported that various cephalosporins reduced the formation of capsule in iron-depleted *Klebsiella pneumoniae*. It is well established that K1 production is one of the mechanisms by which bacteria counteract the bactericidal activity of serum [11, 25, 28], and the possible connection between an antibiotic-induced reduction of K1 and the antibiotic-induced increase of serum sensitivity that has been described [30, 33] is obvious.

We conclude from this study that antibiotics, also in concentrations much below the MIC, have pronounced effects on the quantitative composition of the OM and on capsule formation. A more detailed picture of changes of the bacterial surface properties that occur in the presence of antibiotics will perhaps help to understand some of the influences of antibiotics on host-parasite interaction processes in a better way.

Summary

The influence of subinhibitory concentrations of cephaloridine, moxalactam, imipenem, and ciprofloxacin on the degree of polymerization of the LPS-0-side chain and on the outer membrane (OM) protein pattern of *E. coli* was investigated by SDS-PAGE. In addition, the effects of antibiotics on the content of LPS, phospholipids (PLs), protein, and capsular K1 polysaccharide in the cell envelope were studied by determination of KDO, PL-phosphate, amino acids (AA), or rocket immunoelectrophoresis, respectively. Imipenem, cephaloridine, and ciprofloxacin induced a dose-dependent reduction of the production of capsular K1 polysaccharide by more than 50%. Furthermore, imipenem, moxalactam, and ciprofloxacin reduced the PL/AA ratio in a dose-dependent fashion. This was accompanied by an increase of the relative amount of unsaturated fatty acids. Only ciprofloxacin increased the LPS/AA ratio. The amount of peptidoglycan bound to the OM measured by determination of diaminopimelic acid was increased up to 42% by the antibiotics in a dose-dependent way. The antibiotic-induced alterations of the quantitative composition of the cell envelope of *E. coli* were not accompanied by qualitative changes in the LPS and OM protein patterns.

Acknowledgments. We are grateful to Miss Susanne Wendt and Miss Brigitte Andres for excellent technical assistance, and to Mrs. Ursula Heuzeroth for typing the manuscript.

References

1. Bortolussi R, Ferrieri P, Björkstén B, Quie PG (1979) Capsular K1 polysaccharide of *Escherichia coli:* relationship to virulence in newborn rats and resistance to phagocytosis. Infect Immun 25:293–298
2. Braun V, Wolff H (1975) Attachment of lipoprotein to murein (peptidoglycan) of *Escherichia coli* in the presence and absence of penicillin FL 1060. J Bacteriol 123:888–897
3. Dougherty TJ, Saukkonen JJ (1985) Membrane permeability changes associated with DNA gyrase inhibitors in *Escherichia coli.* Antimicrob Agents Chemother 28:200–206
4. Essig P, Martin HH, Gmeiner J (1982) Murein and lipopolysaccharide biosynthesis in synchronized cells of *Escherichia coli* K12 and the effect of penicillin G, mecillinam, and nalidixic acid. Arch Microbiol 132:245–250
5. Folch J, Less M, Sloane-Stanley GH (1957) A simple method for isolation and purification of total lipids from animal tissue. J Biol Chem 226:497–505
6. Friedman H, Warren GH (1976) Antibody-mediated bacteriolysis: enhanced killing of cyclacillin-treated bacteria. Proc Soc Exp Biol Med 153:301–304
7. Gemski P, Cross AS, Sadoff JC (1980) K1 antigen-associated resistance to the bactericidal activity of serum. FEMS Microbiol Lett 9:193–197
8. Gmeiner J, Kroll HP, Martin HH (1978) The covalent rigid-layer lipoprotein in cell walls of *Proteus mirabilis.* Eur J Biochem 83:227–233
9. Gmeiner J, Martin HH (1976) Phospholipid and lipopolysaccharide in *Proteus mirabilis* and its stable protoplast L-form. Eur J Biochem 67:487–494
10. Horne D, Hakenbeck R, Tomasz A (1977) Secretion of lipids induced by inhibition of peptidoglycan synthesis in streptococci. J Bacteriol 132:704–717
11. Howard CJ, Glynn AA (1971) The virulence for mice of strains of *Escherichia coli* related to the effects of K antigens on their resistance of phagocytosis and killing by complement. Immunology 29:767–777
12. James R (1975) Identification of an outer membrane protein of *Escherichia coli,* with a role in the coordination of deoxyribonucleic acid replication and cell elongation. J Bacteriol 124:918–929
13. Kadurugamuwa JL, Anwar H, Brown MRW, Zak O (1985) Effect of subinhibitory concentrations of cephalosporins on surface properties and siderophore production in iron-depleted *Klebsiella pneumoniae.* Antimicrob Agents Chemother 27:220–223
14. Kadurugamuwa JL, Anwar H, Brown MRW, Zak O (1985) Protein antigens of encapsulated *Klebsiella pneumoniae* surface exposed after growth in the presence of subinhibitory concentrations of cephalosporins. Antimicrob Agents Chemother 28:195–199
15. Karch H, Leying H, Opferkuch W (1984) Analysis of electrophoretically heterogeneous lipopolysaccharides of *E. coli* by immunoblotting. FEMS Microbiol Lett 22:193–196
16. Karkhanis YD, Zeltner JY, Jackson JJ, Carlo DJ (1978) A new and improved microassay to determine 2-keto-3-deoxyoctonate in lipopolysaccharide of gram-negative bacteria. Anal Biochem 85:595–601
17. Kroll HP, Bhakdi S, Taylor PW (1983) Membrane changes induced by exposure of *Escherichia coli* to human serum. Infect Immun 42:1055–1066
18. Leying H, Suerbaum S, Kroll HP, Karch H, Opferkuch W (1986) Influence of β-lactam antibiotics and ciprofloxacin on composition and immunogenicity of *Escherichia coli* outer membrane. Antimicrob Agents Chemother 30:475–480
19. Leying H, Karch H, Kroll HP, Opferkuch W (1985) The influence of β-lactam antibiotics including monobactam on the outer and inner membrane of *Escherichia coli.* In: Adam D, Hahn H, Opferkuch W (eds) The influence of antibiotics on the host-parasite relationship II. Springer, Berlin Heidelberg New York, pp 48–56
20. Lowry OW, Roberts NR, Leiner KY, Wu ML, Farr AL (1954) The quantitative histochemistry of brain. I. Chemical methods. J Biol Chem 207:1–17
21. Lugtenberg B, Meijers J, Peters R, Van der Hoek, Van Alphen L (1975) Electrophoretic resolution of the major outer membrane protein of *E. coli* K12 into four bands. FEBS Lett 58:254–258
22. Markwell MAK, Haar SM, Bieker LL, Tolbert WE (1978) A modification of the Lowry procedure to simplify protein determinations in membrane and lipoprotein samples. Anal Biochem 87:206–210

23. Marr AG, Ingraham JL (1962) Effect of temperature on the composition of fatty acids in *Escherichia coli.* J Bacteriol 84:1260–1267
24. Ofek J, Beachey EW, Eisenstein BI, Alkan ML, Sharon N (1979) Suppression of bacterial adherence by subminimal inhibitory concentrations of β-lactam and aminoglycoside antibiotics. Rev Infect Dis 1:832–837
25. Opal S, Cross A, Gemski P (1982) K antigen and serum sensitivity of rough *Escherichia coli.* Infect Immun 37:956–960
26. Opferkuch W, Büscher KH, Karch H, Leying H, Pawelzik M, Schumann U, Wiemer C (1985) The effect of sublethal concentrations of antibiotics on the host-parasite relationship. Zentralbl Bakteriol Mikrobiol Hyg [A] 13 [Suppl]:165–177
27. Opferkuch W, Büscher KH, Leying H, Klimetzek V (1987) Interaction of *Escherichia coli* and macrophages: alteration by treatment of bacteria with β-lactam antibiotics. Zentralbl Bakteriol Mikrobiol Hyg A 266:116–126
28. Pluschke G, Mayden J, Achtman M, Levine RP (1983) Role of the capsule and the O antigen in resistance of O18:K1 *Escherichia coli* to complement-mediated killing. Infect Immun 42:907–913
29. Svanborg-Edén C, Sandberg T, Stenqvist K, Ahlstedt S (1979) Effects of subinhibitory amounts of ampicillin, amoxycillin and mecillinam on the adhesion of *E. coli* bacteria to human urinary tract epithelial cells: a preliminary study. Infection 7 [Suppl]:452–455
30. Taylor PW, Kroll HP, Tomlinson S (1982) Effect of subinhibitory concentrations of mecillinam on expression of *E. coli* surface components associated with serum resistance. Drugs Exp Clin Res 8:625–631
31. Weeke B (1973) Rocket immunoelectrophoresis. Scand J Immunol 2 [Suppl 1]:37–46
32. Westphal O, Jann K (1965) Bacterial lipopolysaccharides. Extraction with phenol-water and further applications of the procedure. Methods Carbohydr Chem 5:83
33. Wiemer CWC, Kubens B, Opferkuch W (1985) Influence of imipenem on the serum resistance of Enterobacteriaceae. Rev Infect Dis 7:426–431

Pseudomonas aeruginosa: Alterations Induced by Low Concentrations of 4-Quinolones

M. T. LABRO [1], A. BRYSKIER [2], C. BABIN-CHEVAYE [1], and J. HAKIM [1]

Introduction

Since the introduction of nalidixic acid in 1962, several compounds of this class (4-quinolones and in particular the fluoroquinolones), have been synthesized. These molecules have been shown to display an increased antibacterial potency and a broader spectrum. However, concerning potential direct interaction with the host defense system – in particular polymorphonuclear neutrophils (PMNs) – few data have been reported [3, 4, 8] and they do not indicate a significant increase in PMN function. On the contrary, several authors have shown that low concentrations of quinolones may alter bacteria in such a manner that these altered pathogens are significantly more sensitive than control ones to PMN killing [8, 9, 13]. The aim of our work was to analyze the effects of a low concentration of 4-quinolones on *Pseudomonas aeruginosa,* a strain which has lately emerged as an important pathogen with increasing resistance to antimicrobial agents.

Materials and Methods

4-Quinolones: Three fluoroquinolones (ciprofloxacin, Bayer; ofloxacin, Roussel Uclaf; pefloxacin, Rhône Poulenc) were compared with nalidixic acid and oxolinic acid. The compounds were first dissolved (1000 μg) in 300 μl HCl 1*M*; then 300 μl NaOH 1*M* and 400 μl sterile H_2O were added. Further dilutions were performed in trypticase soy broth (TSB) (Biomérieux) to reach the desired concentrations. For oxolinic acid and nalidixic acid, the dissolution was obtained in 300 μl NaOH 1*M*, with further adjunction of 700 μl H_2O.

Pseudomonas aeruginosa was obtained from a clinical isolate (septicemia). The MICs were determined in TSB by a macrodilution method with two inocula (10^5 and 10^7 CFUs/ml) (Table 1). For the experiments reported here, an inoculum of 10^7 CFUs was used. The bacteria were grown overnight in broth supplemented or not by the different 4-quinolones (2 × MIC-1/128 MIC). The following day the bacteria were extensively washed, at least three times, in Hank's buffered solution (HBS). Gram staining was performed on an aliquot of bacterial broth. For morphological alteration studies at least 4 different experiments were performed, and 10 different fields of more than 100 bacteria were counted on each slide.

[1] INSERM U. 294 et Laboratoire d'Hématologie et d'Immunologie CHU Xavier Bichat, 46, rue Henri Huchard, 75018 Paris, France
[2] Laboratoire de Microbiologie, 95100 CHG d'Argenteuil, France

The Influence of Antibiotics on the Host-Parasite Relationship III
Edited by G. Gillissen, W. Opferkuch, G. Peters, and G. Pulverer

Table 1. *Pseudomonas aeruginosa* clinical isolate (septicemia): MICs of 4-quinolone (mg/l) inoculum

	10^5 CFUs/ml	10^7 CFUs/ml
Nalidixic acid	>128	>128
Oxolinic acid	32	64
Pefloxacin	4	8
Ofloxacin	2	2
Ciprofloxacin	0.5	1

Bacterial mass was determined as the weight of an aliquot of 1 ml bacterial suspension, optical density (OD) 478 nm about 1, after centrifugation, removal of supernatant, and drying in sterile atmosphere. In parallel, dilutions and plating of the bacterial suspension were performed to obtain the number of CFUs, and the dried weight was correlated to this number to have the mean bacterial mass of filament or bacteria.

Sensitivity to In Vitro Systems

Sensitivity to citrate buffer pH 6 and to crude granule extract (CGE) of PMNs, which contains O_2-dependent killing systems, was assayed on microplate. Bacteria [100 µl diluted 10^{-5}; OD 0.1] were exposed for 1 h at 37 °C to 100 µl HBS, citrate buffer pH 6.4, or several preparations of CGE [12] diluted in citrate buffer. The CFUs were obtained by subsequent dilutions and plating. The survival was expressed as the percentage of CFUs at 60 min compared with initial counts.

Sensitivity to Oxygen Species. The xanthine (1.25 m*M*), xanthine oxidase (0.25 and 0.05 units/ml, final concentration) system was used to generate oxidant molecules. The bacteria (100 µl, OD 0.1) were exposed for 1 h at 37 °C to these mixtures or to control HBS. The survival was obtained by dilutions and plating of oxidant-exposed bacterial suspension compared with initial counts.

Results

After an overnight exposure to low concentrations of quinolones, *P. aeruginosa* showed morphological alterations. These were of four types: round and swollen cells, alterations in cell structure such as ghost cells, irregular staining or shapes, elongated cells, and filamentous cells. We were able to define a relationship between concentration of quinolones and percentage of morphological alterations. For example (Fig. 1 a–f) at 2 MIC, 1 MIC, and 0.5 MIC, ofloxacin induced some elongated cells and round cells but no filaments; at 0.25 MIC the maximal percentage of elongation (23%) was observed and long filaments (16%) were also present. At decreasing concentrations, elongation and filamentation were reduced and at 0.03 MIC the morphological aspect was similar to that of control

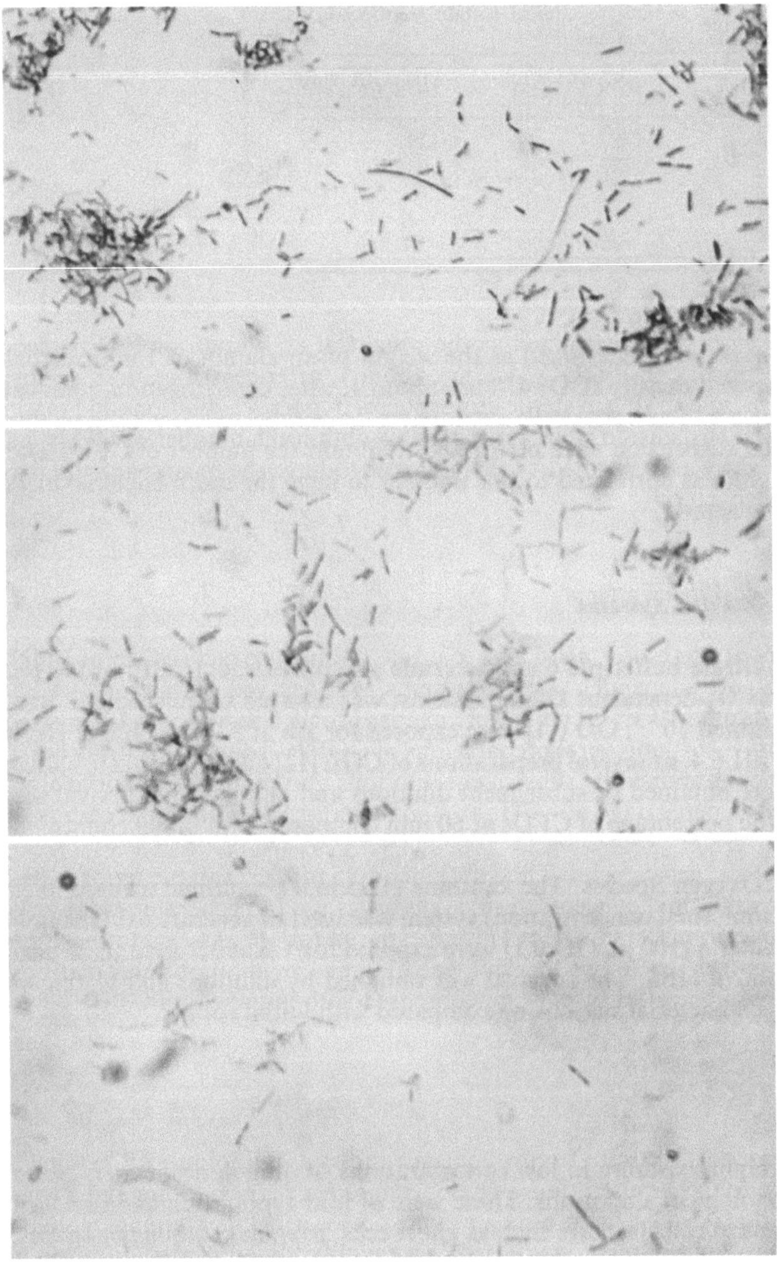

a–c

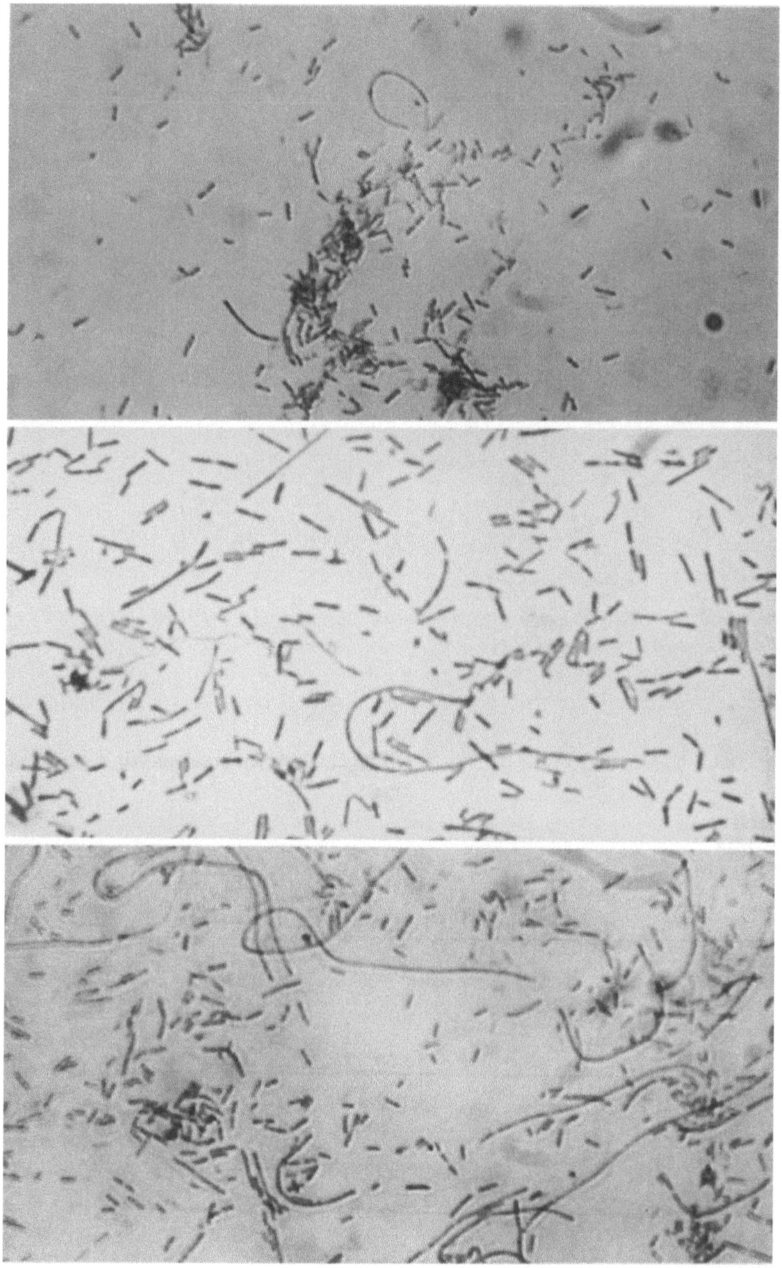

d–f

Fig. 1 d–f. *Pseudomonas aeruginosa* after overnight exposure to ofloxacin: **a** 2 MIC, **b** MIC, **c** 0.5 MIC, **d** 0.25 MIC, **e** 0.125 MIC, **f** 0.06 MIC, × 1000

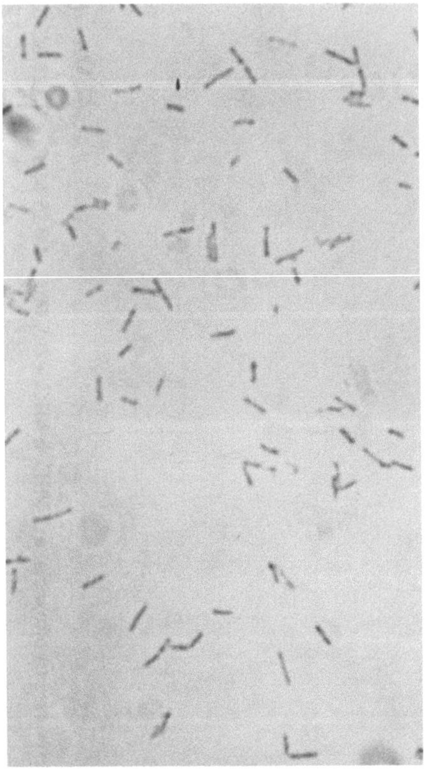

Fig. 2. Control *Pseudomonas aeruginosa,* × 1000

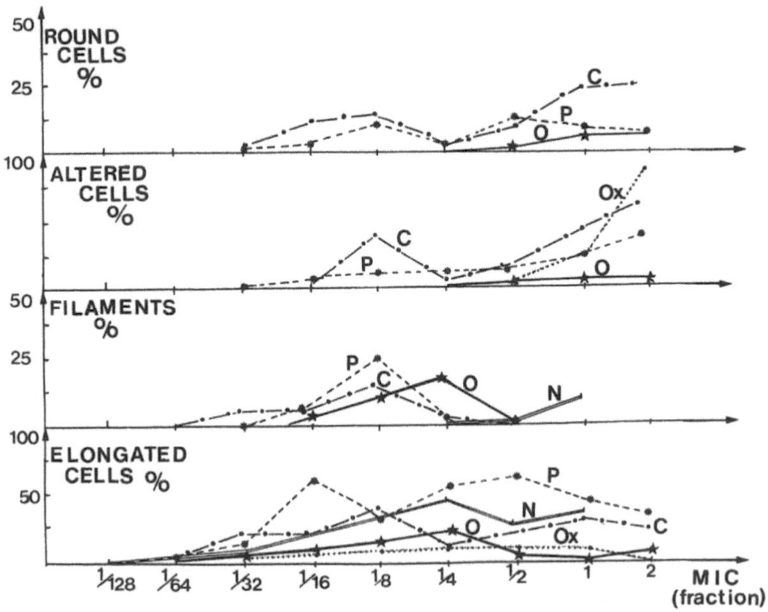

Fig. 3. Effects of 4-quinolones on *P. aeruginosa. P,* pefloxacin; *C,* ciprofloxacin; *O,* ofloxacin; *N,* nalidixic acid; *OX,* oxolinic acid

Table 2. Morphological alterations of *P. aeruginosa* induced by 4-quinolones

	Fractions of MIC								
	2	1	1/2	1/4	1/8	1/16	1/32	1/64	1/128
Ofloxacin									
Elongated	8	2	6	23	16	9	6	0	0
Filament	0	0	1	16	6	0	0	0	0
Round	13	4	5	7	4	1	2	0	0
Altered	5	5	3	2	0	0	0	0	0
Ciprofloxacin									
Elongated	24	31	16	11	34	25	25	8	0
Filament	0	0	0	2	13	5	5	0	0
Round	21	20	5	2	10	8	0	0	0
Altered	68	46	15	2	32	1	2	1	0
Pefloxacin									
Elongated	32	46	60	57	32	57	19	5	8
Filament	0	0	0	0	26	6	1	0	0
Round	5	7	12	3	9	3	2	0	0
Altered	18	8	5	5	6	3	1	1	0
Oxolinic acid									
Elongated	0	13	13	13	3	–	–	8	2
Filament	0	0	0	3	0	–	–	0	0
Round	0	0	8	5	3	–	–	0	0
Altered	80	6	1	1	0	–	–	0	0
Nalidixic acid									
Elongated	–	32	25	40	–	–	10	5	3
Filament	–	12	3	1	–	–	0	0	0
Round	–	3	1	2	–	–	0	0	0
Altered	–	2	1	0	–	–	0	0	0

Results are expressed as percentages of the whole *P. aeruginosa* population.

P. aeruginosa (Fig. 2). A similar concentration dependency was observed with other quinolones (Table 2, Fig. 3) with the following differences: ciprofloxacin, which was the most bactericidal, induced a greater percentage of round and altered cells at 2 and 1 MIC (Fig. 4) and ciprofloxacin and pefloxacin induced more filamentous and elongated cells (Fig. 5 a, b). In particular two waves for induction of elongated cells were seen above and below the filament-inducing concentrations. Oxolinic acid induced a high number of altered cells at 2 MIC (128 mg/liter), but compared with other quinolones few elongated and filamentous cells were observed. For each molecule, a concentration could be defined which induced the highest percentage of filament. We propose to name this value the most filament-inducing concentration (MFIC). It was equal to 0.25 MIC for ofloxacin and oxolinic acid and to 0.125 MIC for pefloxacin and ciprofloxacin. As a consequence, the mean bacterial mass was increased at this concentration and this was more important for ciprofloxacin or pefloxacin-altered bacteria (mean increase, 879% and 563%, respectively) (Table 3).

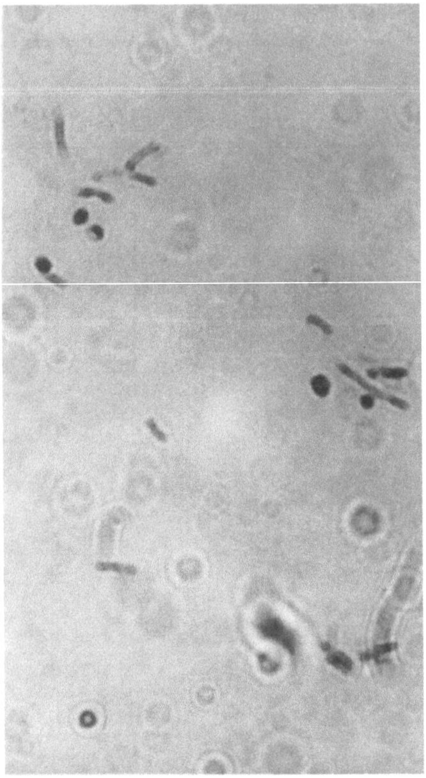

Fig. 4. *Pseudomonas aeruginosa* after overnight exposure to ciprofloxacin 2 MIC, ×1000

Table 3. Increase in bacterial mass after growth in the presence of 4-quinolones

Quinolones	Fractions of MIC				
	1/2	1/4	1/8	1/16	1/32
Ofloxacin (four experiments)	141	194±39.5	194±90	89±12.3	97±17.7
Ciprofloxacin (three experiments)	250±78	345	879±128	394	–
Pefloxacin (three experiments)	222±67	217±46	563±337	158±34	150
Oxolinic acid (one experiment)	–	228	–	220	133
Nalidixic acid (one experiment)	150	116	–	124	95

Mean weight of *P. aeruginosa* ± SD: $3.65 \pm 0.71\ 10^{-9}$ mg (11 experiments). Results are expressed as mean ± SD percentage of increase in bacterial mass (quinolones treated/control *P. aeruginosa*).

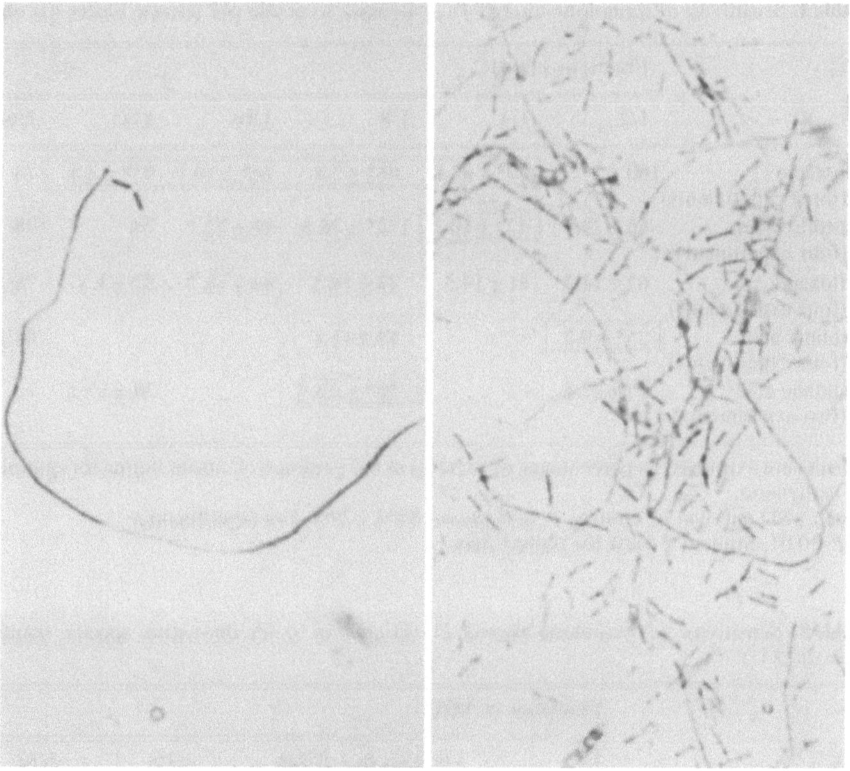

a b

Fig. 5 a, b. *Pseudomonas aeruginosa* after overnight exposure to 0.125 MIC ciprofloxacin **a** and pefloxacin **b**, × 1000

The sensitivity of these altered bacteria to PMN killing was assessed in vitro but did not differ from that of control bacteria (data not shown) when the survival was expressed in terms of CFU survival. But when the bacterial mass was taken into account, all the quinolone-altered bacteria were destroyed significantly more than control *P. aeruginosa*.

The sensitivity of the bacteria was assessed in vitro with three different methods which explore the main killing mechanisms of the PMN phagolysosome, namely acidic pH, bactericidal enzymes, and O_2-dependent systems.

The crude granule extract of PMN has been shown to contain a factor which stimulates the growth of *P. aeruginosa* [7]. Indeed, we observed that control *P. aeruginosa* survival was 216% compared with the initial count; the survivals of the quinolone-exposed bacteria were similar to those of the control except for oxolinic-treated *P. aeruginosa* at 0.25 MIC (MFIC) (data not shown).

On the contrary, the mild acidic pH (6.4) which does not kill control *P. aeruginosa* was very effective for the killing of quinolone-treated *P. aeruginosa* except pefloxacin-treated bacteria (Table 4). Ofloxacin-treated bacteria showed an increased sensitivity in a wide range of concentrations, while ciprofloxacin-treated bacteria showed a very narrow range of sensitivity just above the MFIC.

Table 4. Sensitivity of quinolone-altered *P. aeruginosa* to acidic pH (citrate buffer pH 6)

	Fractions of MIC						
	1/2	1/4	1/8	1/16	1/32	1/64	1/128
Ofloxacin (three experiments)	100	59* ± 28.8	68* ± 7.8	66* ± 10.7	67* ± 2.8	78	107
Ciprofloxacin (four experiments)	66 ± 29.1	43* ± 10.2	172* ± 28.8	96 ± 12.7	78	78	–
Pefloxacin (four experiments)	63 ± 24.2	81 ± 14.3	74 ± 18.3	64 ± 18.7	82 ± 3.5	78 ± 8.5	86 ± 10.6
Oxolinic acid (four experiments)	25* ± 9.2	–	89 ± 11.1	–	–	68 ± 17.1	104 ± 22.4
Nalidixic acid (two experiments)	77 ± 27.5	–	76* ± 2.8	–	78 ± 17.3	–	73 ± 24.7

Results are expressed as percentages of survival in the presence of citrate buffer for quinolone-altered/control *P. aeruginosa*.
Mean ± SD survival of control *P. aeruginosa*: 86% ± 29% (14 experiments).
* $P<0.01$, Student's *t*-test for paired data.

Table 5. Sensitivity of quinolone-altered *P. aeruginosa* to O_2-derivative species (xanthine–xanthine oxidase: 0.25 U)

	Fractions of MIC					
	1/2	1/4	1/8	1/16	1/32	1/64
Ofloxacin (three experiments)	258	165 ± 58.2	208 ± 106.8	87 ± 41.7	146 ± 24.7	75 ± 0.7
Ciprofloxacin (four experiments)	308 ± 110.8	290 ± 85.4	179 ± 61.3	61 ± 24.7	110 ± 42.4	133 ± 94
Pefloxacin (four experiments)	100	123 ± 75.1	337 ± 148.4	115 ± 58.9	173 ± 153.7	198
Nalidixic acid (three experiments)	170 ± 26.9	115 ± 53.1	–	–	95 ± 35.8	–
Oxolinic acid (four experiments)	175 ± 21.2	–	161 ± 85.3	–	–	57 ± 47.2

Results are expressed as percentages of survival for quinolone-altered/control bacteria (mean ± 1 SD). Mean survival ± SEM for control *P. aeruginosa*: 18.4% ± 2,7% (19 experiments).

Finally, the exposure to the xanthine-xanthine oxidase system revealed an interesting feature not previously reported. The quinolone-altered bacteria showed an increased resistance to the oxidative killing mechanism (Tables 5, 6). This was observed after exposure of bacteria to high concentrations of quinolones and was of particular importance in ciprofloxacin-treated bacteria.

Table 6. Sensitivity of quinolone-altered *P. aeruginosa* to O_2-derivative species (xanthine oxidase: 0.05 U)

	Fractions of MIC					
	1/2	1/4	1/8	1/16	1/32	1/64
Ofloxacin (three experiments)	380	131 ± 23.8	163 ± 49.3	107 ± 41.6	85 ± 31.1	100
Ciprofloxacin (five experiments)	159 ± 78.1	361 ± 44.7	88 ± 11.2	78 ± 9.8	100	88 ± 17.7
Pefloxacin (four experiments)	85 ± 55.3	96 ± 40.6	91 ± 58.8	105 ± 85.6	119 ± 12	143 ± 79.9
Nalidixic acid (four experiments)	233 ± 61.5	87 + 55.1	–	–	–	81 ± 55.3
Oxolinic acid (four experiments)	220 ± 34.1	–	130 ± 27.4	–	39 ± 25.7	–

Mean survival ± SEM for control *P. aeruginosa*: 37.6% ± 5.36% (19 experiments). Results are expressed as percentages of survival for quinolone-altered/control bacteria (mean ± 1 SD).

Discussion

Despite the fact that quinolones have been known for more than 20 years, the precise mechanism of their action is still unclear. Interaction with DNA-gyrase [11] or directly with DNA [10] has been proposed as the main effective mechanism, while other authors have claimed that the bactericidal action of these molecules could lie in other interactions with bacteria [1, 2]. The results reported here show that, although their chemical structure is quite similar, their mechanism of action appears different at least for their effect on *P. aeruginosa*.

First, the ability to induce filament or elongation is qualitatively and quantitatively different. Ciprofloxacin and pefloxacin appear to be very strong inducers of filamentation compared with the other fluoroquinolone, ofloxacin. The filaments are induced in a very narrow range of concentrations, with a peak appearing for the MFIC, which differs according to the molecules. The interest of this new index in understanding the mechanism of action of the 4-quinolones requires further study with the newest molecules.

Second, a similar effect was noted for induction of sensitivity to acidic pH which could reflect alterations of bacterial cell walls with increased permeability to protons. This effect was clearly more important for ofloxacin compared with the other two fluoroquinolones.

Third, a very striking point was the increased resistance to oxygen-derivative species not yet reported for bacterial antibiotic-induced alterations. In particular, beta-lactams seem to induce an increased sensitivity of *P. aeruginosa* to the oxygen-dependent killing mechanism (Labro et al. 1987 a, b) [5, 6]. It was of interest to note that this effect was observed with high concentrations of quinolones, where probably the most important DNA-alterations are induced. Since the bactericidal mechanism of O_2-derivative species is still a matter of hypothesis (lipid peroxidation or DNA damage ...), the use of quinolones could be helpful in clarifying this problem. Biochemical analyses are in progress to understand the observed phenomena.

Summary

We studied the effects of three fluoroquinolones (ofloxacin, OX; ciprofloxacin, CX; pefloxacin, PX) compared with oxolinic acid (OA) and nalidixic acid (NA) in a resistant strain of *Pseudomonas aeruginosa* [minimal inhibitory concentrations (MICs) 2, 1, 8, 64, and 128 mg/liter respectively]. After an overnight culture in the presence of subinhibitory concentrations of these molecules, *P. aeruginosa* showed elongated and filamentous cells in a dose-dependent manner. In particular, it was possible to define a new index, the most filament inducing concentration (MFIC). Increase in bacterial mass was correlated with this index. The bactericidal effect of whole human blood was similar for control or quinolone-treated bacteria when expressed as a percentage of colony-forming unit (CFU) survivors, but in proportion to bacterial mass the killing of treated bacteria was significantly increased. The quinolone-treated and control bacteria were exposed to several in vitro systems [acidic pH, crude granule extract (CGE) of polymorphonuclear neutrophils (PMNs) and oxidative species]. The sensitivity of quinolone-treated bacteria did not differ from that of control ones for CGE but an increased sensitivity to acidic pH was noted in particular after OX treatment. A striking point was the increased resistance to the oxidant of these altered bacteria. These data could be of interest in understanding the underlying mechanisms of bactericidal action of 4-quinolones.

References

1. Cohen J, Mc Connell JS (1986) Release of endotoxin from bacteria exposed to ciprofloxacin and its prevention with polymyxin B. Eur J Clin Microbiol 5(1):13–17
2. Diver JM, Wise R (1986) Morphological and biochemical changes in *Escherichia coli* after exposure to ciprofloxacin. J Antimicrob Chemother 18 [Suppl D]:31–41
3. Duncker D, Ullmann U (1984) Einfluß von Ciprofloxacin, Enoxacin und Norfloxacin auf die Phagozytose humaner neutrophiler Granulozyten, gemessen mit der Chemilumineszenz. FAC 3–5:633–635
4. Forsgren A, Bergkvist PI (1985) Effect of ciprofloxacin on phagocytosis. Eur J Clin Microbiol 4(6):575–577
5. Labro MT, Babin-Chevaye C, Hakim S (1987a) Ceftriaxone-induced alteration of Pseudomonas aeruginosa in relation to the bactericidal function of human neutrophils. Proceedings of the 15th ICC Istanbul, July 19–24, vol 1. Berkada B, Kuemmerle HP (eds) pp 782–784
6. Labro MT, Babin-Chevaye C, Hakim S (1988) Influence of subinhibitory concentrations of ceftriaxone on opsonization and killing of pseudomona aeruginosa by human neutrophils. J Antimicrob Chemother 22:341–352
7. Modrzakowski MC, Dosch-Meier D, Hodinka RL (1983) Effect of rat polymorphonuclear leukocyte granule components on the growth and survival of *Pseudomonas aeruginosa* and *Salmonella typhimurium*. Can J Microbiol 29:1339–1343
8. Pulverer G, Peters G (1986) Investigations on ofloxacin: antibacterial activity and influence on the immune system. Infection 14 [Suppl 4] 245–247

9. Roskowski W, Ciborowski P, Ko HL, Schumacher-Perdreau F, Rozkowski K, Jeljaszewicz J, Pulverer G (1985) The effect of subinhibitory concentrations of selected antibiotics on bacteria-phagocyte interaction. In: Adam D, Hahn H, Opferkuch W (eds) The influence of antibiotics on the host-parasite relationship, II. Springer, Berlin Heidelberg New York, pp 179–186
10. Shen LL, Pernet AG (1985) Mechanism of inhibition of DNA gyrase by analogues of nalidixic acid: the target of the drug is DNA. Proc Natl Acad Sci USA 82:307–311
11. Smith JT (1984) Awakening the slumbering potential of the 4-quinolones antibacterials. Pharm J 233:299–305
12. Watanabe Y, Tawara S, Mine Y, Kikuchi H (1986) Synergism of cephalosporins at subinhibitory concentrations and polymorphonuclear leukocytes on phagocytic killing of *Escherichia coli* and its mode of action. J Antibiot (Tokyo) 39:294–303
13. Williams P (1987) Sub MICs of cefuroxime and ciprofloxacin influence interaction of complement and immunoglobulins with *Klebsiella pneumoniae*. Antimicrob Agents Chemother 31(5):758–762

Interference of Tunicamycin-Induced Staphylococcal Lectin Dysfunction with Specific Adherence Mechanisms and Immune Responses *

J. Beuth, H. L. Ko, R. Pfeiffer, A. Yassin, Y. Ohshima, and G. Pulverer

Introduction

Staphylococcus saprophyticus is a coagulase-negative, novobiocin-resistant staphylococcus which is a frequent cause of urinary tract infections, especially in young women [7]. Infection with this microorganism may also involve the upper urinary tract and reduce the concentration capacity of the kidney [5]. *S. saprophyticus* has been shown to adhere in greater numbers to uroepithelial cells and periurethral cells than to other types of cells, e.g., skin and buccal cells [3]. Accordingly, this microorganism is not known as a human pathogen in organ systems other than the urogenital tract [4].

The capacity of bacteria to adhere to eukaryotic cells is dependent upon physicochemical factors such as surface charge, hydrophobic interactions [3], and the presence of characteristic lectin receptors [1]. However, microbial lectins play the dominant role in the specific adherence process. Subinhibitory concentrations of certain antibiotics (e.g., tunicamycin) were found to interfere with the protein glycosylation [6]. Since the organophilic distribution of infectious diseases apparently can be mediated by lectins, a receptor blockade [1] or dysfunction necessarily results in diminished organ colonization. Recent experiments from our laboratories have shown that microorganism-induced stimulation of PMNs (polymorphonuclear granulocytes) obviously is a specific carbohydrate-dependent process, too. Thus, blockade of bacterial lectins with specific glycoconjugates or experimentally induced lectin dysfunction greatly decreased the stimulation of PMNs, suggesting that lectin-like receptors apparently mediate the stimulation of PMNs [2].

In the present study we have examined whether oligosaccharides found on staphylococcal surface glycoproteins (lectins) have changed adhesion properties after interference of the antibiotic tunicamycin with the glycosylation procedure.

* This study was supported by the Deutsche Forschungsgemeinschaft
Institute of Hygiene, University of Cologne, Goldenfelsstr. 19–21, 5000 Cologne 41, Federal Republic of Germany

The Influence of Antibiotics on the Host-Parasite Relationship III
Edited by G. Gillissen, W. Opferkuch, G. Peters, and G. Pulverer

Materials and Methods

Bacteria

Urinary isolates of *S. saprophyticus* (strain S1, kindly provided by Prof. Heczko, Cracow, Poland) were cultivated in tryptic soy broth (Becton-Dickinson, Heidelberg, FRG) for 24 h at 37 °C, centrifuged, resuspended in phosphate-buffered saline (PBS, Flow Laboratories GmbH, Meckenheim, FRG), washed twice, and adjusted to the turbidity of McFarland No. 5. The purity was checked on sheep blood agar and the identity was confirmed by colonial morphology, gram staining, catalase and coagulase test, and novobiocin susceptibility [8].

Adherence Assays

To establish the minimal inhibitory concentration (MIC) of the antibiotic tunicamycin (Sigma Chemicals Co., St. Louis, United States), bacteria (5×10^5/ml) were incubated overnight in a serial dilution of 100–0.39 µg tunicamycin/ml. For certain investigations, *S. saprophyticus* was incubated for 18–22 h with sub-MICs of tunicamycin (25 and 12.5 µg/ml), washed twice, suspended in PBS, and the turbidity adjusted according to McFarland No. 5. Adherence tests were performed as previously described [10]. Briefly, bacteria were mixed with uroepithelial cells, collected from pooled urine specimens at a 5000:1 ratio, and incubated at 37 °C for 15 min in 1 ml RPMI 1640 (Gibco, Karlsruhe, FRG). These conditions were found to be optimal in preliminary experiments. Unbound bacteria were removed by repeated washing with RPMI 1640 and centrifugation (three times). The number of bacteria adherent per cell was determined by counting the organisms (per 100 uroepithelial cells) under a light microscope (×100) after methanol fixation to glass slides and methylene blue staining.

Human PMN Function

Human PMNs from healthy volunteers of both sexes and different age were separated and prepared as previously described [9]. For the chemiluminescence measurements, luminol (Sigma Chemicals Co.) was dissolved in dimethylsulfoxide and used at a concentration of 2×10^{-5} *M*. The reaction mixture consisted of a PMN suspension (0.25 ml) at a concentration of 1×10^6 cells/ml MEM (Gibco), 0.45 ml Hank's solution (Gibco) containing 2×10^{-5} *M* luminol and 0.05 ml of a *Staphylococcus saprophyticus* suspension (strain S1, tunicamycin treated and untreated control, 1×10^9 bacteria/ml PBS). Chemiluminescence measurements were carried out at 37 °C (LKB 1251 Luminometer, Turku, Finland) and recorded as millivolts. The significance of the data *(P)* was calculated by Student's *t*-test.

Results

To demonstrate the lectin-dependent mechanisms of bacterial adhesion requiring intact glycoproteins (with respect to bacterial lectins of glycoprotein character),

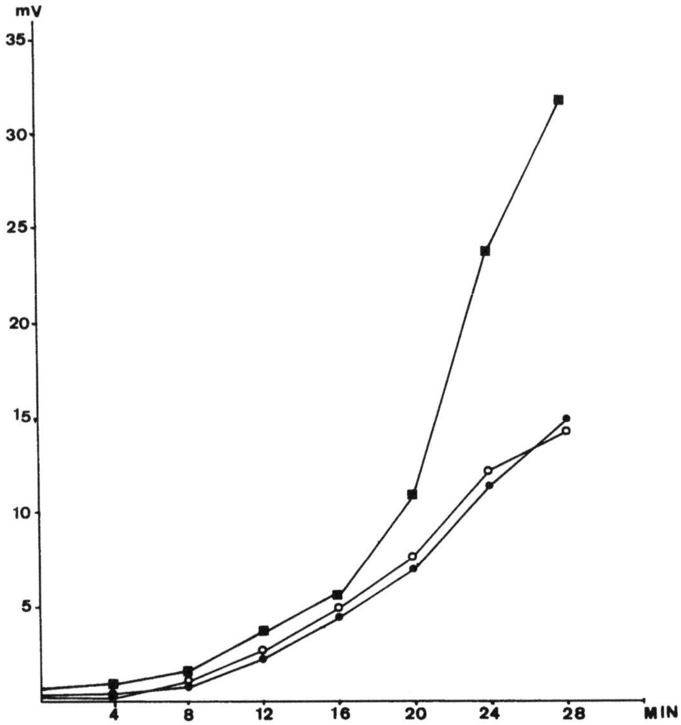

Fig. 1. Induction of chemiluminescence from human PMNs after stimulation with *S. saprophyticus* strain S1 (■, untreated and tunicamycin(*TM*)-treated; ●, 25 µg/ml; ○, 12.5 µg/ml). mV range after 28 min: native strain, 34.69 (SD ± 3.57); TM-treated strain 25 µg/ml, 16.08 (SD ± 1.07), $P<0.005$ (highly significant); TM-treated strain 12.5 µg/ml, 14.78 (SD ± 1.32), $P<0.005$ (highly significant). The experiments were performed twice in duplicate and showed similar patterns. An individual experiment is presented

we treated *S. saprophyticus* (strain 1) with subinhibitory concentrations of tunicamycin (25 and 12.5 µg/ml; MIC = 50 µg/ml). After incubation with uroepithelial cells the total number of bacteria associated with 100 cells was determined by microscopic observation, and the mean value was calculated for native staphylococci (38.9/cell). Tunicamycin (TM) treatment of the staphylococci substantially decreased the microbial adherence to uroepithelial cells (74.6% decrease for 25 µg TM/ml and 71.5% decrease for 12.5 µg TM/ml). In both cases the depression was significant ($P<0.025$). Thus, tunicamycin induced modifications of oligosaccharide structures obviously resulting in lectin (glycoprotein) dysfunction inhibited staphylococcal adherence to uroepithelial cells.

Human PMNs were evidently stimulated in the presence of luminol with native *S. saprophyticus* (strains S1) whereas tunicamycin treatment of the bacteria significantly ($P<0.005$) decreased the stimulation. The response in chemiluminescence is presented in Fig. 1. This loss of PMN-stimulating potency as well as the drastically reduced adherence to uroepithelial cells apparently is the result of a bacterial lectin dysfunction resulting from the incompleteness in oligosaccharide biosynthesis. Thus, bacterial surface lectins apparently mediate the specific adhesion to host cells and the stimulation of antibacterial immune response (granulocytes).

Discussion

Adhesion to mucosal surfaces is recognized as an important component of pathogenic mechanisms leading to the colonization of host tissue. Generally one can distinguish between specific attachment, mainly due to lectins or specific antibodies, and nonspecific attachment due to other forces of a cell-cell interaction. The majority of microbial surface lectins (adhesins or colonization factors) appear to recognize complex oligomers on eukaryotic cell surfaces. Similar to vertebrate lectins, bacterial adhesins require intact protein and carbohydrate structures for adequate interaction with oligosacharide moieties in the specific recognition process [11]. To evaluate the role of bacterial surface glycoprotein receptors (lectins) in certain infectious diseases, we have utilized subinhibitory concentrations of tunicamycin to modify them in order to assess their importance in the specific adherence process. Our data show that tunicamycin-mediated modification of the surface glycosylation of *S. saprophyticus* strain S1 greatly reduced (more than 70%) staphylococcal adherence to uroepithelial cells. Similar effects could be achieved with a blockade of staphylococcal lectins with specific complementary glycoconjugates, which decreased the microbial adherence to those cells by about 80% (unpublished data). Thus, receptor blockade or antibiotic (tunicamycin) treatment resulting in glycoprotein (lectin) dysfunction inhibited bacterial adherence. Consequently, the antibacterial immune system (e.g., monocytes, humoral factors) of the host might be more effective against these nonadherent bacteria since the adherence process is a prerequisite for invasion and induction of infectious diseases.

Apart from nonspecific adherence mechanisms [11], the specific lectin-mediated adhesion seems to be very important for the PMN-*Staphylococcus* interaction, too. Thus, bacterial lectin dysfunction (after treatment of *S. saprophyticus* with subinhibitory concentrations of tunicamycin) resulted in a substantially decreased stimulation of human PMNs which could be observed as well after microbial lectin blockade with specific glycoconjugates [2]. However, it should be considered that PMNs most likely also have lectin-like surface receptors which may be important for their function. Further studies are needed to elucidate these PMN receptors.

In conclusion, subinhibitory concentrations of antibiotics (e.g., tunicamycin) apparently inhibit the specific (lectin-mediated) adhesion of staphylococci to host cells, which might protect the host from bacterial organ colonization. However, such a treatment may also interfere with (decrease) the receptor-mediated stimulation of PMN function, which is important for the host's resistance to bacterial infections.

Summary

Microbial surface glycoproteins with lectin function are considered to be involved in the specific recognition process associated with infectious diseases. Treatment of *Staphylococcus saprophyticus* (strain S1, which exhibits well-defined surface lectins) with subinhibitory concentrations of the antibiotic tunicamycin was found to block the protein glycosylation of the bacterial surfaces. Since microbial lectins (adhesins) generally are glycoproteins and play an important role in the organophilic distribution of infectious diseases, adhesion of *S. saprophyticus* to human uroepithelial cells was substantially decreased (74.6%) after inhibition of the biosynthesis of N-linked carbohydrate chains, which are important for adequate lectin function. Chemiluminescence measurements of human polymorphonuclear leukocyte (PMN) function yielded results suggesting the importance of lectin-carbohydrate interactions in this process, too. Apparently, the presence of intact cell surface carbohydrate chains is required for a successful completion of the adhesion phase of pathogenic bacteria in infectious diseases and for the induction of PMN stimulation.

References

1. Beuth J, Ko HL, Schroten H, Sölter J, Uhlenbruck G, Pulverer G (1987) Lectin mediated adhesion of *S. pneumoniae* and its specific inhibition. Zbl Bakt Hyg [A] 265:160–168
2. Beuth J, Ko HL, Pulverer G (1988) The role of staphylococcal lectins in human granulocyte stimulation. Infection 16:46–48
3. Colleen S, Hovelius B, Wislander A, Mardh PA (1979) Surface properties of *S. saprophyticus* and *S. epidermidis* as studied by adherence tests and two-polymer, aqueous phase systems. Acta Pathol Microbiol Scand [B]87:321–328
4. Gunnarson A, Mardh PA, Lundblad A, Svenson S (1984) Oligosaccharide structures mediating agglutination of sheep erythrocytes by *S. saprophyticus*. Infect Immun 45:41–46
5. Hovelius B, Mardh PA, Bygren P (1979) Urinary tract infections caused by *Staphylococcus saprophyticus*. J Urol 122:645–647
6. Irimura T, Gonzales R, Nicolson GL (1981) Effects of tunicamycin on B 16 metastatic melanoma cell surface glycoproteins. Cancer Res 41:3411:3418
7. Jordan PE, Iravani A, Richard GA, Baer H (1980) Urinary tract infection caused by *Staphylococcus saprophyticus*. J Infect Dis 142:510–515
8. Kloos WE, Schleifer KH (1975) Simplified scheme for routine identification of human *Staphylococcus* species. J Clin Microbiol 1:82–88
9. Pulverer G, Roszkowski W, Ko HL, Roszkowski K, Jeljaszewicz J (1986) Tierexperimentelle Untersuchungen zur Beeinflussung des Immunsystems durch Ofloxacin. Infection 14:40–44
10. Teti G, Chiofalo MS, Tomasello F, Fava C, Mastroeni P (1987) Mediation of *S. saprophyticus* adherence to uroepithelial cells by lipoteichoic acid. Infect Immun 55:839–842
11. Uhlenbruck G (1987) Bacterial lectins: mediators of adhesion. Zbl Bakt Hyg [A]263:497–508

An In Vitro Model to Investigate the Influence of Antibiotics on Bacterial Susceptibility to Surface Phagocytosis by Human Polymorphonuclear Leukocytes *

C. G. Gemmell

The importance of bacterial adherence followed by invasion has been recognized in infective endocarditis wherein the bacteria must first adhere to the cardiac valve before colonization and invasion can occur [21]. Specific adherence of *Staphylococcus aureus* as well as *S. epidermidis* to endothelial cells and to artificial valvular prostheses has been demonstrated [6]. Some insight into the mechanism of invasion has recently been gained from the finding that endothelial cells may ingest *S. aureus* [17]. Fibronectin too has been shown to potentiate endothelial adherence but not phagocytic ingestion [8]. Likewise *S. epidermidis* is a common and innocuous inhabitant of human skin which can become an opportunistic pathogen of transiently or permanently implanted plastic prostheses such as intravascular catheters [18], CSF shunts [22], peritoneal dialysis catheters [24], orthopaedic devices [26], cardiac pacemakers [15] and prosthetic valves [23]. *S. epidermidis* is able to adhere to and to grow on the surfaces of such prostheses in vitro [2]. Later an extracellular slime substance is produced in which the staphylococci become enmeshed [19]. It has been suggested that this extracellular slime substance may also act as a virulence determinant in foreign body infections by interfering with some of the host defences [7] such as the lymphoproliferative response of mononuclear cells to polyclonal stimuli. In addition the slime was shown to inhibit polymorphonuclear leucocyte (PMNL) chemotaxis, to stimulate degranulation [11] and to impair ingestion of preopsonized bacteria ([10] Gemmell, unpublished observations). However, these studies do not accurately reflect the normal clinical situation in which *S. epidermidis* is present as a biofilm on a plastic surface. Therefore the encounter between these bacteria and PMNLs in vivo is likely to take place in a stationary phase or adherent to a surface [9]. Almost 40 years ago it was shown [27] that "surface phagocytosis" is involved in host defence against *Streptococcus pneumoniae*. This bacterium could be cleared from the lung prior to the development of specific anticapsular antibodies normally necessary for opsonophagocytosis. Surface phagocytosis allowed the host to overcome pneumococcal infection without these opsonins.

More recently a laboratory model of surface phagocytosis was developed whereby adherent *Staphylococcus aureus* and *Pseudomonas aeruginosa* could be handled by PMNLs on plastic, agar or glass surfaces [13]. It was shown that opsonization was not necessary for successful ingestion and killing by PMNLs. The

* Part of this study was supported by Upjohn Inc., Kalamazoo, USA
Department of Bacteriology, University of Glasgow, Royal Infirmary, Glasgow G4 OSF, United Kingdom

The Influence of Antibiotics on the Host-Parasite Relationship III
Edited by G. Gillissen, W. Opferkuch, G. Peters, and G. Pulverer

technology of this study involved the use of radiolabelled bacteria based on the assay developed earlier by Verhoef et al. [25]. In our laboratory we have used clinical isolates *Staphylococcus epidermidis* as indicator organisms of adherence to plastic and collagenous surfaces followed by their phagocytosis by PMNLs [4]. The strains used had been isolated from cases of peritonitis in patients maintained on chronic ambulatory peritoneal dialysis (CAPD) and were variable with respect to slime production according to the methods developed by Christensen et al. [2].

Thereafter it was deemed important to assess the effect of various antistaphylococcal antibiotics on bacterial adherence and subsequent opsonophagocytosis. These studies were prompted by the earlier observations from this laboratory and others that the susceptibility of staphylococci to phagocytosis can be potentiated by pre-exposure of the bacteria to low concentrations of certain antibiotics [5, 16]. Clindamycin and fusidic acid were more effective in this respect by inhibiting protein A expression on the surface of *S. aureus*. Protein A has been recognized as an inhibitor of opsonophagocytosis [20] and its removal may be important to our understanding of the treatment of staphylococcal infections of artificial prostheses.

Briefly we used the method developed by Lee et al. [13] with a number of modifications such as a ten-fold-reduction in the numbers of bacteria used as the inoculum to individual wells of polystyrene tissue culture plates. By allowing the radiolabelled bacteria to remain in contact with the solid surface for 3 h it was possible thereafter to measure the degree of bacterial adherence from the residual radioactivity found in saline washes of the wells as follows:

1. Bacteria grown with [^{3}H]adenine for 15 h at 37 °C in Mueller Hinton broth
2. Washed three times with saline and standardized to 1×10^7/ml
3. Bacteria (in 1 ml) allowed to attach to plastic for 3 h
4. Plastic washed three times with saline
5. Radioactivity measured in washings to estimate percentage bacteria adherent to plastic
6. Ten percent human serum added to opsonize bacteria for 15 min
7. Addition of 5×10^5 PMNLs to adherent bacteria
8. Incubation with shaking for up to 45 min
9. Treatment with trypsin to remove PMNLs
10. Collection of washings and centrifugation at low speed to measure PMNL-associtated bacteria

In this way the relative adherence of four strains of *S. epidermidis* was analysed (see Table 1). By comparison a strongly slime-producing strain (KH11) isolated from a catheter-associated infection is included. In addition we looked at the ability of these bacteria to adhere to the same polystyrene plates covered with a thin layer of dried collagen. Variation in adherence to both surfaces was recognized amongst the strains (high and low), which showed no correlation with slime production. The adherence of these strains of *S. epidermidis* was reasonably consistent from experiment to experiment and was used to examine their susceptibility to opsonophagocytosis by human PMNLs. Purified PMNLs prepared according to the method of Böyum [1] were used in these studies. Human serum was used

Table 1. Comparison of different strains of *S. epidermidis* with respect to their adherence to plastic and collagen

Strain	% Adherence to	
	Plastic	Collagen
Murray	31	25
Logan	20	15
Thomson	71	49
Tait	20	36
KH11	53	56

Table 2. Opsonic requirements of *S. epidermidis*[a] with respect to surface phagocytosis by PMNs

Time	% Uptake by PMNs	
	Without serum	With serum
15 min	12	33
30 min	25	46.5
45 min	9.5	27.5

[a] Strain Murray used in study.

at a concentration of 10% (V/V) to determine whether opsonization was necessary to ensure phagocytic ingestion of *S. epidermidis*. Contrary to the earlier studies [13, 14] with *S. aureus*, we found that *S. epidermidis* and latterly *S. aureus* required serum opsonization before surface phagocytosis could take place (see Table 2).

Having monitored the elements of normal surface phagocytosis of *S. epidermidis*, our attention was then directed to follow adherence and opsonophagocytosis of bacteria grown in the presence of sub-MIC levels ($^1/_8$, ¼ and ½ MIC) of two antistaphylococcal antibiotics (clindamycin, vancomycin). The bacteria had been exposed during growth at 37 °C to each drug for 15 h before assessment of their ability to adhere to polystyrene and their susceptibility to opsonophagocytosis. The results of such experiments are summarized in Tables 3–6.

Table 3. Adherence to and subsequent phagocytosis of *S. epidermidis* from plastic following growth in the presence of sub-MIC levels of clindamycin

Cultural conditions	% Adherence of strain Logan	% Bacteria phagocytosed in 10 min
No antibiotic	43	15
$^1/_2$ MIC clindamycin	14	12
$^1/_4$ MIC clindamycin	10	5.6
$^1/_8$ MIC clindamycin	21	10.3

Table 4. Adherence to and subsequent phagocytosis of *S. epidermidis* from plastic following growth in the presence of sub-MIC levels of clindamycin

Cultural conditions	% Adherence of *strain Tait*	% Bacteria phagocytosed in 10 min
No antibiotic	15	21
$^1/_2$ MIC clindamycin	21	20
$^1/_4$ MIC clindamycin	20	19
$^1/_8$ MIC clindamycin	21	17

Table 5. Adherence of *S. epidermidis* to plastic following growth in the presence of sub-MIC levels of vancomycin

Cultural conditions	% Adherence of	
	Strain Murray	Strain Tait
No antibiotic	44	31
$^1/_2$ MIC vancomycin	27	9
$^1/_4$ MIC vancomycin	31	30
$^1/_8$ MIC vancomycin	42	33

Table 6. Surface phagocytosis of *S. epidermidis* strains: influence of vancomycin at subgrowth inhibitory concentrations

Cultural conditions	% Phagocytosis[a] of	
	Strain Murray	Strain Tait
No antibiotic	32.0	10.0
$^1/_2$ MIC vancomycin	27.0	19.5
$^1/_4$ MIC vancomycin	32.5	27.0
$^1/_8$ MIC vancomycin	33.0	25.5

[a] Measured after 10 min interaction with PMNs.

Table 7. Surface phagocytosis of *S. aureus*: influence of vancomycin at subgrowth inhibitory concentrations

	S. aureus[a] (Cowan 1)	*S. aureus*[b] (Morris)
Effect of adherence	Inhibition at $^1/_2$ MIC	None
Effect on surface phagocytosis	Stimulation at $^1/_2$ and $^1/_4$ MIC	None

[a] Cowan 1 strain rich in protein A.
[b] Morris strain rich in polysaccharide capsule.

There are obvious differences between each strain used (Logan and Tait) when the bacteria were exposed to sub-MIC clindamycin. One strain (Logan) displayed reduced adherence to plastic and some reduction in susceptibility to surface phagocytosis (probably due to reduced members of available target bacteria on the plastic surface) under these circumstances. The other strain (Tait) showed no differences in adherence or susceptibility to phagocytosis with this antibiotic.

By comparison when vancomycin was used as the test drug both bacterial strains tested showed a reduced ability to adhere to the plastic at ½ MIC but not at higher dilutions of the drug. Only strain Tait showed increased susceptibility to phagocytosis following exposure to ½, ¼ and $^1/_8$ MIC vancomycin. Microscopic examination of the coagulase-negative staphylococci after growth in the presence of each drug did not provide an explanation for these differences. It did not appear as though their ability to elaborate surface slime was affected by exposure to the drug. More subtle changes in the hydrophobic/hydrophilic nature of the cell surface might be more critical since we are concerned only with the very earliest phase of colonization of the plastic surface before the bacteria have had time to synthesize extracellular slime substance.

Changes in their surface topography are also likely to account for the differences seen between two strains of *S. aureus* used in a similar assay. One strain (Cowan 1) is rich in protein A and the other (Morris) is encapsulated. Vancomycin failed to alter the adherence or susceptibility of strain Morris to surface phagocytosis. On the other hand strain Cowan 1 displayed reduced adherence and increased susceptibility to phagocytosis in the presence of the drug (see Table 7).

Discussion

Phagocytosis of staphylococci adherent to a surface may provide an in vitro model to study plastic foreign body infections in man. We have looked only at the early stages of bacterial colonization and its interrelationship with phagocytic cells. However, when *S. epidermidis* was allowed to grow on the plastic surface for up to 18 h [11], slime production was not apparent by 6 h whereas visible slime was seen after 12 h. In this study slime production correlated with the development of resistance to surface phagocytosis. Our studies have shown that bacterial resistance to phagocytosis may also occur early in the colonization process and that exposure to antibiotics at low concentrations prior to contact with the plastic surface may alter both the degree of bacterial adherence and the susceptibility of the staphylococci to surface phagocytosis. Intracellular killing was not measured in the present studies. Since there is evidence of a local granulocyte defect at the site of implantation of a foreign body in animals [28], there is merit in exploring this phenomenon further using such a laboratory model. In this respect the effect of appropriate antibiotics on the efficacy of surface phagocytosis would be worthy of study especially in the light of knowledge that intracellular accumulation of some antibiotics can occur to the benefit of the phagocytic cell killing process [3, 12]. It will be important, however, to mimic as far as possible the situation as it pertains to the use of artificial prostheses in man. In this respect the correct form of polystyrene substrate should be used to measure bacterial adherence and opsonophagocytosis. A greater understanding of the pathogenesis and management of infections associated with the use of prosthetic valves or intravenous catheters should emerge.

Summary

1. *Staphylococcus epidermidis* is more adherent than *S. aureus* to plastic surfaces.
2. Different strains of *S. epidermidis* show different degrees of adherence to plastic.

3. Growth in the presence of low concentrations of antistaphylococcal drugs can alter the intensity of plastic adherence.
4. Changes in adherence do not correlate with changes in susceptibility to surface phagocytosis.
5. Surface phagocytosis can be potentiated or depressed by pre-exposure of the bacteria to antibiotics.
6. Changes do not appear to be related to slime production.

References

1. Böyum A (1968) Isolation of mononuclear cells and granulocytes from human blood. Scand J Clin Lab Invest 21 [Suppl 97]:77–89
2. Christensen GD, Simpson WA, Bisno AL, Beachey EH (1982) Adherence of slime-producing strains of *Staphylococcus epidermidis* to smooth surfaces. Infect Immun 37:318–326
3. Easmon CSF (1979) The effect of antibiotics on the intracellular survival of *Staphylococcus aureus* in vitro. Br J Exp Pathol 60:24–28
4. Gemmell CG, Marshall E (1987) Surface phagocytosis of *Staphylococcus epidermidis:* influence of exposure to certain antibiotics. In: Proceedings of third European congress of clinical microbiology. The Hague, Holland abstr 62
5. Gemmell CG, O'Dowd A (1983) Regulation of protein A biosynthesis in *Staphylococcus aureus* by certain antibiotics: its effect on phagocytosis by leukocytes. J Antimicrob Chemother 12:587–597
6. Gould K, Ramirez-Ronda CH, Holmes RK, Sanford JP (1975) Adherence of bacteria to heart valves in vitro. J Clin Invest 56:1364–1370
7. Gray ED, Peters G, Verstegen M, Regelmann WE (1984) Effect of extracellular slime substance from *Staphylococcus epidermidis* on the human cellular response. Lancet i:365–367
8. Hamill RJ, Vann JM, Proctor RA (1986) Phagocytosis of *Staphylococcus aureus* by cultured bovine aortic endothelial cells: model for postadherence events in endovascular infections. Infect Immun 54:833–836
9. Hayashi K, Lee DA, Quie PG (1986) Chemiluminescent response of polymorphonuclear leukocytes to *Streptococcus pneumoniae* and *Haemophilus influenzae* in suspension and adhered to glass. Infect Immun 52:397–400
10. Johnson GM, Lee DA, Regelmann WE, Gray ED, Peters G, Quie PG (1986) Interference with granulocyte function by *Staphylococcus epidermidis* slime. Infect Immun 54:13–20
11. Johnson GM, Regelmann WE, Gray ED, Peters G, Quie PG (1987) Staphylococcal slime and host defences: effects on polymorphonuclear granulocytes. Zbl Bakt Mikrobiol Hyg Suppl 16:33–44
12. Klempner M, Styrt B (1981) Clindamycin uptake by human neutrophils. J Infect Dis 144:472–479
13. Lee DA, Hoidal JR, Clawson CC, Quie PG, Peterson PK (1983) Phagocytosis by polymorphonuclear leukocytes of *Staphylococcus aureus* and *Pseudomonas aeruginosa* adherent to plastic, agar or glass. J Immunol Methods 63:103–114
14. Lee DA, Hoidal JR, Garlich DH, Clawson CC, Quie PG, Peterson PK (1984) Opsonin – independent phagocytosis of surface adherent bacteria by human alveolar macrophages. J Leukocyte Biol 36:689–701
15. Lemire GG, Morin JE, Dobell ARC (1975) Pacemaker infections: a 12-year review. Can J Surg 18:181–184
16. Milatovic D, Braveny I, Verhoef J (1983) Clindamycin enhances opsonization of *Staphylococcus aureus*. Antimicrob Agents Chemother 24:413–417
17. Ogawa SK, Yurberg ER, Hatcher VB, Levitt MA, Lowy FD (1985) Bacterial adherence to human endothelial cells in vitro. Infect Immun 50:218–224
18. Peters G, Locci R, Pulverer G (1981) Microbial colonization of prosthetic devices. II Scanning electron microscopy of naturally infected intravenous catheters. Zent Bakt Mikrobiol Hyg I Abt Orig B 173:293–299

19. Peters G, Locci R, Pulverer G (1982) Adherence and growth of coagulase-negative staphylococci on surfaces of intravenous catheters. J Infect Dis 146:479–482
20. Peterson PK, Verhoef J, Sabath LD, Quie PG (1977) Effect of protein A on staphylococcal opsonization. Infect Immun 15:760–764
21. Scheld WM (1984) Pathogenesis and pathophysiology of infective endocarditis. In: Sande MA, Kaye D, Root RM (eds) Endocarditis. Churchill-Livingstone, New York, pp 1–32
22. Schoenbaum SC, Gardner P, Shillito J (1975) Infection of cerebrospinal fluid shunts: epidermiology, clinical manifestations and therapy. J Infect Dis 131:543–552
23. Speller DCE, Mitchell RG (1973) Coagulase-negative staphylococci causing endocarditis after cardiac surgery. J Clin Pathol 16:517–522
24. Vas SI (1983) Microbiologic aspects of chronic ambulatory peritoneal dialysis. Kidney Int 23:83–92
25. Verhoef J, Peterson PK, Quie PG (1977) Kinetics of staphylococcal opsonization attachment, ingestion and killing by human polymorphonuclear leukocytes: a quantitative assay using (^{3}H) thymidine-labelled bacteria. J Immunol Methods 14:303–311
26. Wilson PD, Salvati EA, Aglietti P, Kutner LT (1973) The problem of infection in endoprosthetic surgery of the hip joint. Clin Orthop 96:213–221
27. Wood WB, Smith MR, Watson B (1946) Studies on the mechanism of recovery in pneumococcal pneumonia IV. The mechanism of phagocytosis in the absence of antibody. J Exp Med 84:387–402
28. Zimmerli W, Lew PD, Waldvogel FA (1984) Pathogenesis of foreign body infection. Evidence for a local granulocyte defect. J Clin Invest 73:1191–1200

Growth Rate, Iron Depletion, and a Sub-Minimal Inhibitory Concentration of Penicillin G Affect the Surface Hydrophobicity of *Staphylococcus aureus**

P. A. G. Domingue [1,2], E. Schwarzinger [3], and M. R. W. Brown [1]

Introduction

The surface composition of bacteria is important in interactions with the host [6, 11, 50] and with antibiotics [7, 8]. The surface is altered by the growth environment [6, 16, 50] so that bacteria become typical of it. Thus bacteria grown in vitro and in vivo reflect both genotypic and phenotypic changes [6, 14, 20, 51]. More attention to in vivo characteristics would enhance understanding of infectious processes, and in vitro design should account for this. We report on batch-culture conditions that approximate to in vivo conditions and that alter surface hydrophobicity (SH).

Growth rate per se significantly alters envelope composition [6, 21, 53], including penicillin-binding proteins [57], and *Staphylococcus aureus* usually has reduced doubling times in vivo [Zak and Sande, cited in 14 (p 179); 23, 29].

Nutrient depletion also affects surface composition and evidence obtained directly, without subculture, shows that bacteria grow under conditions of iron depletion in humans [2, 3, 9, 30, 49].

The hydrophobic properties of protein molecules are primarily attributed to side chains of phenylalanine, tyrosine and tryptophan residues and to a folding of the polypeptide chain to give tertiary and quaternary structures [17]. In membrane teichoic acid or lipopolysaccharide, hydrophobicity is conferred by the presence of lipid moieties. The degree of SH of various bacteria correlated positively with the degree of adherence to different types of animal cells [34, 62, 66]. In natural environments at least, hydrophobic adhesins are partly responsible for adherence and also for scavenging surface-localised nutrients [27, 28].

Environmental factors such as growth phase, nutrition or the presence of antibiotics alter SH. Iron deprivation is known to decrease the SH of *Neisseria gonorrhoeae* [33]. The SH of *S. aureus* was suppressed by unknown factors in blood agar but enhanced by brain-heart infusion agar [31, 65]. Exponential-phase *S. aureus* were more hydrophobic than those in the stationary phase [35, 41, 65]. Bacteria

* This work was partly supported by grants from the Medical Research Council and the Cystic Fibrosis Research Trust. PAGD was supported by a grant from the Science and Engineering Research Council.

[1] Microbiology Research Group, Pharmaceutical Sciences Institute, Department of Pharmaceutical Sciences, Aston University, Aston Triangle, Birmingham B4 7ET, United Kingdom
[2] Current address: Department of Biology, University of Calgary, 2500 University Drive N. W., Calgary, Alberta, Canada T2N 1N4
[3] Sandoz Research Institute, Brunner Str. 59, 1235 Vienna, Austria

The Influence of Antibiotics on the Host-Parasite Relationship III
Edited by G. Gillissen, W. Opferkuch, G. Peters, and G. Pulverer

may encounter subinhibitory concentrations of drugs in vivo [4] and the SH of low protein A-producing *S. aureus* strains was increased by subminimal inhibitory concentrations (sub-MICs) of penicillin G, by uncharacterised mechanisms [63]. We report on the influence of growth rate, iron depletion and penicillin G on the SH of *S. aureus*.

Materials and Methods

Bacteria. *S. aureus* NCTC 6571 (Oxford strain; National Collection of Type Cultures, Central Public Health Laboratory, Colindale Avenue, London NW9 5HT, UK) and *S. aureus* 113 (Sandoz Culture Collection, Sandoz Forschungsinstitut, Brunner Straße 59, 1235 Vienna, Austria) were used.

Chemicals and Reagents. Those used and not specified in the text were Analar grade (BDH Chemicals Ltd., Poole, UK). Benzylpenicillin sodium (penicillin G) was obtained from Glaxo Laboratories Ltd., Greenford, UK. All solutions were made up in double-distilled water.

Preparation of Plastic- and Glassware. Treatment has been described elsewhere [26].

Preparation of Iron-Depleted Broth. Two ion-exchange columns (1 in. internal diameter, 500 ml volume; Pharmacia Ltd., Milton Keynes, UK) were each packed with 200 ml bed volumes of Chelex 100 resin (Bio-Rad Laboratories Ltd., Watford, UK) that had been conditioned to pH 7.4 according to the manufacturer's instructions (Bio-Rad Technical Bulletin No. 2020, 1981). 1.4 l of double-strength tryptone soya broth (TSB; Oxoid Ltd., Basingstoke, UK) was reconstituted in chilled, double-distilled water. It was then passed down consecutive columns in the cold, at a rate of 2 ml min^{-1}. The first 200 ml of fluid from each pass was discarded to avoid dilution with the water retained on the columns due to the conditioning. The treated TSB, i.e. cation-depleted TSB, and untreated or control TSB that had also been reconstituted with double distilled water were sterilised together by autoclaving at 115 °C for 20 min.

Cations including or excluding Fe were added back aseptically to treated TSB to restore original levels (TSB + Fe and TSB − Fe respectively). The osmolarities of TSB + Fe, TSB − Fe, untreated TSB and pooled, normal human serum were compared in an osmometer (Knauer Regler, Berlin, FRG) using a calibration curve constructed according to commercial standards (Fiske Associates Inc., Uxbridge, USA). Sufficient amounts of a vitamin supplement [39] (biotin, 0.003 μg ml^{-1}; pantothenic acid, 0.5 μg ml^{-1}; nicotinic acid, 0.5 μg ml^{-1}; thiamine, 0.5 μg ml^{-1}; Sigma Ltd., Poole, UK) were added aseptically so that the TSB + Fe was the equivalent of untreated TSB in morphological, cultural and limited biochemical tests (see Results and Discussion sections).

Spectroscopy. Atomic absorption spectroscopy (Model 560 spectrophotometer; Perkin Elmer Ltd., Beaconsfield, UK) was used to determine pre- and post-treatment levels of iron, calcium, magnesium, zinc and copper, and double-distilled water washings from plastic- and glassware were checked regularly for potential contamination. The levels of each cation were determined from a calibration curve constructed using commercial standards (Spectrosol grade; BDH Ltd.). The operational conditions of the spectrophotometer were as specified by the manufacturer for the cation in question.

Growth Measurements. Bacterial growth was monitored by observing the change in optical density (OD) i.e. extinction at 470 nm (E_{470}). Inocula were always taken from stationary-phase, iron-poor cultures.

Growth Conditions. Iron-rich and iron-poor cocci were grown with a relatively slow doubling time of 48 min ($t_d = 48$ min) by using an inoculum size that gave an initial absorbance of $E_{470} = 0.5$ in 250 ml pre-warmed TSB in a 500-ml flask in an orbital incubator (Gallenkamp Ltd., Loughborough, UK) at a shaking rate of 200 rm and at 37 °C. Relatively fast growth ($t_d = 24$ min) was obtained by the use of an inoculum size that gave an initial $E_{470} = 0.05$ in 250 ml pre-warmed TSB in a 1-l flask at 300 rpm and 37 °C.

Minimal Inhibitory Concentration and Sub-Minimal Inhibitory Concentration of Penicillin G. The minimal inhibitory concentration (MIC) was determined by a tube dilution method [46] using 1 ml volumes of untreated TSB, TSB+Fe and TSB−Fe and an inoculum of 10^6 colony-forming units (CFUs) of overnight, iron-poor bacteria. The tubes were incubated for 18 and 36 h at 37 °C.

The sub-MIC was chosen by growth in untreated TSB, TSB+Fe and TSB−Fe in the presence, from zero time, of different sub-MICs of penicillin. Samples were taken along the growth curve (not shown) and transferred to 5% (v/v) formalin for morphological analysis. The sub-MIC chosen was one which, crucially, did not alter the growth rate as judged by E_{470} results, but did induce morphological changes visible using light microscopy [32].

In one type of experiment, the sub-MIC of penicillin G was added, when required, to logarithmic-phase cells. The addition was at an approximate $E_{470} = 3$ for slow-growing cocci and $E_{470} = 0.5$ for fast-growing cocci. Bacteria were harvested after they had been exposed to penicillin for a further generation. Alternatively, the sub-MIC was present from zero time and samples for contact angles (CAs) were taken along the growth curves of replicate flasks, which were monitored by taking E_{470} readings.

Surface Hydrophobicity. SH was assayed by van Oss et al.'s [62] CA method. When modified as below, the method was reproducible. Cells were harvested, washed three times in 0.85% (w/v) sodium chloride and resuspended in this to a final volume of 25 ml and $E_{470} = 20$. The cells were then vacuum filtered (Millipore Ltd., London, UK) onto 47 mm diameter, 0.2 µm cellulose acetate filter pads (Sartorius Ltd./Baird and Tatlock Ltd., Atherstone, UK) that had previously been washed three times in hot, double-distilled water. After filtration, the pads were glued onto microscope slides with water-soluble glue (Gloy, Henkel Chemicals Ltd., London, UK). They were then placed in petri dish damp chambers and left overnight at 4 °C. The next day, the chambers were uncovered and the pads and adherent bacteria left to dry for 3 h at 22 °C. This period had previously been determined to give a plateau of constant CAs (see Results and Discussion sections). After drying, the pads were placed in position opposite a goniometer (Ealing Scientific Ltd., London, UK) and the angle of contact made between the bacterial lawn and a 20-μl drop of 0.85% (w/v) sodium chloride measured. A minimum of ten observations, i.e. ten CAs, were obtained for each cultural condition and each experiment was performed a minimum of three times.

Results

Reconstitution and Testing of Chelex-Treated TSB. Linear regression analysis of the atomic absorption calibration curves always gave correlation coefficients greater than 0.95. Pre-treatment and post-treatment cation levels are shown in Table 1. Double-distilled water washings of plastic- and glassware were free of contaminating cations and the contribution to iron levels by the vitamin and cation stock solutions was negligible (Table 1). Linear regression analysis of osmometer calibration curves gave correlation coefficients greater than 0.95, and both TSB+Fe and TSB−Fe were isotonic (280 mosmol) with untreated TSB and pooled, normal human serum.

The TSB+Fe was equivalent to the untreated TSB in terms of growth kinetics (Fig. 1), colonial morphology, Gram's stain, clumping factor (CF), staphylocoagulase enzyme [12] and biochemical tests (API Staph; API Ltd., Basingstoke, Hampshire, UK). TSB−Fe cultures demonstrated a more rapid onset of the stationary phase and their plateau was lower (Fig. 1). At this point they also had less pigment, looser pellets upon centrifugation and reduced catalase activity [18]. The results of the staphylocoagulase test were positive for both types of culture, but approximately four times as much was present in TSB+Fe culture supernatants when titres were related to 10^8 CFU ml^{-1} (TSB+Fe, 1:1.48; TSB−Fe, 1:0.40). The CF reaction was positive only in TSB+Fe cultures.

Choice of a Sub-MIC of Penicillin G. The MIC of penicillin G at 18 and 36 h was 0.047 μg ml^{-1} for untreated TSB, TSB+Fe and TSB−Fe cultures of *S. aureus*

Table 1. The cation content of Chelex-treated and untreated TSB and iron content of vitamin and cation stock solution

Molarity $\times 10^{-5}$				
Cation	TSB		Vitamins ($10^3 \times$ stock)	Cation ($250 \times$ stock)
	Untreated	Treated		
Fe	5.73	0.125	0.0125	0.107
Cu	0.0998	0.0281	–	–
Mg	39.20	0.0417	–	–
Ca	28.30	0.218	–	–
Zn	5.91	1.720	–	–

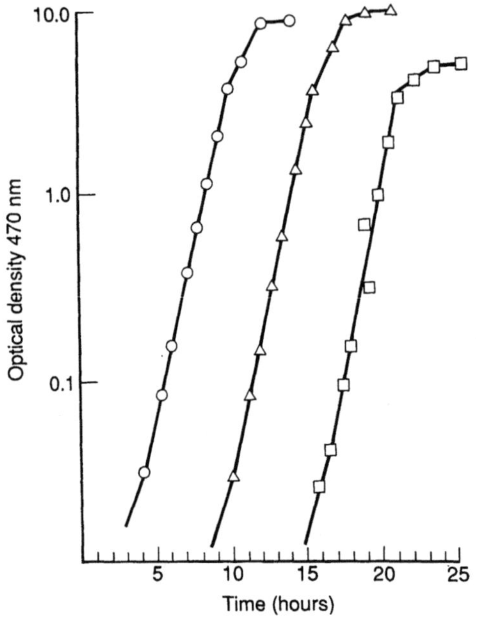

Fig. 1. Growth of *S. aureus* NCTC 6571 in TSB of varying iron content. The curves are superimposable, but have been separated for clarity and do not imply different lag phases. ○, untreated TSB; △, TSB+Fe; □, TSB−Fe

Table 2. Percentage of *S. aureus* NCTC 6571 showing morphological changes in the presence of 1/16 MIC of penicillin G (mean of ten high-power fields)

TSB+Fe		TSB−Fe	
No antibiotic	1/16 MIC	No antibiotic	1/16 MIC
4.00	56.98	2.80	62.12

NCTC 6571. Morphological changes, evident as giant cocci or incompletely divided cocci, were present in 1/16 MIC 6 h after inoculation and were quantified microscopically (Table 2). The growth rate was not altered by 1/16 MIC and therefore this sub-MIC was used throughout the study. The MIC for *S. aureus* 113 was 0.3 $\mu g\ ml^{-1}$ and, taking the same criterion, its sub-MIC of 0.03 $\mu g\ ml^{-1}$ was determined.

Growth Kinetics. Differences in initial OD, broth-volume: flask-size ratios and shaking rates resulted in relatively slow ($t_d = 48$ min) and relatively fast ($t_d = 24$ min) growing cocci. Some were harvested in the mid-log arithmic to early stationary phase (Fig. 2) whilst others were analysed throughout the growth cycle (see below). The growth rate was not affected by penicillin G or iron deprivation but the latter caused a lower stationary phase onset for the slow-growing cocci.

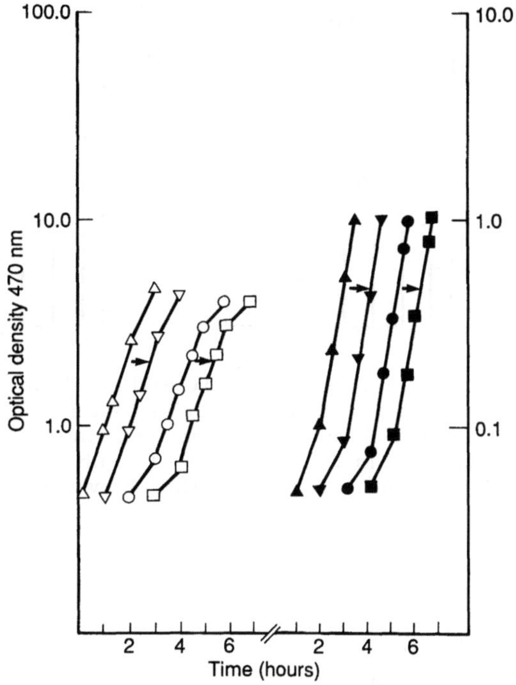

Fig. 2. Slow ($t_d = 48$ min; *open symbols*) and fast ($t_d = 24$ min; *filled symbols*) growth of *S. aureus* NCTC 6571. Different growth rates were induced by alterations in initial ODs and aeration (see text). *Arrows* denote time of addition of penicillin G. △, TSB + Fe with no antibiotic; ▽, TSB + Fe with 1/16 MIC penicillin G; ○, TSB − Fe with no antibiotic; □, TSB − Fe with 1/16 MIC penicillin G ($t_d = 48$ min). ▲, TSB + Fe with no antibiotic; ▼, TSB + Fe with 1/16 MIC penicillin G; ●, TSB − Fe with no antibiotic; ■, TSB − Fe with 1/16 MIC penicillin G ($t_d = 24$ min)

Table 3. Influence of drying time upon CAs of *S. aureus* NCTC 6571

Drying time (h)	$t_d = 48$ min		$t_d = 24$ min	
	Untreated TSB with no antibiotic	Untreated TSB with 1/16 MIC	Untreated TSB with no antibiotic	Untreated TSB with 1/16 MIC
1	12.88° ± 2.71	18.40° ± 1.60	36.50° ± 3.00	46.71° ± 2.80
2	20.58° ± 1.83	31.71° ± 4.57	48.25° ± 6.50	55.00° ± 2.50
3	30.43° ± 1.40	48.60° ± 1.60	60.00° ± 1.83	66.50° ± 4.44
3.5	29.28° ± 1.70	49.10° ± 2.30	51.30° ± 2.14	65.20° ± 2.80
4	Repeated cracking		–	–

Values are means of a minimum of ten separate determinations ± SD.

Contact Angles. The method was characterised with respect to the drying times of the pads. It was apparent that a 3-h drying period was optimal (Table 3). Initial CA experiments showed that the trend and the drying time needed to reach a plateau of constant angles for *S. aureus* were in accord with published findings [1, 10].

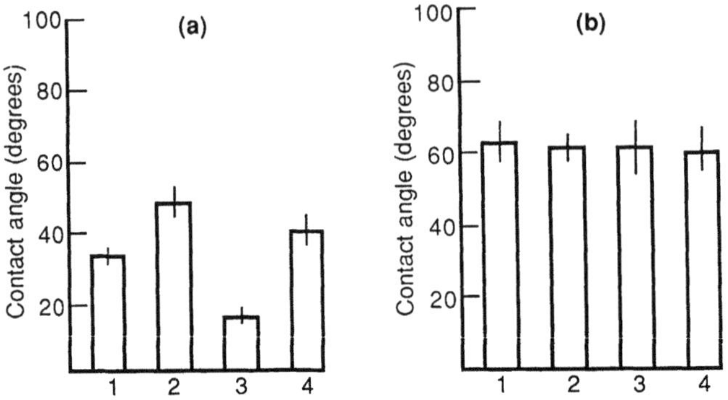

Fig. 3 a, b. SH of *S. aureus* NCTC 6571 (t_d=48 and 24 min) in TSB+FE and TSB−Fe and in the absence and presence of 1/16 MIC of penicillin G as determined by the CA method. **a** t_d= 48 min, **b** t_d=24 min. *Bars* represent standard deviations, values are means of a minimum of ten separate determinations. *1*, TSB+Fe with no antibiotic; *2*, TSB+Fe with penicillin G; *3*, TSB−Fe with no antibiotic; *4*, TSB−Fe with penicillin G

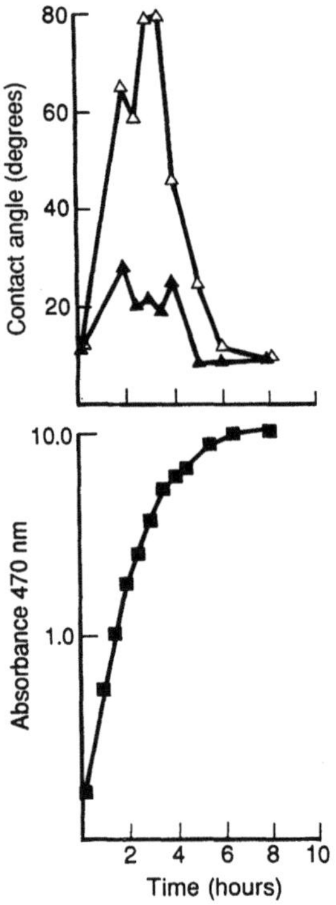

Fig. 4. Changes in SH *S. aureus* along the growth curve (t_d= 48 min): the influence of penicillin G. Note that only one representative growth curve (■) is shown. ▲, *S. aureus* 113 without penicillin G; △, *S. aureus* 113 with penicillin G

Significant differences between the eight coccal types harvested in the logarithmic phase were detected. In the slow-growing model, Fe− cocci were markedly less hydrophobic than Fe+ cocci, and penicillin G significantly increased the relative hydrophobicity of both, despite treatment for only one generation before harvest (Fig. 3 a). However, fast-growing cocci uniformly had a relatively high

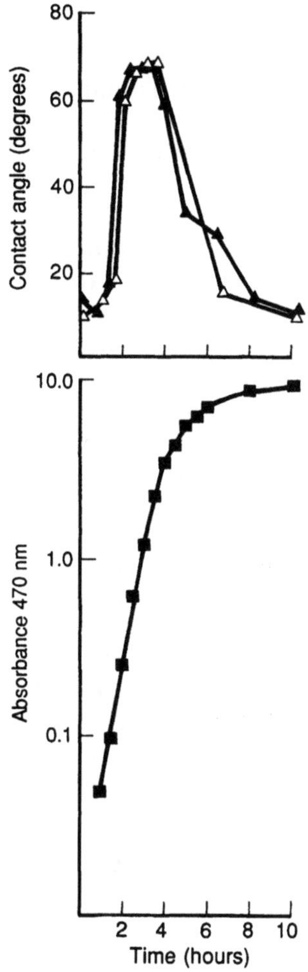

Fig. 5. Changes in SH of *S. aureus* along the growth curve ($t_d = 24$ min): lack of influence of penicillin G. Note that only one representative growth curve (■) is shown. ▲, *S. aureus* 113 without penicillin G; △, *S. aureus* 113 with penicillin G

surface hydrophobicity regardless of iron status or penicillin G treatment (Fig. 3 b).

In other experiments, it was possible to analyse the growth curves and pinpoint the appearance of these trends. The slow-growing cocci had a low SH throughout, except in the presence of penicillin G when there was a rapid increase within two generations of the start of exponential growth, rising to a maximum within approximately three generations. This maximum value was approximately 3.5 times that of maximum CAs obtainable with controls (Fig. 4). In contrast, the fast-growing cocci had a high relative SH, regardless of penicillin status, and this trend commenced approximately two generations into logarithmic growth (Fig. 5). For all cocci, the plateau of maximum SH was maintained for approximately one generation after growth departed from linear.

Discussion

Bacterial iron uptake mechanisms have been well characterised, but in gram-negative bacteria [24, 44, 45]. Very little is known about those in staphylococci although they exhibit an iron-dependent physiology [5, 36–38, 47, 48, 54, 55].

Chelex 100 has previously been shown to be efficient at removing cations from brain-heart infusion broth [13]. The method developed here for the production of TSB − Fe was successful in that TSB + Fe supported growth of *S. aureus*, indistinguishable from that in untreated TSB in terms of growth kinetics, resuits of enzymic and morphological tests and a simple biochemical screen. Yet, the omission of iron in the reconstituted medium had a significant effect, although it did not affect growth rate. Alterations in yield, the loss of pigment and decrease in catalase activity for iron-poor cocci have been previously noted [47, 54, 55].

There are several methods of determining a sub-MIC [4]. The one chosen here was one that induced significant morphological changes compared with controls, but neither lysis nor a change in growth rate. Thus it was possible to examine the SH of *S. aureus* under conditions approximating to in vivo in those respects.

The final CAs were much higher than those previously published for *S. aureus* [62] but the latter were obtained for oxygen-limited cultures. The maximum SH in *S. aureus* occurred as a function of exponential growth. This confirms the findings in a radioactive palmitic acid partition assay, when, just before onset of exponential-phase growth, there was an abrupt 4- to 5-fold increase in SH. As the stationary phase was approached, SH reached a plateau and then slowly decreased throughout the stationary phase [35]. It has been confirmed elsewhere that growth rate influences SH profoundly in a range of environmental bacteria. They became more hydrophobic during exponential growth [60] and also at high dilution rates in a chemostat [59]. The effect of iron deprivation upon SH is little characterised but it decreased SH in *N. gonorrhoeae* [33] and in this report the effect has been shown to extend to *S. aureus*. The effect of a sub-MIC of penicillin G in increasing SH confirms previous findings established by hydrophobic interaction chromatography [63] and may represent a novel action of penicillin.

Phagocytosis is a multi-step surface phenomenon that can be described in physico-chemical terms and occurs mainly due to differences in surface free energies of bacteria and phagocytes [43, 52, 61]. The first step results in attachment of the bacterium to phagocyte membrane receptors via an energy-dependent process. There are receptors for non-specific interactions such as SH which can be regarded as an earlier, more primitive system [34]. There are also receptors that undergo specific ligand-ligand or antibody-complement (C′) interactions that are saturable and possibly represent evolved mechanisms. It is possible that the predicted sequences of phagocyte-prey interactions governed by genetically more ancient mechanisms such as SH are modulated by evolved, specific binding mechanisms. If SH measurements are to be of use in understanding the in vivo interaction between host and parasite, then they must be related to the SH of the human phagocyte. The CA assay is not only a significant assay for determining bacterial SH [42, 58] but also has the advantage of not using hydrocarbons or high sodium chloride concentrations that can perturb mammalian membranes, and phagocytes have been found to have CAs of between 18° and 19° [56, 62].

In non-opsonised systems, the virulent, encapsulated *S. aureus* M was less prone to phagocytosis and had a lower CA than avirulent non-capsulated strains. Most significantly, the CAs of virulent bacteria were lower than those of phagocytes [62], i.e. the relative interfacial tensions of the bacterium and phagocyte were important. Bacteria with a lower CA, i.e. a lower interfacial tension, than phagocytes were not easily ingested. Other human blood cells had the same CA as the neutrophils. The binding of specific antisera during opsonisation increased *S. aureus* SH to give a CA greater than 18°, and the presence of C′ ensured maximum attainable SH. C′ alone had no action on the SH [62]. An increase in SH was also caused by normal human serum and purified IgG, and was dose-dependent for IgG [40]. SH was also increased by fibrin and fibrinogen [40, 62] which made ingestion easier [62]. Thus, one result of successful opsonisation is an increase in bacterial SH relative to that of the phagocyte. Penicillin G increased the SH of *S. aureus* [63], but did not affect neutrophil SH [62]. IgA reduced *S. aureus* SH, which is significant, as the role of IgA may be to protect mucosal surfaces by reducing bacterial adherence [62]. Perhaps the reported interference of opsonisation by protein A [15] is because it binds IgG at the F_c region, exposing the hydrophilic F_{ab} portion to the neutrophil. The results reported here for non-opsonised CAs predict that in the slow-growing model, iron-depleted *S. aureus,* with their CA of 16.44°, would be less easily phagocytosed than the rest in non-opsonised systems. Penicillin G, even at 1/16 MIC, would enhance the engulfment of iron-depleted *S. aureus* NCTC 6571 by increasing its hydrophobicity.

Approximately 90% of clinical isolates of *S. aureus* have an SH higher than that of non-clinical isolates [31, 65]. The SH appeared to be related to the protein A content as protein A-rich *S. aureus* strains Cowan I and 17970 had a higher relative SH than *S. aureus* strains that produced less protein A. However, other surface structures such as the fibronectin-binding protein and other protease-sensitive components probably contribute to SH because such enzymic digestion drastically reduces SH [31] and because some protein A-negative *S. aureus* strains have the same high relative SH values as high-level protein A producers [25, 63]. Possession of a capsule renders *S. aureus* strains hydrophilic [25, 62].

Significantly, abnormally high neutrophil SH values have been reported in diabetics prone to recurrent infections [19, 62] and in a group of children with recurrent middle ear and upper respiratory tract infections [22].

The knowledge of the SH properties of *S. aureus* has been exploited in the creation of a hydrophobised wound dressing that actively removes *S. aureus* from wounds, thereby speeding up healing [64].

Summary

In *S. aureus,* a slow growth rate of the magnitude found in in vivo allowed a sub-MIC of penicillin G and iron depletion profoundly to alter SH as measured by Cs. Penicillin G increased SH whilst iron depletion decreased SH compared with that in controls. In contrast, a fast growth rate abolished the effects of both penicillin G and iron in that all phenotypes had a similarly high SH.

Acknowledgment. M.R.W.B. is grateful to Dr. Jurgen Drews for generously providing excellent facilities for sabbatical research at Sandoz Forschungsinstitut, Vienna, where some of the experiments were carried out.

References

1. Absolom DR, Lamberti FV, Policova Z, Zingg W, van Oss CJ, Neumann AW (1983) Surface thermodynamics of bacterial adhesion. Appl Environ Microbiol 46:90–97
2. Anwar H, Brown MRW, Day A, Weller PH (1984) Outer membrane antigens of mucoid *Pseudomonas aeruginosa* isolated directly from the sputum of a cystic fibrosis patient. FEMS Microbiol Lett 24:235–239
3. Anwar H, Shand GH, Ward KH, Brown MRW, Alpar KE, Gowar J (1985) Antibody response to acute *Pseudomonas aeruginosa* infection in a burn wound. FEMS Microbiol Lett 29:225–230
4. Atkinson BA, Amaral L (1982) Sublethal concentrations of antibiotics, effects on bacteria and the immune system. CRC Crit Rev Microbiol 9:101–138
5. Bergeron RJ, Elliott GT, Kline SJ, Ramphal R, St. James III L (1983) Bacteriostatic and fungistatic action of catecholamide iron chelators. Antimicrob Agents Chemother 24:725–730
6. Brown MRW, Williams P (1985) The influence of environment on envelope properties affecting survival of bacteria in infections. Ann Rev Microbiol 39:527–556
7. Brown MRW, Williams P (1985) Influence of substrate limitation and growth phase on sensitivity to antimicrobial agents. J Antimicrob Chemother 15 [Supp A]:7–14
8. Brown MRW, Gilbert P, Klemperer RMM (1979) Influence of the bacterial cell envelope on combined antibiotic action. In: Williams JD (ed) Antibiotic interactions. Academic London, pp 72–76
9. Brown MRW, Anwar H, Lambert PA (1984) Evidence that mucoid *Pseudomonas aeruginosa* in the cystic fibrosis lung grows under iron-restricted conditions. FEMS Microbiol Lett 21:113–117
10. Busscher HJ, Weerkamp AH, van der Mei HC, van Pelt AWJ, de Jong HP, Arends J (1984) Measurement of the surface free energy of bacterial cell surfaces and its relevance for adhesion. Appl Environ Microbiol 48:980–983
11. Costerton JW, Marrie TJ (1983) The role of the bacterial glycocalyx in resistance to antimicrobial agents. In: Easmon CSF, Jeljaszewicz J, Brown MRW, Lambert PA (eds) Medical microbiology, vol 3. Academic, London, pp 63–85
12. Cowan ST, Steel KJ (1974) Identification of medical bacteria, 2nd edn. Cambridge University Press, Cambridge
13. Cowart RE, Marquadt MP, Foster BC (1980) The removal of iron and other trace elements from a complex bacteriological medium. Microbios Lett 13:117–122
14. Dalhoff A (1985) Differences between bacteria grown in vitro and in vivo. J Antimicrob Chemother 15 [Suppl A]:175–195
15. Dossett JH, Kronvall G, Williams RC Jr, Quie PG (1969) Antiphagocytic effects of staphylococcal protein A. J Immunol 103:1405–1410
16. Ellwood DC, Tempest DW (1972) Effects of environment on bacterial wall content and composition. Adv Microb Physiol 7:83–117
17. England E (1986) Hydrophobic interaction chromatography. Lab Pract January:64–67
18. Fung DYC, Petrishko DT (1973) Capillary tube catalase test. Appl Microbiol 26:631–632
19. Galdiero F, Romano-Carratelli C, Folgore A, Nuzzo I (1983) Phagocytosis in diabetic subjects: increase in hydrophobicity of granulocyte cytoplasmic membrane. Experentia 39:1041–1042
20. Gemmell CG (1985) In vivo consequences of the interaction between antibiotic-damaged pathogens and host animal defences. In: Adam D, Hahn H, Opferkuch W (eds) The influence of antibiotics on the host-parasite relationship. II. Springer, Berlin Heidelberg New York, pp 259–266
21. Gilbert P, Brown MRW (1978) Influence of growth rate on the gross cellular composition of *Pseudomonas aeruginosa* and its resistance to 3- and 4-chlorophenol. J Bacteriol 133:1066–1072

22. Gillman CF, Bernstein JM, van Oss CJ (1976) Decreased phagocytosis associated with increased surface hydrophobicity of neutrophils of children with chronic infections. Fed Proc 35:227
23. Gladstone GP, Glencross JG (1960) Growth and toxin production of Staphylococci in cellophane sacs in vivo. Br J Exp Pathol 41:313:333
24. Griffiths E (1983) Availability of iron and survival of bacteria in infection. In: Easmon CSF, Jeljaszewicz J, Brown MRW, Lambert PA (eds) Medical microbiology, vol 3. Academic, London, pp 153–177
25. Jonsson P, Wadstrom T (1983) High surface hydrophobicity of *Staphylococcus aureus* as revealed by hydrophobic interaction chromatography. Curr Microbiol 8:347–353
26. Kadurugamuwa JL, Anwar H, Brown MRW, Shand GH, Ward KH (1987) Media for study of growth kinetics and envelope properties of iron-deprived bacteria. J Clin Microbiol 25:849–855
27. Kefford B, Kjelleberg S, Marshall KC (1982) Bacterial scavenging: utilisation of fatty acids localised at a solid/liquid interface. Arch Microbiol 133:257–260
28. Kjelleberg S, Humphrey BA, Marshall KC (1983) Initial stages of starvation and activity of bacteria at surfaces. Appl Environ Microbiol 46:978–984
29. Lam C, Georgopoulos A, Laber G, Schutze E (1984) Therapeutic relevance of penicillin-induced hypersensitivity of *Staphylococcus aureus* to killing by polymorphonuclear leukocytes. Antimicrob Agents Chemother 26:149–154
30. Lam C, Turnowsky F, Schwarzinger E, Neruda W (1984) Bacteria recovered without subculture from infected human urines expressed iron-regulated outer membrane proteins. FEMS Microbiol Lett 24:255–259
31. Ljungh A, Hjerten S, Wadstrom T (1985) High surface hydrophobicity of autoaggregating *Staphylococcus aureus* strains isolated from human infections studied with the salt aggregation test. Infect Immun 47:522–526
32. Lorian V (1980) Effects of subminimum inhibitory concentrations of antibiotics on bacteria. In: Lorian V (ed) Antibiotics in laboratory medicine. Williams and Wilkins, Baltimore, pp 342–408
33. Magnusson K-E, Kilhstrom E, Norquist A, Davies J, Normark S (1979) Effect of iron on surface charge and hydrophobicity of *Neisseria gonorrhoeae*. Infect Immun 26:402–407
34. Magnusson K-E, Dahlgren C, Maluszynska GM, Kihlstrom E, Skogh T, Stendahl O, Soderlund G, Ohman L, Walan A (1985) Non-specific and specific recognition mechanisms of bacterial and mammalian cell membranes. J Disp Sci Technol 6:69–89
35. Malmqvist T (1983) Bacterial hydrophobicity measured as partition of palmitic acid between the two immiscible phases of cell surface and buffer. Acta Pathol Microbiol Immunol Scand [B] 91:69–73
36. Marcelis JH, den Daas-Slagt HJ, Hoogkamp-Korstanje JAA (1978) Iron requirement and chelator production of Staphylococci, *Streptococcus faecalis* and Enterobacteriaceae. Antonie van Leeuwenhoek 44:257–267
37. Maskell JP (1980) The functional interchangeability of enterobacterial and staphylococcal iron chelators. Antonie van Leeuwenhoek 46:343–351
38. Miles AA, Khimji PL (1975) Enterobacterial chelators of iron: their occurrence, detection and relation to pathogenicity. J Med Microbiol 8:477–490
39. Miller RD, Fung DYC (1973) Amino acid requirements for the production of enterotoxin B by *Staphylococcus aureus* S-6 in a chemically defined medium. Appl Microbiol 25:800–806
40. Miorner H, Myhre E, Bjork L, Kronvall G (1980) Effect of specific binding of human albumen, fibrinogen and immunoglobulin G on surface characteristics of bacterial strains as revealed by partition experiments in polymer phase systems. Infect Immun 29:879–885
41. Miorner H, Albertsson P-A, Kronvall G (1982) Isoelectric points and surface hydrophobicity of gram-positive cocci as determined by cross-partition and hydrophobic affinity partition in aqueous two phase systems. Infect Immun 36:227–234
42. Mozes N, Rouxhet PG (1987) Methods for measuring hydrophobicity of microorganisms. J Microbiol Methods 6:99–112
43. Mudd EBH, Mudd S (1933) The process of phagocytosis. The agreement between direct observation and deductions from theory. J Gen Physiol 16:625–636

44. Neilands JB (1981) Microbial iron compounds. Annu Rev Biochem 50:715–731
45. Neilands JB (1982) Microbial envelope proteins related to iron. Annu Rev Microbiol 36:285–309
46. Reeves DS, Phillips I, Williams JD, Wise R (1978) Laboratory methods in antimicrobial chemotherapy. Churchill Livingstone, London
47. Schade AL (1963) Significance of serum iron for the growth, biological characteristics and metabolism of *Staphylococcus aureus*. Biochem Z 338:140–148
48. Schade AL, Myers NH, Reinhart RW (1968) Carbohydrate metabolism and production of diffusible active substances by *Staphylococcus aureus* grown in serum at iron levels in excess of siderophilin iron-saturation and below. J Gen Microbiol 52:253–260
49. Shand GH, Anwar H, Kadurugamuwa J, Brown MRW, Silverman SH, Melling J (1985) In vivo evidence that bacteria in urinary tract infection grow under iron-restricted conditions. Infect Immun 48:35–39
50. Smith H (1977) Microbial surfaces in relation to pathogenicity. Bacteriol Rev 41:475–500
51. Smith H (1980) The effect of environmental conditions in vivo and in vitro on the determinants of microbial pathogenicity. In: Smith H, Skehel JJ, Turner MJ (eds) The molecular basis of microbial pathogenicity. Chemie, Dahlem, pp 159–172
52. Stendhal O (1983) The physiochemical basis of surface interaction between bacteria and phagocytic cells. In: Easmon CSF, Jeljaszewicz J, Brown MRW, Lambert PA (eds) Medical microbiology, vol 3. Academic, London, pp 137–152
53. Tempest DW, Wouters JM (1981) Properties and performance of microorganisms in chemostat culture. Enzyme Microb Technol 3:283–290
54. Theodore TS, Schade AL (1965) Growth of *Staphylococcus aureus* in media of restricted and unrestricted inorganic iron availability. J Gen Microbiol 39:75–83
55. Theodore TS, Schade AL (1965) Carbohydrate metabolism of iron-rich and iron-poor *Staphylococcus aureus*. J Gen Microbiol 40:385–395
56. Tufano MA, Romano-Carratelli C, Sommese L, Bentivoglio C, Galdiero F (1985) Modifications of surface properties in some enteropathogenic serogroups of *Escherichia coli*. Microbiologica 8:181–190
57. Turnowsky F, Brown MRW, Anwar H, Lambert PA (1983) Effect of iron limitation of growth rate on the binding of penicillin G to the penicillin binding proteins of mucoid and non-mucoid strains of *Pseudomonas aeruginosa*. FEMS Microbiol Lett 17:243–245
58. van Loosdrecht MCM, Lyklema J, Norde W, Schraa G, Zehnder AJB (1987) The role of bacterial cell wall hydrophobicity in adhesion. Appl Environ Microbiol 53:1893–1897
59. van Loosdrecht MCM, Lyklema J, Norde W, Schraa G, Zehnder AJB (1987) Electrophorectic mobility and hydrophobicity as a measure to predict the initial steps of bacterial adhesion. Appl Environ Microbiol 53:1898–1901
60. van Loosdrecht MCM, Norde W, Zehnder AJB (1987) Influence of cell surface characteristics on bacterial adhesion to solid supports. In: Neijssel OM, van der Meer RR, Luyben KCAM (eds) Proceedings of the European congress on biotechnology, vol 4. Elsevier, Amsterdam
61. van Oss CJ (1978) Phagocytosis as a surface phenomenon. Annu Rev Microbiol 32:19–39
62. van Oss CJ, Gillman CF, Neuman AW (1975) Phagocytic engulfment and cell adhesiveness. Dekker, New York
63. Wadstrom T, Hjerten S, Jonnson P, Tylewska S (1981) Hydrophobic surface properties of *Staphylococcus aureus, Staphylococcus saprophyticus* and *Streptococcus pyogenes*. In: Jeljaszewicz J (ed) Staphylococci and Staphylococcal infections. Fischer, Stuttgart, pp 441–447
64. Wadstrom T, Bjornberg S, Hjerten S (1985) Hydrophobised wound dressings in the treatment of experimental *Staphylococcus aureus* infections in the young pig. Acta Pathol Microbiol Immunol Scand [B] 93:359–363
65. Wadstrom T, Brown A, Ljungh A, Rozgonyi F, Hjerten S (1985) Comparative hydrophobicity studies of *Staphylococus aureus* and coagulase-negative Staphylococci in the salt aggregation test (SAT) and binding to various hydrophobic biomaterials. Abstr Annu Meeting Am Soc Microbiol 26:B48
66. Xiu JH, Magnusson K-E, Stendahl O, Edebo L (1983) Physiochemical surface properties and phagocytosis by polymorphonuclear leucocytes of different serogroups of Salmonella. J Gen Microbiol 129:3075–3084

Reduced Wall Degradation of Staphylococci After Pretreatment with Bacteriostatic Antibiotics *, **

J. Wecke [1], M. Lahav [2], P. Blümel [1], and P. Giesbrecht [1]

Introduction

The cellular immune system is known to be not capable of degrading the cell wall of certain pathogenic bacteria such as streptococci and staphylococci [5, 6, 15, 16].

Such undegraded bacterial wall material may induce chronic inflammatory processes [14, 2]. An important reason for the low degradability of this bacterial wall material seems to be the high degree of *O*-acetylation of the murein: In previous studies it was shown that bone marrow-derived macrophages degraded de-*O*-acetylated wall material of staphylococci much faster than normal *O*-acetylated wall material [18]. An inhibitory effect of these *O*-acetyl groups was also demonstrated to exist toward the degradative action of lysozyme [7]. The degree of *O*-acetylation increased after application of certain bacteriostatic antibiotics such as chloramphenicol [9]. In addition, bacteriostatic antibiotics were capable of inducing huge amounts of cell wall material in staphylococci [3, 4]. All these effects of bacteriostatic antibiotics seem to be important factors in strengthening the resistance of staphylococcal walls against degradation by the immune system. In the present study we investigated the degradability of staphylococci treated with erythromycin as bacteriostatic antibiotic in a defined system of bone marrow-derived macrophages, in order to see whether or not this drug would cause degradation resistance and, by this, would also increase the risk of chronic inflammatory processes.

Material and Methods

Isolation and Cultivation of Macrophages

Animals. Female BALB/c mice (Zentralinstitut für Versuchstierzucht, Hannover, FRG) 6–8 weeks old were used in all experiments.

---

* Dedicated to Prof. Dr. Wohlfarth-Bottermann on the occasion of his 65th birthday.

** This study was supported by a grant from the Deutsche Forschungsgemeinschaft.

[1] Robert Koch-Institute of the Federal Health Office, Nordufer 20, 1000 Berlin 65, Federal Republic of Germany
[2] The Hebrew University, Hadassah Medical Center, Jerusalem, Israel

The Influence of Antibiotics on the Host-Parasite Relationship III
Edited by G. Gillissen, W. Opferkuch, G. Peters, and G. Pulverer

Macrophages. Bone marrow cells were isolated from the femur and tibia of mice. The cells were seeded on hydrophobic Petriperm dishes (Heraeus, Hanau, FRG). Dulbecco's modified minimum essential medium (D-MEM, Biochrom, FRG) containing 5% calf serum, 15% horse serum, and 20% L-cell supernatant as colony-stimulating factor was used. The cells were cultivated in 5% CO_2 at 37 °C, and refed every other day starting at day 5.

Bacteria. *Staphylococcus aureus* strain SG 511 from the culture collection of the Robert Koch-institute was used. The bacteria were transferred from 1.5% peptone agar plates to bottles containing 1.5% peptone water (Bacto Peptone, Difco) +0.5% sodium chloride, and cultivated for 16 h at 37 °C (stationary phase-culture).

Erythromycin Treatment

Stationary phase suspensions of staphylococci were diluted with fresh peptone medium to give an optical density (OD) at 578 nm of 1.0. Erythromycin base (Schering AG, Berlin (West), FRG) was added to the bacterial suspension (final concentration of erythromycin, 1 mg/liter). After growth for 4 h at 37 °C under constant shaking the bacteria were harvested by centrifugation (Sorvall, RC 2B) at 10000 × g for 15 min.

Opsonization

Before phagocytosis, staphylococci were opsonized with bacterial wall-specific antiserum produced by rabbits (25% antiserum, 20 min in phosphate butter, incubation at 20 °C).

Labeling Experiments

The cell wall of staphylococci was specifically labeled with [^{14}C]*N*-acetyl-glucosamine (Amersham-Buchler, FRG) during the erythromycin treatment or for 4 h in the case of untreated bacteria during the stationary phase of growth starting at an OD of 1.0.

De-O-Acetylation

The removal of *O*-acetyl groups was performed as previously described by 0.05 *N* NaOH, 1 h, 37 °C [11]. The removal of *O*-acetyl groups was controlled by Fourier transform infrared spectroscopy [7].

Phagocytosis

Phagocytosis was performed with bone marrow-derived macrophages 10–11 days old. The opsonized staphylococci were added to the adherent macrophages (approximately 100 bacteria/macrophage). After 30 min ingestion the macrophages were washed three times with D-MEM-medium. To determine the ingestion rate, samples were removed from the medium after ingestion and from the washing liquids and counted in a β-counter (Tricarb 460 C, Packard, United States). After 3 h of digestion the label released from macrophages to the supernatant was measured. The medium was then completely replaced by medium containing antibiotics (100 U/ml penicillin + 100 µg/ml streptomycin). Further digestion lasted for 1, 2, 3, and 4 days respectively. Each fraction of a phagocytosis experiment was performed with three or four parallel dishes. One and the same dish were used for both the radiochemical experiments and the electron microscopic analysis.

Electron Microscopy

The adherent macrophages were fixed with 2.5% glutardialdehyde (Serva, Heidelberg, FRG) in 0.1 *M* cacodylate buffer pH 7.2 for 16 h at 4 °C. After washing with cacodylate buffer the macrophages were postfixed with 1.5% osmium tetroxide (Serva, Heidelberg, FRG) + 1.65% potassium dichromate (Merck, Darmstadt, FRG) in 0.1 *M* cacodylate buffer pH 7.0 for 1 h at 20 °C. After washing again with the same buffer the macrophages were poststained with 0.5% uranylacetate in distilled water for 1 h at 20 °C. All further steps for thin sectioning were used as described previously [19].

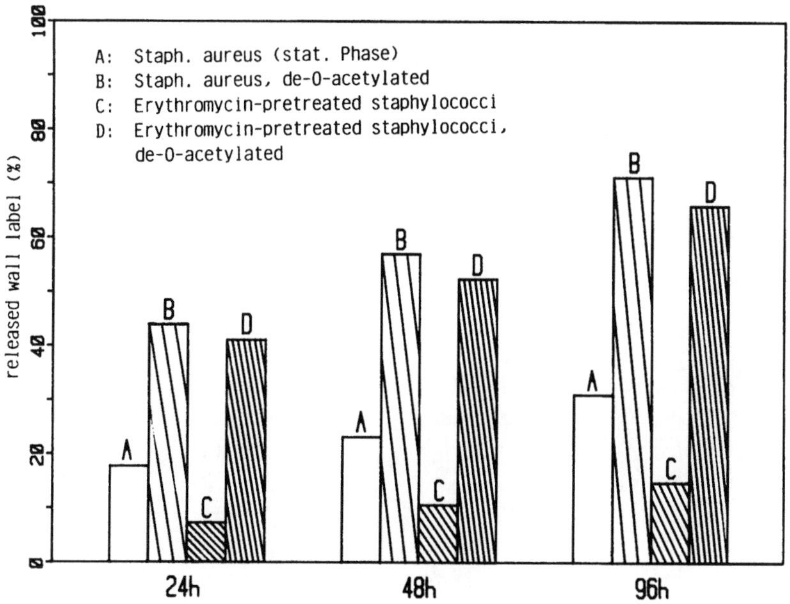

Fig. 1. Wall degradation with and without erythromycin pretreatment and de-*O*-acetylation of staphylococci within macrophages, in terms of release of specific wall label

Results

In order to determine quantitatively the degradation of labeled staphylococcal cell walls pretreated with erythromycin and ingested by macrophages, the release of their specific wall label from the macrophages was measured after different digestion times. This release was considerably reduced by the drug as compared with untreated staphylococci (cf. Fig. 1 C with Fig. 1 A). However, after removal of *O*-acetyl groups from the murein of untreated staphylococci the release of wall label increased remarkably (cf. Fig. 1 A with Fig. 1 B). The difference of degradation was even higher in the case of erythromycin-treated staphylococci (cf. Fig. 1 C with Fig. 1 D): Degradation after de-*O*-acetylation of the wall murein was

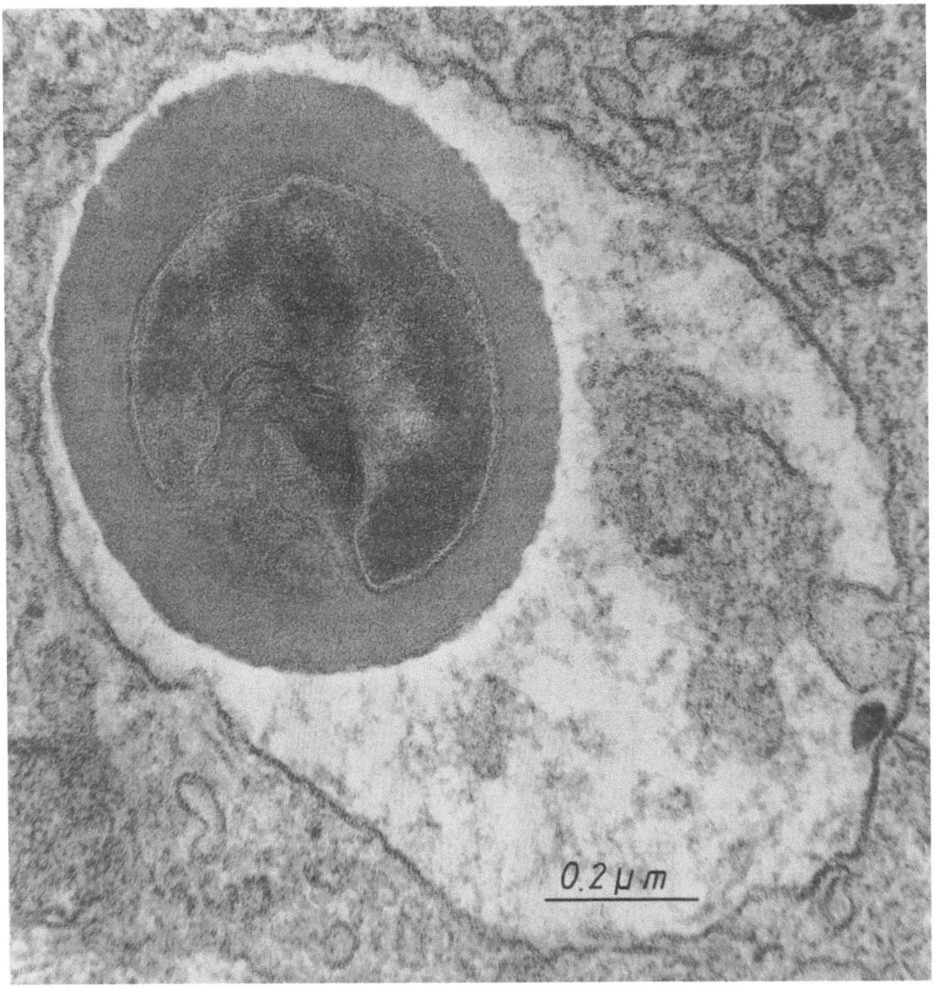

Fig. 2. Erythromycin-pretreated staphylococcal cell after 1 day of digestion within a macrophage. No indication for wall degradation can be detected

five times higher than the *O*-acetylated erythromycin-treated staphylococci, thus reaching the degree of degradability of de-*O*-acetylated control cell walls.

More detailed information about the degradation mechanism was obtained from electron microscopic investigations.

The digestion of erythromycin-pretreated staphylococci was examined after different periods. After 1 day of digestion within the macrophages no changes in the bacterial ultrastructure could be detected (Fig. 2) and after 2 days only minor changes were observed. The thickened cell wall revealed sometimes only a layered structure. While the cell walls of the ingested bacteria seemed to be intact at that time, the bacterial cytoplasm appeared to be degraded in some cases. After 4 days of digestion the majority of the bacterial cytoplasm was degraded while the cell walls still showed only minor changes.

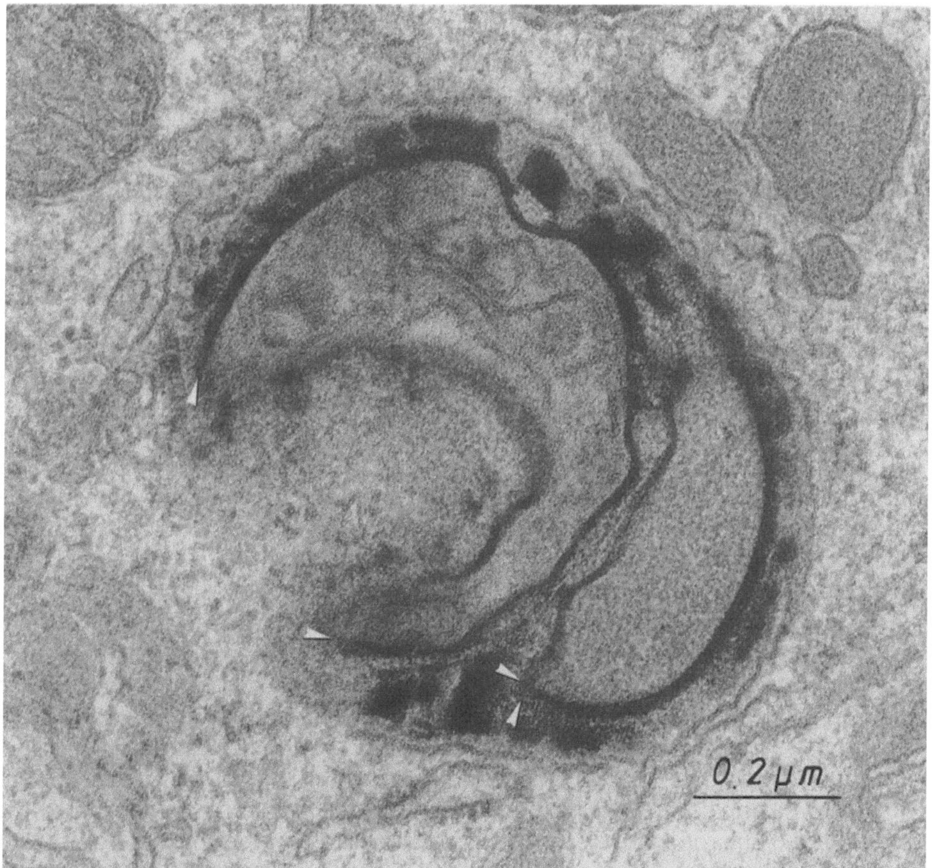

Fig. 3. Erythromycin-pretreated staphylococcal cell after de-*O*-acetylation of its cell wall, ingested in a macrophage; after 1 day of digestion rather large parts of the peripheral wall are dissolved. However, a well-defined inner part of the cell wall, continuing into the cross wall, proved to be resistant (*arrows*)

A completely different picture was found to result in bacterial cells having been de-*O*-acetylated before phagocytosis. In both the cytoplasm and the cell wall, first indications of degradation were already observed after 4 h of digestion. Astonishingly, degradation of the cell wall started from the periphery of the cell. During further progress of the digestion, the cell walls of the de-*O*-acetylated staphylococci degraded very quickly. Figure 3 illustrates the situation after 1 day of degradation. The peripheral part of the cell wall material appeared to be decomposed into big pieces. But a rather small inner part of the cell wall was more resistant to degradation. This more resistant part of the peripheral wall continued into the outer layers of the cross wall, while the inner part of the cross wall was completely dissolved.

After longer digestion times only small remnants of treated bacteria were to be seen.

Discussion

This study has demonstrated that treatment of staphylococci with a bacteriostatic antibiotic may enhance the degradation resistance of the bacterial wall to the lytic attack by bone marrow-derived macrophages. An increased number of *O*-acetyl groups in the murein, induced by erythromycin treatment of the bacteria, was apparently responsible for this effect. Previous studies had provided evidence that treatment of staphylococci with chloramphenicol or erythromycin raised the degree of *O*-acetylation as determined by gas chromatography and Fourier transform infrared spectroscopy [1, 8]; this *O*-acetylation of bacterial cell walls after chloramphenicol treatment was significantly higher than that of normal stationary phase cells and could be correlated with the degradability of the walls against lysozyme in an in vitro system [9, 10].

Also peptidoglycans of certain strains of *Neisseria gonorrhoeae* were shown to differ substantially in their sensitivities to lysozyme, which correlated well with the respective degrees of *O*-acetylation [12]. Furthermore, in these bacteria the rate of degradation of *O*-acetylated peptidoglycan by normal human serum and human polymorphonuclear leukocytes proved to be up to four times lower than that of non-*O*-acetylated peptidoglycan [13].

Basically, the degradation of bacterial cell walls by the cellular immune system can be achieved by two different processes: (1) the action of bacterial wall autolytic enzymes starting in the region between the cytoplasmic membrane and the cell wall proper ("attack from the inside") [17] and (2) the wall-lytic action of the macrophage enzymes which is considered to start the attack on the cell wall from the outside of the bacteria. Our electron micrographs suggest that wall degradation of erythromycin-treated staphylococci was predominantly carried out by the action of the macrophage. Consequently, one has to consider the possibility that the reduced degradability of staphylococcal cell walls after treatment with bacteriostatic antibiotics may induce chronic inflammatory processes, especially if some immunological deficiencies exist.

Summary

Evidence is presented from radiochemical and electron microscopic investigations that treatment of staphylococci with erythromycin makes the bacterial cell walls less readily degradable within bone marrow-derived macrophages. Removal of *O*-acetyl groups from the murein of staphylococci pretreated with erythromycin resulted in a fivefold increase of cell wall degradation, thus reaching the degree of degradability of de-*O*-acetylated control cell walls. These findings indicate that the increased number of *O*-acetyl groups induced by certain bacteriostatic antibiotics may be responsible for the resistance of staphylococcal walls to the lytic attack of the host cellular immune system.

References

1. Burghaus P, Johannsen L, Naumann D, Labischinski H, Bradaczek H, Giesbrecht P (1983) The influence of different antibiotics on the degree of *O*-acetylation of staphylococcal cell walls. In: Hakenbeck R, Höltje J-V, Labischinski H (eds) The target of penicillin. Walter de Gruyter, Berlin, pp 317–322
2. Fleming TJ, Wallsmith DE, Rosenthal RS (1986) Arthropathic properties of gonococcal peptidoglycan fragments: implications for the pathogenesis of disseminated gonococcal disease. Infect Immun 52:600–608
3. Giesbrecht P, Ruska H (1968) Über Veränderungen in der Feinstruktur von Bakterien unter der Einwirkung von Chloramphenicol. Klin Wochenschr 46:575–582
4. Giesbrecht P, Wecke J, Reinicke B (1976) On the morphogenesis of the cell wall of staphylococci. Int Rev Cytol 44:225–318
5. Ginsburg I (1979) The role of lysosomal factors of leukocytes in the biodegradation and storage of microbial constituents in infectious granulomas. In: Jacque P, Dingle J (eds) Lysosomas in applied biology and therapeutics. North Holland, Amsterdam, pp 327–406
6. Ginsburg I, Sela MN (1976) The role of leukocytes and their hydrolases in the persistence, degradation, and transport of bacterial constituents in tissues: relation to chronic inflammatory processes in staphylococcal, streptococcal, and mycobacterial infections and in chronic periodontal diseases, CRC Crit Rev Microbiol 44:249–332
7. Johannsen L (1986) Über den Einfluß der *O*-Acetylierung des Mureins von *Staphylococcus aureus* auf die Abbaubarkeit bakterieller Zellwände durch zellwandlytische Enzymsysteme. Dissertation, Free University of Berlin
8. Johannsen L, Labischinski H, Burghaus P, Giesbrecht P (1983 a) Acetylation in different phases of growth of staphylococci and their relation to cell wall degradability by lysozyme. In: Hakenbeck R, Höltje J-V, Labischinski H (eds) The target of penicillin. Walter de Gruyter, Berlin, pp 261–266
9. Johannsen L, Labischinski H, Reinicke B, Giesbrecht P (1983 b) Changes in the chemical structure of walls of *Staphylococcus aureus* grown in the presence of chloramphenicol. FEMS Microbiol Lett 16:313–316
10. Johnson KG, Campbell JN (1972) Effect of growth conditions on peptidoglycan structure and susceptibility to lytic enzymes in cell walls of *Micrococcus sodonensis*. Biochemistry 11:277–286
11. Logardt I-M, Neujahr HY (1975) Lysis of modified walls from *Lactobacillus fermentum*. J Bacteriol 124:73–77
12. Rosenthal RS, Blundell JK, Perkins HR (1982) Strain-related differences in lysozyme sensitivity and extent of O-acetylation of gonococcal peptidoglycan. Infect Immun 37:826–829
13. Rosenthal RS, Folkening WJ, Miller D, Swim SC (1983) Resistance of O-acetylated gonococcal peptidoglycan to human peptidoglycan-degrading enzymes. Infect Immun 40:903–911

14. Schwab JH, Cromartie WJ, Ohanian SH, Craddock JG (1967) Association of experimental chronic arthritis with the persistence of group A streptococcal cell-walls in the articular tissue. J Bacteriol 94:1728–1735
15. Schwab JH, Ohanian SH (1967) Degradation of streptococcal cell wall antigens in vivo. J Bacteriol 94:1346–1352
16. Stimpson SA, Lerch RA, Cleland DR, Yarnall DP, Clark RL, Cromartie WJ, Schwab JH (1987) Effect of acetylation on arthropathic activity of group A streptococcal peptidoglycan-polysaccharide fragments. Infect Immun 55:16–23
17. Wecke J, Lahav M, Ginsburg I, Giesbrecht P (1982) Cell wall degradation of *Staphylococcus aureus* by lysozyme. Arch Microbiol 131:116–123
18. Wecke J, Kwa E, Johannsen L, Giesbrecht P, Lahav M, Ginsburg I (1986a) O-acetylation of staphylococcal cell walls as an important factor for their degradability within bone marrow-derived macrophages. In: Seidl PH, Schleifer KH (eds) Biological properties of peptidoglycan. Walter de Gruyter, Berlin, pp 198–202
19. Wecke J, Lahav M, Ginsburg I, Kwa E, Giesbrecht P (1986b) Inhibition of wall autolysis of staphylococci by sodium polyanethole sulfonate "liquoid". Arch Microbiol 144:110–115

Influence of Subinhibitory Concentrations of Ceftriaxone on Opsonic Requirements of *Pseudomonas aeruginosa*

M. T. Labro, C. Babin-Chevaye, and J. Hakim

Introduction

We have previously reported that ceftriaxone (CRO), an oxi-imino-amino 2 thiazolyl cephalosporin, does not significantly alter the functions of human polymorphonuclear neutrophils (PMNs) [6]. At subinhibitory concentrations, however, CRO alters *Staphylococcus aureus* and *Klebsiella pneumoniae* in such a way that these CRO-treated bacteria become more sensitive to PMN killing and in particular to a non-O_2-dependent killing system [7]. Since Bassler et al. [1] have reported that CRO cooperates with PMNs for the killing of *Pseudomonas aeruginosa,* it was of interest to analyze whether subinhibitory concentrations of CRO could alter this bacterial strain.

Materials and Methods

Ceftriaxone was kindly provided by Laboratoires Produits Roche (Neuilly, France). It was diluted 100 mg/liter in Hank's buffered solution and further diluted in Trypticase Soy Broth (TSB) (Bio Mérieux, France) to reach the desired concentrations.

Pseudomonas aeruginosa was kindly provided by Dr. A. Bryskier (Argenteuil, France). It was a clinical isolate from septicemia, resistant to serum bactericidal activity and slime producer. The minimum inhibitory concentration (MIC) for ceftriaxone was determined in TSB by the standard dilution test. It was greater than 128 mg/liter. The bacteria were grown overnight in TSB supplemented or not by CRO (10 mg/liter). The next day, the bacteria were washed, adjusted to an optical density of 0.1 (approximately 10^8 CFUs/ml), and opsonized (or not) in 25% normal human serum (NHS), decomplemented serum (DNHS), or antibody-depleted serum (ANHS) by contact with bacteria for 1 h at 25 °C.

Polymorphonuclear neutrophils were obtained from human blood of healthy volunteers by dextran 2% sedimentation and osmotic lysis of residual erythrocytes.

Luminol-amplified chemiluminescence assay (LACL) was recorded in a Packard luminometer; 100 µl PMNs (10^6/ml) was placed in sterile plastic tubes at 37 °C in the apparatus. After the background was recorded (about 1000 counts/

INSERM U 294 and Laboratoire d'Hématologie et d'Immunologie, CHU Xavier Bichat, 46, rue Henri Huchard, 75877 Paris Cédex 18, France

The Influence of Antibiotics on the Host-Parasite Relationship III
Edited by G. Gillissen, W. Opferkuch, G. Peters, and G. Pulverer

10^5 PMNs-30 s), 50 μl bacteria (OD, 0.1) were added. The counts were recorded every 4 min for 40 min. The LACL peak and the CL (Chemiluminescence) index were determined. The CL index was defined as the ratios of the counts for CRO-treated bacteria/counts for control bacteria.

Results

After an overnight culture in TSB supplemented with CRO, *P. aeruginosa* displayed filamentous forms. As a consequency, the bacterial mass was increased ($\times 5.0 \pm 0.1$ mean $\pm$ SD for seven experiments) and the incorporation of ^{14}C-radiolabeled aminoacids was also increased ($\times 4.4 \pm 0.5$).

In the LACL test the PMNs from 21 donors could be separated into two groups depending on the peak CL induced by control *P. aeruginosa* (Fig. 1). The limit was arbitrarily fixed at 5×10^6 counts/10^5 PMNs/30 s. The difference between the two groups of PMNs (high responder, HR, and low responder, LR) became even more striking when the opsonic requirements of the bacteria were studied (Table 1). In each PMN group, the maximal response was observed with stimulation by NHS-opsonized bacteria. When the serum was depleted from antibodies (ANHS), the response was not significantly different for HR PMNs (89%

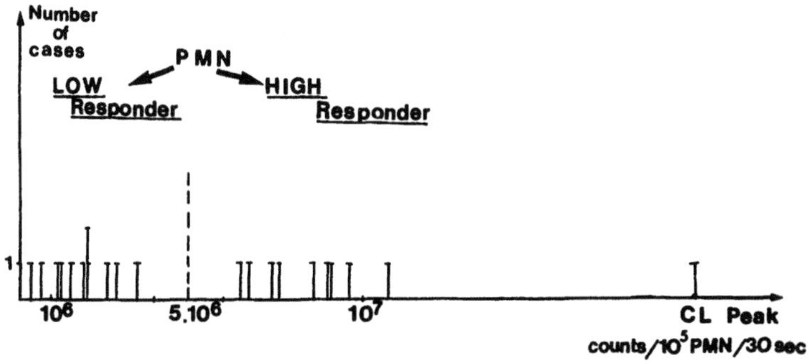

Fig. 1. Classification of PMNs (21 donors) according to the CL peak after stimulation by control *P. aeruginosa*. LR PMNs 11 cases; HR PMNs, 10 cases

Table 1. Chemiluminescence response of PMNs after stimulation by control *P. aeruginosa* depending on opsonization

PMN group	No.	NHS	DNHS	ANHS
High responder	34% ± 7% (5)[a]	100% (10)	65% ± 11% (8)	89% ± 5% (7)
Low responder	27% ± 5.8% (3)	100% (11)	30% ± 8.7% (3)	45% ± 3.7%[b] (5)[b]

Results are expressed as mean ±1 SD of the percentage of CL response obtained by *P. aeruginosa* unopsonized or opsonized by DNHS or ANHS compared with NHS opsonization. NHS, normal human serum; DNHS, decomplemented serum; ANHS, antibody-depleted human serum.

[a] Number of experiment.

[b] $P < 0.01\%$, Student's *t*-test for paired data.

Table 2. Increase in chemiluminescence response of PMNs after stimulation by CRO-treated *P. aeruginosa* depending on opsonization

PMN group		No.	NHS	DNHS	ANHS
High responder	Peak[a]	(5)[b] 410% ± 76.2%	(10) 252% ± 18.9%	(8) 240% ± 48.7%	(7) 120% ± 14.8%
	Index[a]	470% ± 145.3%	253% ± 24.3%	260% ± 53%	134% ± 19.9%
Low responder	Peak[a]	(3) 272% ± 107.9%	(11) 249% ± 33.9%	(3) 171% ± 43.3%	(5) 257% ± 61.8%
	Index[a]	291% ± 87.3%	248% ± 29.3%	169% ± 35.3%	261% ± 49.1%

Results are expressed as mean ±1 SD for the percentage of the response obtained after stimulation by CRO-treated *P. aeruginosa*/response obtained after stimulation by control *P. aeruginosa*.
NHS, normal human serum; DNHS, decomplemented serum; ANHS, antibody-depleted human serum.
[a] For definition, see "Materials and methods".
[b] Number of experiments.

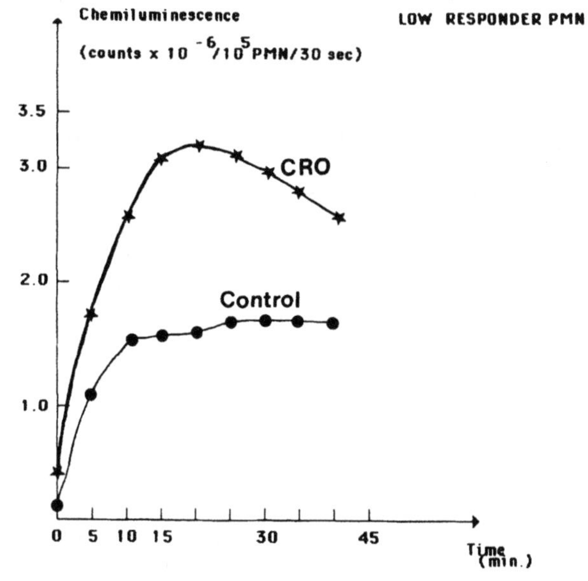

Fig. 2. Chemiluminenscence response of HR PMNs after stimulation by control or CRO-treated *P. aeruginosa*

±5% of NHS opsonization) while LR PMNs gave a significant decreased response compared with NHS opsonization. Complement was important for stimulation and in particular in LR PMNs. Non-opsono-dependent stimulation occurred in each group but the response, compared with NHS opsonization, was decreased by about 70%.

The CRO-treated and NHS-opsonized *P. aeruginosa* induced an increased response of PMNs (by about 150%) whatever the PMN group (Table 2, Figs. 2, 3). Moreover, the shape of the curve was different for control and CRO-treated *P. aeruginosa* (Figs. 2, 3). Control bacteria induced a CL peak at $21 \pm 2_{min}$ (LR PMNs) and $22 \pm 3.1_{min}$ (HR PMNs) (mean ± SD for 11 and 10 experiments re-

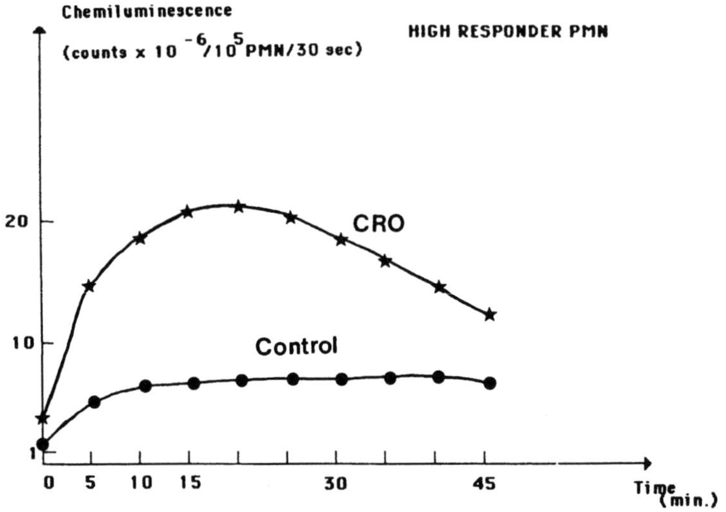

Fig. 3. Chemiluminescence response of HR PMNs after stimulation by control or CRO-treated *P. aeruginosa*

spectively); this response was prolonged for 30–40 min. The CRO-treated bacteria induced a sharp increase but the time to peak was similar to that of control bacteria stimulation, $19 \pm 0.8_{min}$ versus 21 and $20 \pm 1.7_{min}$ versus 22 for LR and HR PMNs respectively. After the peak was reached, a rapid decrease was observed. When the CRO-treated *P. aeruginosa* was opsonized in ANHS, a significant increased response was observed in the LR PMN group only. This result suggests that new receptors for complement were accessible after CRO alteration and permitted a greater activation of LR PMNs. The maximal response already obtained in the case of HR PMNs was no longer amplified by new complement receptors. When the CRO-treated bacteria were opsonized in decomplemented serum, although the response was decreased compared with NHS opsonization, the stimulation of PMNs was greater than that induced by control bacteria. The enhancement was around 70% in the LR PMN group and 150% in the HR PMN group. These results show that "new antigens" are demasked by CRO pretreatment, which permits a better fixation of natural antibodies. When the bacteria were not opsonized, CRO pretreatment led to some modifications of the *P. aeruginosa* cell-wall, which rendered these bacteria able to induce an increased oxidative response in particular in HR-PMN compared with control *P. aeruginosa*.

Discussion

The data have clearly shown that interaction of low concentrations of antibiotics alter the bacterial morphology [8, 9], metabolism [12], and interestingly the sensitivity of these altered pathogens to the host defense system [2, 10, 11]. Ceftriaxone, a 2 aminothiazolyl cephalosporin, does not significantly alter PMN bactericidal function [3, 6] but cooperates with PMN and serum for the killing of *S. aureus* and *P. aeruginosa* [1]. Furthermore, *S. aureus* or *K. pneumoniae* grown in sub-MIC concentrations of ceftriaxone display an increased sensitivity to PMN bactericidal function [7]. The results reported here confirm and extend to *P. aeruginosa* the work of Roszkowski et al. [13] concerning the ability of PMNs from different donors to kill *S. aureus* and to respond by an oxidative burst to stimulation by this bacterium. It was possible to classify the PMNs from 21 donors into 2 groups depending on the CL peak response, high and low responder PMNs. These two groups were also different concerning the opsonic requirements for *P. aeruginosa*. In particular, antibody opsonization was not needed in the HR PMN group for a maximal response. This also seems to correlate with different phagocytic and bactericidal abilities of the PMNs (data not shown). In this work we also report that *P. aeruginosa*, a strain resistant to ceftriaxone, is altered after growth in presence of a low concentration of ceftriaxone. In particular filamentation and increase in bacterial mass and incorporation of ^{14}C-amino acids are observed. Moreover, modifications of the cell wall are evidenced by an increased deposit of opsonins (antibody and complement), which leads to an increased stimulation of PMN oxidative response. On the other hand, some alterations of the cell wall permit an increased non-opsono-dependent stimulation of PMN membrane. Such alterations of bacterial cell wall have also been reported for ceftriaxone interaction with *K. pneumoniae* and exposure of "new antigens" has been proved by Kadurugamuwa et al. [4, 5]. The consequences of these alterations on PMN bactericidal function have been studied [7] and we have shown that CRO-treated *P. aeruginosa* displays a greater sensitivity to PMN killing and is significantly more susceptible to O_2-dependent killing than control bacteria. The molecular mechanisms of these modifications are under study.

Summary

Pseudomonas aeruginosa [minimum inhibitory concentration (MIC) > 128 mg/liter] becomes filamentous after overnight exposure to a low concentration (10 mg/liter) of ceftriaxone, a 2-amino thiazolyl cephalosporin. The ability of these filaments to induce an oxidative burst in human neutrophils (PMNs), as assessed in a luminol-amplified chemiluminescence (LACL) assay, was compared with that of control untreated bacteria. The results showed that, according to their response to control bacteria, PMNs may be classified into low (LR-PMNs) and high (HR-PMNs) responders. Filaments opsonized with normal human serum induced an increased response (about 150%) in both PMN groups. On the contrary, filaments opsonized with antibody-depleted serum induced an increased response in the LR-PMN group only. Filaments, unopsonized or treated with decomplemented serum, stimulated the PMN response more efficiently than control bacteria. This effect was greater in the LR-PMN than in the HR-PMN group.

It may be concluded that ceftriaxone alters *P. aeruginosa* cell wall in such a way that "neoantigens" or complement receptors become more accessible to serum opsonins, leading to an increased opsonodependent stimulation of PMNs.

Furthermore, other cell wall modifications permit an increased non-opsono-dependent stimulation of PMNs.

References

1. Bassler M, Blaschke H, Just M, Daschner FD (1982) Effect of ceftriaxone on *Pseudomonas aeruginosa* and *Staphylococcus aureus* in broth, serum and in combination with human polymorphonuclear leukocytes. Chemotherapy 28:390–396
2. Gemmel CG (1984) Potentiation of phagocytosis of pathogenic bacteria by exposure to low concentrations of antibiotics. J Antimicrob Chemother 13:407–409
3. Grassi GG, Fietta A, Sacchi F, De Rose V (1984) Influence of ceftriaxone on natural defence system. Am J Med 77:37–41
4. Kadurugamuwa JL, Anwar H, Brown MRW, Zak O (1985a) Protein antigens of encapsulated *Klebsiella pneumoniae* surface exposed after growth in the presence of subinhibitory concentrations of cephalosporins. Antimicrob Agents Chemother 28:195–199
5. Kadurugamuwa JL, Anwar H, Brown MRW, Zak O (1985b) Exposure of protein antigens and reduction of siderophore production after growth of gram-negative bacteria in subinhibitory concentration of cephalosporins. In: Adam D, Hahn H, Opferkuch W (eds) The influence of antibiotics on the host parasite relationship. Springer, Berlin Heidelberg New York, pp 36–47
6. Labro MT, Babin-Chevaye C, Pochet Y, Hakim J (1987a) Interaction of ceftriaxone with human polymorphonuclear neutrophil function. J Antimicrob Chemother 20:849–855
7. Labro MT, Babin-Chevaye C, Pochet Y, Hakim J (1987b) Consequency of ceftriaxone-induced alterations of bacteria on neutrophil bactericidal function. J Antimicrob Chemother 20:857–869
8. Lorian V (1978) Effects of subinhibitory concentrations of antibiotics on bacteria. Curr Chemother 1:72–78
9. Lorian V (1985) Low concentrations of antibiotics. J Antimicrob Chemother 15 [Suppl A]:15–26
10. Lorian V (1986) Effect of low antibiotic concentration on bacteria: effects on ultrastructure, their virulence and susceptibility to immunodefenses. In: Lorian V (ed) Antibiotics in laboratory medicine. Williams and Wilkins, Baltimore, pp 596–668
11. Lorian V, Atkinson B (1984) Bactericidal effect of polymorphonuclear neutrophils on antibiotic-induced filaments of gram negative bacilli. J Infect Dis 149:719–727
12. Mychajlonka M, Mac Dowell TD, Shockman GD (1980) Inhibition of peptidoglycan, ribonucleic acid and protein synthesis in tolerant strains of *Streptococcus mutans*. Antimicrob Agents Chemother 17:572–582
13. Roszkowski W, Ciborowski P, Ko HKL, Schumacher-Perdreau F, Roszkowski K, Jeljaszewicz J, Pulverer G (1985) The effect of subinhibitory concentration of selected antibiotics on bacteria-phagocyte interaction. In: Adam D, Hahn H, Opferkuch W (eds) The influence of antibiotics on the host parasite relationship II. Springer, Berlin Heidelberg New York, pp 178–187

Traditional Chinese Medicines and Drugs in Relation to the Host-Defense Mechanism

N. SATOMI [1], A. SAKURAI [1], R. HARANAKA [2], and K. HARANAKA [1]

Introduction

Pseudomonas aeruginosa infection is observed mostly under immunosuppressive conditions. We have clarified that the combined use of antibiotics and specific antibodies is effective against mouse *P. aeruginosa* infection in vivo [1–5]. From our previous experiments, traditional Chinese medicines and crude drugs are known to cause stimulation of the reticuloendothelial system [6]. Kiger et al. [7] found that *P. aeruginosa* treatment (10^8 killed organisms) had a capacity to induce release of tumor-necrotizing factor in the serum of bacille Calmette-Guérin (BCG)-pretreated mice to the same extent as lipopolysaccharide (LPS) treatment. Our experiments on tumor necrosis factor (TNF) have demonstrated the production of TNF as well as its associated severe toxicity [8–10]. Recently, recombinant human TNF has been mass produced and many actions of this factor have become clear. We have found that by employing traditional Chinese medicines as priming agents, the toxic symptoms after administration of LPS could be reduced.

In the present experiments, several Chinese medicines were used to activate the host-defense mechanism. In addition, the contribution of TNF in a state of systemic infection was also examined.

Materials and Methods

Animals. DDY strain female mice weighing 28–35 g (Shizudokyo, Shizuoka, Japan) were used for experimental infection and for the production of mouse TNF. Japanese Albino rabbits (Kanamarudobutu, Tokyo, Japan) were used for the production of anti-mouse TNF antibody.

Bacteria. *Pseudomonas aeruginosa* NC-5 was provided by the Type Culture Collection Room at our Institute. This strain has a strong virulence to mice. The LD_{50} of this bacterium by intraperitoneal inoculation together with 2.5% mucin was 7.5×10^2.

[1] Department of Internal Medicine, Institute of Medical Science, University of Tokyo 4-6-1, Shirokanedai, Minato-ku, Tokyo 108, Japan
[2] Department of Biochemistry, Nihon University School of Medicine, 30-1, Ooyaguchi-Kamimachi, Itabashi-ku, Tokyo 173, Japan

The Influence of Antibiotics on the Host-Parasite Relationship III
Edited by G. Gillissen, W. Opferkuch, G. Peters, and G. Pulverer

Antibiotics. Astromycin (ASTM) (provided by Kyowa Hakko Kogyo, Tokyo, Japan), cefbuperazone (CBPZ) (provided by Kakenseiyaku, Tokyo, Japan), and aztreonam (AZT) (provided by Eisai, Tokyo, Japan) were used.

Drugs. Lentinan [a polysaccharide from *Lentinus edodes* (Berk.) Sing.] was provided by Yamanouchi Pharmaceutical (Tokyo, Japan). Xiao-chai-hu-tang, Shi-quan-da-bu-tang, and Bu-zhong-yi-qi-tang were obtained from Tsumura (Tokyo, Japan). Urinastatin was provided by Mochida Pharmaceutical (Tokyo, Japan). Cortisone acetate (Banyu Pharmaceutical, Tokyo, Japan) and reduced glutathione (GSH) (Yamanouchi Pharmaceutical) were also used.

Tumor Necrosis Factor and Anti-TNF Antibody. Two milligrams per mouse of formalin-killed *Propionibacterium acnes* was administered intraperitoneally 9 days prior to injection of LPS (10 μg/mouse) from *Escherichia coli* O 111 : B4*w* (Difco Lab., MI, United States). Blood was collected 2 h after the LPS administration. Purification was carried out as described previously [11]. A rabbit was immunized with the purified mouse TNF. The IgG fraction of the anti-mouse TNF serum was used. Recombinant human TNF was provided by Dainippon Pharmaceutical (Osaka, Japan).

Modes of Administration. Urinastatin was administered (1300 U/mouse) at the same time as the bacterial challenge. ASTM (300 μg/mouse) and/or CBPZ (1.5 mg/mouse) were administered subcutaneously at the same time and at 12 h after the inoculation of *P. aeruginosa*. Lentinan (40 μg/mouse) was administered intraperitoneally every other day for a total of four times prior to the *P. aeruginosa* inoculation. Xiao-chai-hu-tang (50 mg/mouse), Shi-quan-da-bu-tang (50 mg/mouse), and Bu-zhong-yi-qi-tang (50 mg/mouse) were administered to mice in their drinking water for 2 weeks before the bacterial inoculation. Recombinant human TNF (1000 U/mouse) or anti-mouse TNF IgG (300 U/mouse) was administered subcutaneously at the same time as the bacterial inoculation. Cortisone acetate (0.1 mg/mouse) or GSH (30 mg/mouse) was also injected subcutaneously at the same time as the bacterial challenge.

Bacterial Challenge. *Pseudomonas aeruginosa* NC-5 was incubated in heart infusion broth for 18 h. Bacteria were suspended in 2.5% bacteriological mucin (Difco) and inoculated intraperitoneally. Each group consisted of five mice. Evaluations of the therapeutic effect were made on the basis of the number of mice surviving 5 days after the inoculation.

Phagocytosis. Macrophages from the spleen were prepared as described previously [2]. Each combination of macrophage, antibiotics, and TNF was mixed and incubated with bacteria. The number of surviving bacteria was calculated by colony counting. Macrophages were also collected from Xiao-chai-hu-tang-primed mice.

Chemiluminescence. The chemiluminescence of whole spleen cells from control or Chinese medicine-primed mice was measured using a Lumi counter 1000 (Niti-on Medical and Physical Instruments, Chiba, Japan) as described elsewhere [12].

Results

Therapeutic Effects of Combination Therapy. The results for combination therapy with antibiotics are summarized in Fig. 1. ASTM or CBPZ had no therapeutic effect against *P. aeruginosa* infection at the present dosage; however, with a combination of these antibiotics, synergistic effects were observed. When urinastatin was also added to such combination therapy, the therapeutic effects were further improved. Urinastatin itself had a therapeutic effect against *P. aeruginosa* infection.

Figure 2 shows the results for the therapeutic effect of Chinese medicines and lentinan. Pretreatment with these medicines had a significant effect against the lethal challenge of *P. aeruginosa* infection.

The influence of TNF on the infectious state was examined. Administration of recombinant human TNF increased the lethality of *P. aeruginosa* challenge. In contrast, administration of anti-mouse TNF IgG showed a strong protective ac-

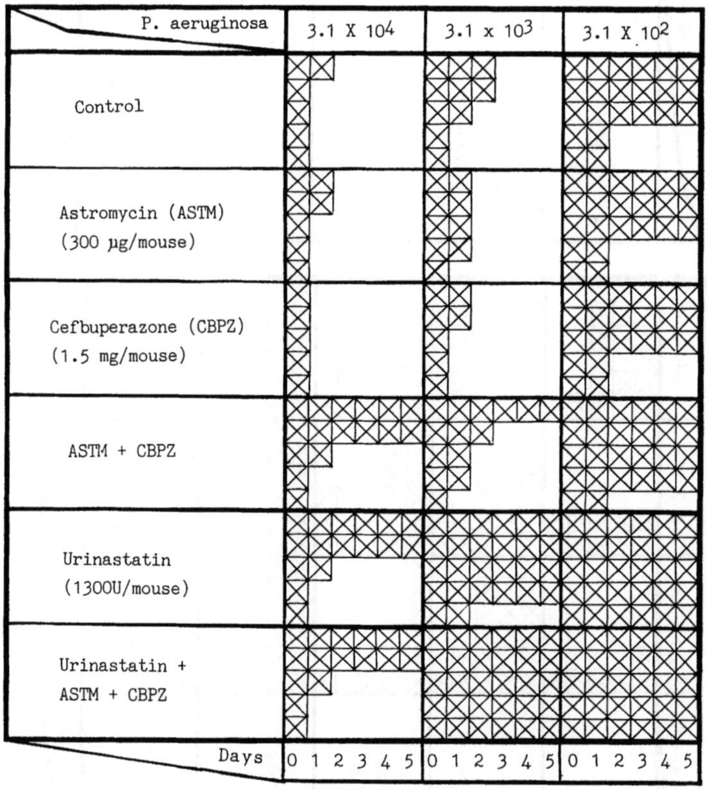

Fig. 1. Combination therapy with antibiotics and/or urinastatin against *P. aeruginosa* infection. Astromycin (ASTM; 300 µg/mouse) and/or cefbuperazone (CBPZ; 1.5 mg/mouse) were administered s.c. at the same time and 12 h after inoculation of *P. aeruginosa*. Urinastatin (1300 U/mouse) was administered at the same time as the bacterial challenge. Evaluations of the therapeutic effect were made on the basis of the number of mice surviving

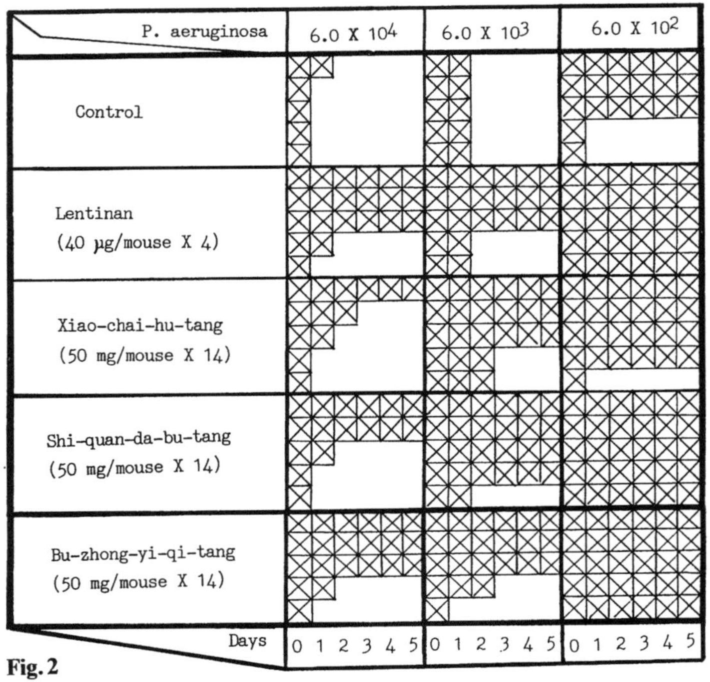

Fig. 2

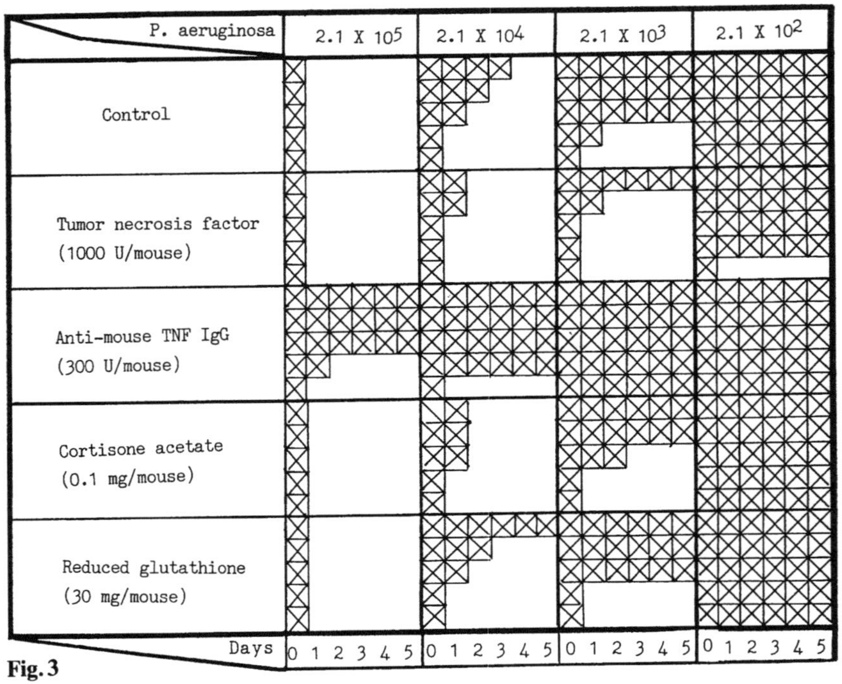

Fig. 3

Fig. 2. Therapeutic effects of Chinese medicines and lentinan. Lentinan (40 μg/mouse) was administered i.p. every other day a total of four times. The Chinese medicines (50 mg/mouse) were administered p.o. for 2 weeks before the bacterial challenge

Fig. 3. Effects of host factor against *P. aeruginosa* infection. Recombinant human tumor necrosis factor (TNF; 1000 U/mouse) was administered s.c. at the same time as the bacterial challenge. Anti-mouse TNF IgG (300 U/mouse), cortisone acetate (0.1 mg/mouse), or GSH (30 mg/mouse) was administered s.c. at the same time as the bacterial challenge

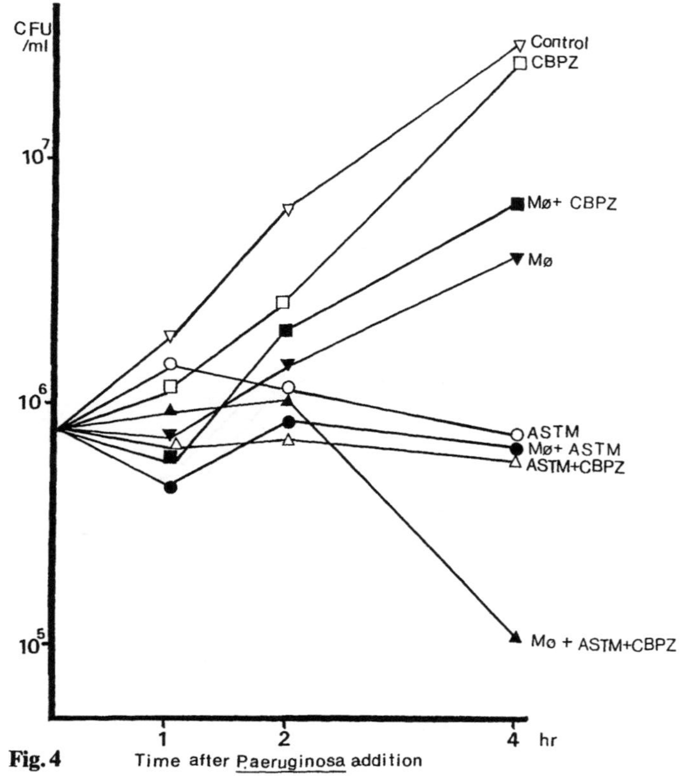

Fig. 4

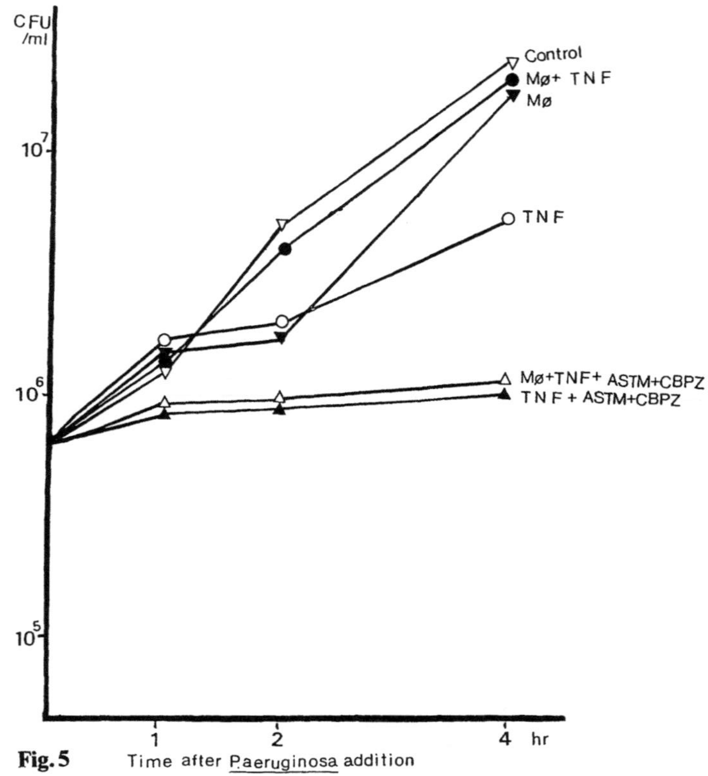

Fig. 5

Fig. 4. Results of macrophage phagocytosis against *P. aeruginosa* in combination with antibiotics. One-fifth of the MIC of ASTM and/or CBPZ was added to the phagocytic system. Macrophage: *P. aeruginosa* = 1 : 10

Fig. 5. Influence of TNF on phagocytosis. TNF (final 100 U) was added to the phagocytic system

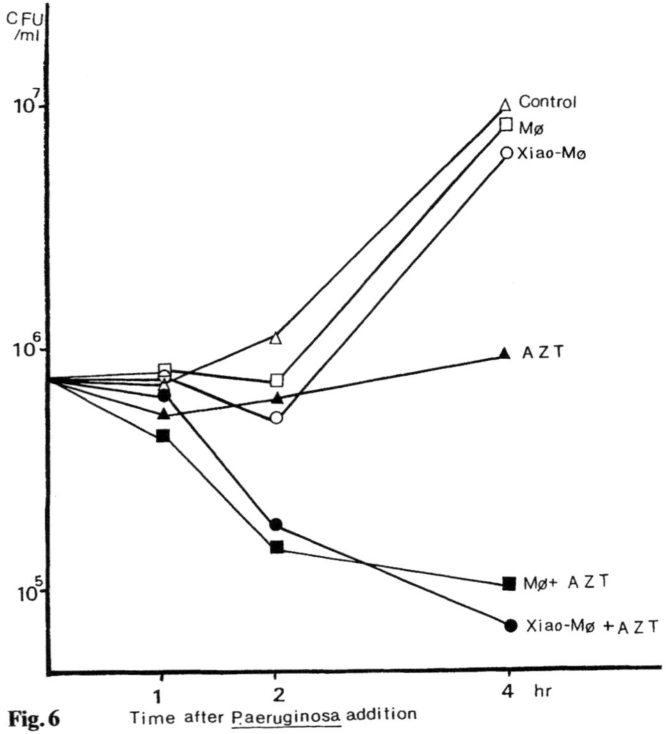

Fig. 6

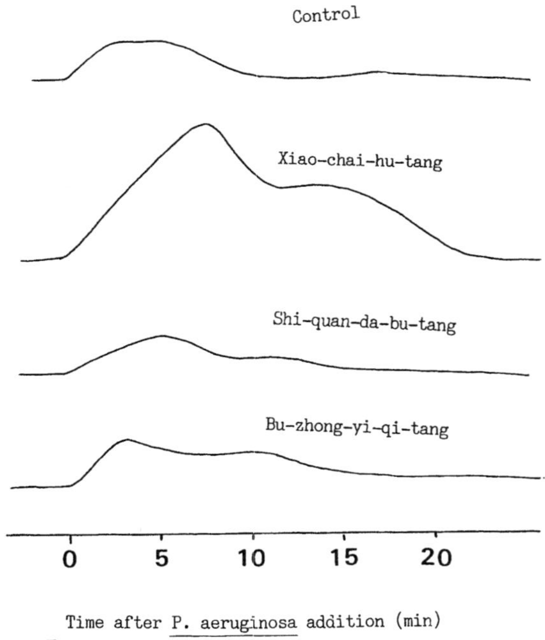

Fig. 7

Fig. 6. Phagocytic reaction of macrophages from control mice and macrophages from Xiao-chai-hu-tang-primed mice. AZT (1/5 MIC) was added

Fig. 7. Chemiluminescence patterns from whole spleen cells. Spleen cells from control or Chinese medicine primed mice were examined using a Lumi counter 1000

Table 1. Results for ASTM and CBPZ by the checkerboard technique

Cefbuperazone (μg/ml)	Astromycin (μg/ml)									
	0	0.39	0.78	1.56	3.12	6.25	12.5	25	50	100
0	+	+	+	+	+	+	+	−	−	−
0.39	+	+	+	+	+	+	+	−	−	−
0.78	+	+	+	+	+	+	−	−	−	−
1.56	+	+	+	+	+	+	−	−	−	−
3.12	+	+	+	+	+	+	−	−	−	−
6.25	+	+	+	+	+	−	−	−	−	−
12.5	+	+	+	+	+	−	−	−	−	−
25	+	+	+	+	+	−	−	−	−	−
50	+	+	+	+	−	−	−	−	−	−
100	−	−	−	−	−	−	−	−	−	−

tivity against the lethal bacterial challenge (Fig. 3). Administration of cortisone acetate or GSH did not influence the lethality.

Phagocytosis. The results for macrophage phagocytosis against *P. aeruginosa* in combination with various antibiotics are summarized in Fig. 4. The number of surviving bacteria was significantly decreased in the case of macrophages combined with ASTM and CBPZ. The minimal inhibitory concentrations (MICs) of the antibiotics against *P. aeruginosa* were as follows: ASTM, 25 μg/ml; CBPZ, 100 μg/ml; and AZT, 12.5 μg/ml. Table 1 shows the results for ASTM and CBPZ by the checkerboard technique against *P. aeruginosa* NC-5. Addition of TNF to the phagocytic system did not enhance the phagocytosis even in combination with antibiotics (Fig. 5).

Macrophages from control mice and macrophages from Xiao-chai-hu-tang-primed mice were compared in combination with AZT. There were no statistically significant differences in the phagocytic reaction (Fig. 6). However, the recovery rate of macrophages from one spleen was one-half greater in the Xiao-chai-hu-tang-primed group.

Chemiluminescence. Typical chemiluminescence patterns from whole spleen cells derived from control, Xiao-chai-hu-tang-primed, Shi-quan-da-bu-tang-primed, and Bu-zhong-yi-qi-tang-primed mice are shown in Fig. 7.

Discussion

Pseudomonas aeruginosa infection often occurs in patients undergoing immunosuppressive therapy. We have examined the therapeutic effects of antibody against experimental murine infections [1–5]. From the results obtained, we speculated that the host-defense mechanism (including serum factor) is intimately related to protection against *P. aeruginosa* infection.

Pseudomonas aeruginosa frequently displays resistance to antibiotics. Nevertheless, combinations of antibiotics were found to demonstrate therapeutic effects in vivo (Fig. 1) and in vitro (Figs. 4, 5). It has been reported that synergistic activities of ASTM in combination with β-lactam antibiotics against *P. aeruginosa* are observed in vitro and in vivo [13]. It has also been found that the host-defense mechanisms are stimulated by CBPC [14].

Urinastatin, a urinary trypsin inhibitor, is known to have a protective effect against hemorrhagic shock and endotoxic shock [15]. By administration of urinastatin, the lethality of *P. aeruginosa* infection could be significantly decreased (Fig. 1).

Chinese medicines have often been observed clinically to show efficacy against infection, and it has been suggested that their effectiveness may be derived from some action which they exert on the immune system of the host [16]. Lentinan, which has an antitumor activity, is well known as an immunopotentiating substance [17]. Pretreatment with Chinese medicines (per os) demonstrated protective effects against *P. aeruginosa* infection similar to those of pretreatment with lentinan (Fig. 2).

Tumor necrosis factor has been investigated as a strong biological antitumor substance [18, 19]. Following the recent success of large-scale production of recombinant human TNF, many other functions of this factor have been clarified. Activation of neutrophil functions by TNF has been reported [20, 21]. In contrast, passive immunization against cachectin/TNF protects mice from the lethal effect of endotoxin [22]. Since *P. aeruginosa* is reported to show eliciting activity of TNF [7], the participation of TNF against *P. aeruginosa* infection was examined. One hundred units/mouse of recombinant human TNF ($^1/_{20}$ LD_{50}) was administered at the same time as bacterial challenge. The lethality was found to be increased by this treatment. On the other hand, administration of anti-TNF IgG showed a strong protective activity against the lethality of *P. aeruginosa* infection (Fig. 3). In in vitro experiments, addition of TNF to a phagocytic system of macrophages caused no enhancement of the phagocytosis (Fig. 6). These results suggest that TNF may show a rather negative action in the host-defense mechanism. We have speculated that the antitumor activity of TNF is deeply related to the arachidonic cascade and O_2 radicals [23]. Cortisone acetate and GSH were therefore used in the present experimental model. However, no significant differences were observed (Fig. 3).

We have confirmed that the host-defense mechanism is strongly influenced in *P. aeruginosa* infection. To clarify the underlying reason for the protective activity of Chinese medicines, investigations of phagocytosis and chemiluminescence were carried out. Employing macrophages from Xiao-chai-hu-tang-primed mice, the phagocytosis was examined. There are no differences in surviving bacterial counts with the same number of macrophages; however, the number of macrophages from the spleen was increased by the pretreatment (Fig. 6). In addition, the chemiluminescence was enhanced by the pretreatment (Fig. 7). We have investigated the antitumor activities and TNF producibility of traditional Chinese medicines and crude drugs [24]. Our previous experiments demonstrated the hepatosplenomegaly on pretreatment with Chinese medicines [24]. On the basis of these results, it is speculated that Chinese medicines may enhance the host-defense mechanism by increasing the numbers of phagocytes especially in the reticuloendothelial system of the liver and spleen.

In conclusion, it is considered important to potentiate the host-defense mechanism in *P. aeruginosa* infection by treatment with such agents as Chinese medicines or lentinan. The lethality of *P. aeruginosa* infection can be improved by treatment with urinastatin or anti-TNF antibody.

Summary

Traditional Chinese medicines (Xiao-chai-hu-tang, Shi-quan-da-bu-tang, and Bu-zhong-yi-qi-tang) enhanced the host-defense mechanism in mice which were infected with *Pseudomonas aeruginosa* NC-5 strain. After adiministration of these drugs, hepatosplenomegaly was observed. In in vitro experiments, chemiluminescence was also enhanced. Lentinan or urinastatin exerted a preventative effect against the lethality of *P. aeruginosa.* Administration of anti-TNF (tumor necrosis factor) antibody improved the survival rate in this model. On the basis of these results, it is speculated that the host-defense mechanism (including serum factor) acts strongly against the lethality of *P. aeruginosa* infection.

References

1. Haranaka K, Sugane K, Mashimo K (1975) Combination therapy of anti-endotoxin antibody and gentamicin in the immunosuppressed mice with *Pseudomonas aeruginosa* infection. Jpn J Exp Med 45:207–213
2. Haranaka K, Matsuo M, Mashimo K (1977) The enhancement of phagocytosis and intracellular killing of *Pseudomonas aeruginosa* and its common antigen (OEP) coated latex particles by mouse spleen macrophages to which anti-OEP-IgG and gentamicin have been added. Jpn J Exp Med 47:35–40
3. Haranaka K, Satomi N, Sakurai A, Kunii O (1982) The combined use of antibiotics and specific antibodies against mouse *Pseudomonas aeruginosa* infection in vivo and the phagocytosis of peritoneal exudate cells in vitro. In: Eickenberg HU et al. (eds) The influence of antibiotics on the host-parasite relationship. Springer, Berlin Heidelberg New York, pp 161–167
4. Haranaka K, Matsuo M, Satomi N, Kunii O, Mashimo K (1978) The influence of anti-OEP-IgG and -IgM upon mouse spleen macrophage phagocytic activity against *Pseudomonas aeruginosa* and OEP-coated latex granules. J Jpn Infect Dis Soc 52:482–489
5. Haranaka K, Satomi N, Matsuo M, Kunii O, Mashimo K (1979) Therapeutic effects of anti-OEP-antibodies in the *Psudomonas aeruginosa* (Fisher's seven serotypes) infection of mice and the influence of this antibody upon the phagocytic activity of mice spleen macrophages. J Jpn Infect Dis Soc 53:175–181
6. Haranaka K, Satomi N, Sakurai A, Haranaka R, Okada N, Kobayashi M (1985) Antitumor activities and tumor necrosis factor producibility of traditional Chinese medicines and crude drugs. Cancer Immunol Immunother 20:1–5
7. Kiger N, Khalil A, Mathe G (1980) Tumor-necrotizing serum production by administration of BCG + *Pseudomonas.* Its application in treatment of fibrosarcoma in mice. Recent Results in Cancer Research (RRCR) 75:220–223
8. Haranaka K, Satomi N, Sakurai A, Kunii O (1985) Role of lipid A in the production of tumor necrosis factor and differences in antitumor activity between tumor necrosis factor and lipopolysaccharide. Tohoku J Exp Med 144:385–396
9. Haranaka K, Satomi N, Sakurai A (1984) Differences in tumor necrosis factor productive ability among rodents. Br J Cancer 50:471–478

10. Sakurai A, Satomi N, Haranaka K (1986) Differences in tumor necrosis factor productive ability among rabbits. Jpn J Exp Med 56:247–250
11. Haranaka K, Carswell EA, Williamson BD, Prendergast JS, Satomi N, Old LJ (1986) Purification, characterization, and antitumor activity of nonrecombinant mouse tumor necrosis factor. Proc Natl Acad Sci USA 83:3949–3953
12. Muto S, Igarashi M, Matsumoto Y, Ogino H, Yuki H (1986) A simple and rapid method for the determination of macrophage activating factor involving a new type of apparatus suitable for the measurement of macrophage chemiluminescence. J Immunol Methods 90:51–56
13. Sato K, Yamashita K, Okachi R (1985) In vivo combination effects of astromycin and β-lactam antibiotics against *Pseudomonas aeruginosa*. Jpn J Antibiot 36:1487–1493
14. Suzuki I, Senda H (1985) In vivo activity of cefbuperazone (T-1982) against various experimental infections in mice. J Antibiot (Tokyo) 38:249–258
15. Oda T, Miyawaki T, Sameshima T, Miyao J (1984) Antishock effects of urinary trypsin inhibitor, MR-20 (in Japanese). Anesthesia 33:137–142
16. Yamamoto T, Okada H, Kuroiwa A (1985) Effects of Oriental herbal medicines on immunity in the elderly. In: Oda T et al. (eds) Recent advances in traditional medicine in East Asia. Excerpta Medica, Tokyo, pp 96–105
17. Maeda Y, Chihara G (1971) Lentinan, a new immuno-accelerator of cell-mediated responses. Nature 229:634
18. Carswell EA, Old LJ, Kassel RL, Green S, Fiore N, Williamson B (1975) An endotoxin-induced serum factor that causes necrosis of tumors. Proc Natl Acad Sci USA 72:3666–3670
19. Haranaka K, Satomi N, Sakurai A (1984) Antitumor activity of murine tumor necrosis factor (TNF) against transplanted murine tumors and heterotransplanted human tumors in nude mice. Int J Cancer 34:263–267
20. Shalaby MR, Aggarwal BB, Rindeknecht E, Svedersky LP, Finkle BS, Palladino MA Jr (1985) Activation of human polymorphonuclear neutrophil functions by interferon-γ and tumor necrosis factors. J Immunol 135:2069–2073
21. Tsujimoto M, Yokota S, Vilcek J, Weissmann G (1986) Tumor necrosis factor provokes superoxide anion generation from neutrophils. Biochem Biophys Res Commun 137:1094–1110
22. Beutler B, Milsark IW, Cerami AC (1985) Passive immunization against cachectin/tumor necrosis factor protects mice from lethal effect of endotoxin. Science 229:869–871
23. Satomi N, Sakurai A, Haranaka R, Haranaka K (1988) Preventive effects of several chemicals against lethality of recombinant human tumor necrosis factor. J Biol Response Mod 7:54–64
24. Haranaka K, Satomi N, Sakurai A, Haranaka R, Okada N, Kosodo H, Kobayashi M (1985) Antitumor activities and tumor necrosis factor producibility of traditional Chinese medicines and crude drugs. J Tradit Chin Med 5:271–278

Influence of Antibiotic Therapy of Mice on the Humoral Immune Response Against Sheep Erythrocytes

K.-H. BÜSCHER [1], G. SCHWARZ [2], B. ANDRES [2], S. WENDT, [2] and W. OPFERKUCH [2]

Introduction

Antibiotics may alter the host-parasite relationship by modification of bacterial properties, e.g., expression of capsular polysaccharides or other surface constituents [16–25] or liberation of toxins [8] of lipopolysachharide, etc. On the other hand, they may exert a direct influence on immunocompetent cells [2, 6, 13, 17, 20]. Only limited information is available on the influence of antibiotic treatment in vivo on parameters of the immune system [1, 2, 4–6, 10, 21–24]. Furthermore, the data obtained by different authors are controversial and hardly comparable. Whereas Gillissen [4, 5] described an augmenting effect of 1-day treament of mice with different β-lactam antibiotics on the primary humoral immune response against sheep erythrocytes, Roszkowski et al. [22, 23] found suppressive effects after 7 days of treatment. In this case mezlocillin and cefotaxime showed the most pronounced suppression of the humoral and cellular immune response. The difference between these studies might be due to differences induced by a prolonged action of antibiotics on immunocompetent cells, to differences in the action of antibiotics on the intestinal flora [7, 26, 27], to different stress situations of the mice [11, 15], induced for example by the different number of injections, or to different housing conditions [3, 7, 9]. The first hypothesis seems to be unlikely, because Büscher et al. [1] did not find a suppressive effect of 7-day treatment of Balb/c mice with mezlocillin.

In the present study the effect of long-term treatment of different strains of mice with antibiotics on the humoral immune response and the reactivity of peritoneal macrophages and on the intestinal flora was investigated in order to obtain more information on the molecular and cellular basis of the immunosuppressive effect of antibiotics described by Roszkowski et al. [21–23].

Material and Methods

Reagents. The following antibiotics were used in this study: mezlocillin (Bayer AG, Dortmund, FRG), cefotaxim (Hoechst AG, Frankfurt, FRG), cefodizime (Hoechst AG, Frankfurt, FRG), clindamycin (Upjohn, Heppenheim, FRG), amikazin (Grünenthal GmbH, Stolberg, FRG), and ciprofloxacin (Bayer AG,

[1] E. Merck, Fo Diag KC, U 26, Postfach 4119, 6100 Darmstadt 1, Federal Republic of Germany
[2] Department of Medical Microbiology and Immunology, Ruhr-Universität Bochum, 4630 Bochum, Federal Republic of Germany

The Influence of Antibiotics on the Host-Parasite Relationship III
Edited by G. Gillissen, W. Opferkuch, G. Peters, and G. Pulverer

Dortmund, FRG). Cell culture reagents were obtained from Biochrom KG (Berlin, FRG). All the other reagents used were obtained from Sigma Chemicals (Munich, FRG) or Merck (Darmstadt, FRG) and were of the highest analytical grade available.

Media. Minimum essential medium (MEM)-Hank's phosphate buffer (MHPB), pH 7.2, was prepared from MEM-Hank's (Biochrom) without sodium carbonate. The buffer was supplemented with 1.16 m*M* Na_2HPO_4, 1.19 m*M* $MgCl_2$ according to [14]. Dulbecco's PBS-serum-free (DPBS-S), pH 7.2, was prepared from DPBS (Biochrom) by addition of 1 mg/ml bovine serum albumin, 2.5 mg/ml glucose, 1% v/v nonessential amino acids, 1% v/v essential amino acids, and 1 m*M* L-glutamine.

Animals. Male Balb/c or B6D2F1 mice, 8–12 weeks old, obtained from the Central Institute for Experimental Animals (Hannover, FRG) were used throughout the experiments.

Chemotherapy. Mice (four to seven animals per group) were injected subcutaneously with 0.6 mg cefotaxime, 0.15 mg amikacin, 2.85 mg mezlocillin, 0.35 mg clindamycin, 0.4 mg ciprofloxacin, or 1 mg cefodizime in 0.1 ml 0.9% NaCl twice a day for seven consecutive days. Control mice received the same volume of NaCl.

Humoral Response. Following 7 days treatment with antibiotics, mice received an intraperitoneal injection of 2×10^8 sheep erythrocytes in 0.5 ml NaCl. Four days after the immunization, spleen cells were suspended in MHPB, and the number of direct plaque-forming cells was determined by use of the thin-layer modification of the Jerne plaque assay [14].

Superoxide Production. Superoxide generation was determined by use of the cytochrome c reduction assay [12]. The assay was performed as a microassay. Peritoneal cells were harvested by peritoneal lavage with 5 ml MHPB. The cells were washed twice and adjusted to a density of 1×10^6 cells/ml in DPBS-S. The reaction mixture consisted of 100 µl cell suspension, 50 µl cytochrome c (4 mg/ml), 25 µl DPBS-S or superoxide dismutase (12000 U/ml), and 25 µl of the respective stimulus [phorbol myristate acetate (PMA, 26.65 ng); zymosan (20 µg)]. The samples were incubated at 37 °C in a microtiter plate (Greiner, Solingen, FRG) and the optical density at 550 nm was determined by use of an ELISA-Reader MR600 (Dynatech, Denkendorf, FRG). The amount of superoxide produced was calculated by use of an extinction coefficient of 21.1×10^6 cm^2/mol for reduced cytochrome c.

Intestinal Flora. Fecal samples were taken from the cecum of mice, diluted in 0.9% NaCl, and aliquots were plated onto agar plates. Identification of the bacteria was performed using standard procedures.

Statistics. Student's *t*-test was used for statistical analysis of the data. The significance level was set to $\alpha = 0.01$.

Results

Humoral Immune Response

Treatment of Balb/c mice for 7 days with different antibiotics led to no significant alteration of the humoral immune response against sheep erythrocytes (Table 1). Similar results were obtained when B6D2F1 mice were studied, with the only exception that treatment of those mice with amikazin led to a significant suppression (54%) of the immune response (Table 1). The weight of the spleen was not found to be influenced by antibiotic treatment of either strain of mice (Table 2).

Reactivity of Peritoneal Cells

In order to study the possible influence of antibiotic treatment on the nonspecific defense system, namely macrophages and granulocytes, the production of superoxide anion after stimulation with PMA or zymosan was investigated. The gen-

Table 1. Influence of antibiotic therapy on the humoral immune response against sheep erythrocytes

Treatment	PFC/10^6 spleen cells[a]	
	Balb/c	B6D2F1
Cefotaxim	1698±292	1326±371
Amikazin	ND	1140±403[b]
Mezlocillin	1657±378	1678±795
Clindamycin	2113±231	2532±404
Ciprofloxacin	2300±924	3102±856
Cefodizime	ND	3043±569
–	1595±411	2453±688

ND, not done.
[a] PFC, plaque-forming cells.
[b] $P<0.01$.

Table 2. Influence of antibiotic therapy on the spleen weight of different strains of mice

Antibiotic	Spleen weight (g)	
	Balb/c	B6D2F1
Cefotaxime	0.112±0.015	0.164±0.018
Amikazin	0.110±0.047	0.163±0.032
Mezlocillin	0.109±0.022	0.137±0.025
Clindamycin	0.104±0.016	0.146±0.034
Ciprofloxacin	0.117±0.019	0.144±0.031
Cefodizime	0.102±0.007	0.256±0.111
–	0.104±0.018	0.137±0.022

Table 3. Influence of antibiotic therapy on the superoxide production by peritoneal cells from B6D2F1 mice

Antibiotic	Superoxide production (nmol $O_2^-/10^6$ macrophages × 1 h) in response to		
	DPBS	PMA	Zymosan
Cefotaxime	0.90±0.76	10.90±3.10	12.44±4.56
Amikazin	1.19±0.57	11.31±5.43	8.36±1.19
Mezlocillin	0.91±1.16	11.76+5.58	9.65±0.95
Clindamycin	0.50±0.90	10.86±2.27	9.07±1.36
Ciprofloxacin	0.33±0.90	11.88±3.57	9.21±2.13
Cefodizime	1.63±0.92	15.39±2.57	10.10±1.26
–	1.13±0.58	12.37±4.65	9.60±1.58

Table 4. Influence of antibiotic therapy on the superoxide production by peritoneal cells from Balb/c mice

Antibiotic	Superoxide production (nmol $O_2^-/10^6$ macrophages × 1 h) in response to		
	DPBS	PMA	Zymosan
Cefotaxime	0.80±0.27	10.62±1.79	6.72±0.80
Amikazin	1.58±0.35	13.39±3.93	8.83±2.05
Mezlocillin	1.19±0.35	14.15±5.35	8.98±1.16
Clindamycin	1.62±0.29	13.93±2.93	7.30±1.17
Ciprofloxacin	0.88±0.21	11.80±2.97	7.08±1.13
–	1.38±0.37	12.22±2.07	7.58±1.93

Table 5. Influence of antibiotic treatment of B6D2F1 mice on the composition of the intestinal flora

Bacteria	Composition of the intestinal flora after treatment with[a]						
	Cefotaxime	Amikazin	Mezlocillin	Clindamycin	Ciprofloxacin	Cefodizime	–
Enterobacteriaceae	–	0.0002	14.5	95.5	0.02	1.1	0.3
Staphylococcus	1.1	0.07	0.01	0.3	1.4	3.2	0.05
Streptococcus	0.1	3.0	4.6	1.2	23.9	89.3	9.0
Bacillus	0.06	5.7	–	–	–	–	–
Neisseriaceae	0.03	–	0.1	–	–	–	–
Bacteroides/ Sphaerophorus group	73.1	73.3	71.9	0.4	28.9	3.6	22.7
Lactobacillus	10.2	14.3	0.6	2.6	37.8	–	–
Clostridium	–	–	0.5	–	–	–	–
Eubacterium	15.4	3.7	4.5	0.08	7.9	–	64.4
Anaerobic cocci	–	0.01	3.5	0.02	–	2.8	3.6
Total number bacteria/g faeces	2.5×10^8	$3.0 - 10^8$	9.2×10^8	1.0×10^9	1.0×10^8	5.0×10^7	3.9×10^8

[a] Percentage of total number bacteria/g faeces.

eration of superoxide anion by peritoneal macrophages of different strains of mice treated with antibiotics was not altered in comparison with controls (Tables 3, 4). These data indicate that antibiotic treatment in vivo has no effect on the activity and function of the membrane-bound NAD(P)H-oxidase or the mannose receptor of phagocytes.

Intestinal Flora

The treatment of mice with antibiotics led to marked alterations in the relative composition of the intestinal flora (Tables 5, 6). The effects are dependent not only on the antibiotic used but also on the respective strain of mice. Whereas cefotaxime induced an increase in the number of Enterobacteriaceae in feces of Balb/c mice, this antibiotic led to a decrease in B6D2F1 mice (Tables 5, 6). The consequence of these alterations for the immune system is still unclear.

Table 6. Influence of antibiotica treatment of Balb/c mice on the composition of the intestinal flora

Bacteria	Composition of the intestinal flora after treatment with[a]					
	Cefotaxime	Amikazin	Mezlocillin	Clindamycin	Ciprofloxacin	–
Enterobacteriaceae	1.1	0.005	3.2	0.08	0.00003	0.002
Staphylococcus	0.2	0.006	–	–	0.02	0.06
Streptococcus	7.8	8.2	1.3	8.5	8.8	7.0
Bacillus	–	0.01	–	–	–	–
Bacteroides/Sphaerophorus group	57.3	82.4	31.8	52.8	74.1	69.1
Lactobacillus	3.1	–	–	–	–	–
Clostridium	–	–	60.6	7.2	1.0	–
Eubacterium	30.4	9.2	3.0	28.2	16.2	23.8
Anaerobic cocci	–	–	–	0.8	–	–
Total number of bacteria/g faeces	1.1×10^9	6.6×10^8	2.0×10^9	1.5×10^9	1.5×10^{10}	8.8×10^8

[a] Percentage of total number of bacteria/g faeces.

Discussion

Roszkowski et al. [21–24] described marked alterations of parameters of the immune system of Balb/c mice after 7 days of treatment with different antibiotics. Whereas cefotaxime, amikacin, mezlocillin, and piperacillin had a suppressive effect on the delayed-type hypersensitivity reaction as well as on the primary and secondary humoral immune response, clindamycin had no effect and ciprofloxacin even enhanced the humoral immune response. These authors found a total suppression of the humoral immune response after treatment of mice with at least 1.7 mg mezlocillin/day [22, 23]. In contrast, we could not find any significant suppression [$P > 0.01$) with doses up to 5.7 mg mezlocillin/day ([1]; Table 1). Only amikacin exerted an immunosuppressive effect in Balb/c mice. No reduction of the spleen weight (Table 2) or loss of hair as described by Roszkowski et al. [22]

could be found with either antibiotic and strain of mice. Furthermore, we could not detect any influence of antibiotic treatment on the response of mouse peritoneal cells to stimulation with PMA or zymosan (Tables 3, 4).

The composition of the intestinal flora of mice is known to be modified after anibiotic therapy [26]. Furthermore, the intestinal flora might exert an influence on the immune system [26, 27]. In this study, we found marked alterations of the intestinal flora, but these modifications were dependent on the antibiotic and strain of mice investigated (Tables 5, 6). There was no relationship between changes of the composition of the intestinal flora and the humoral immune response against sheep erythrocytes [Tables 1, 5, 6).

The reason for the discrepancy between the results described by Roszkowski et al. [22–24] and ours is yet unclear. One might speculate that the difference is due to different housing conditions and/or different patterns of the intestinal flora of the animals, but this hypothesis needs further investigation.

Summary

Antibiotics may alter the immune system of mammals either by modulating the function of immunocompetent cells or by affecting the microbiological flora of the organism, which may result in the liberation of immunomodulatory substances of the bacterial membrane. The published data concerning the effect of antibiotic treatment in vivo are only limited and controversial. In this study the effect of treatment of different strains of mice (Balb/c, B6D2F1) with amikazin, mezlocillin, cefotaxime, cefodizime (HR 221), clindamycin, or ciprofloxacin on the humoral immune response, the reactivity of peritoneal macrophages, and the colonization of the intestinal tract was investigated. No significant ($P > 0.01$) effect of antibiotic therapy with the exception of amikazin on the humoral immune response of Balb/c and B6D2F1 mice could be found. In addition, no alteration of the splenic mass could be detected after therapy of either strain of mice. Furthermore, no influence on superoxide generation of peritoneal cells in response to PMA or zymosan was found. Although antibiotic treatment led to marked alterations in the composition of the intestinal flora, this could not be correlated with alterations of the investigated parameters of the immune system.

References

1. Büscher KH, Andres B, Wendt S, Opferkuch W (1986) Einfluß von Mezlocillin auf die humorale Immunantwort in vivo. FAC 5-3:443
2. Finch R (1980) Immunomodulating effects of antimicrobial agents. J Antimicrob Chemother 6:691
3. Fortmeyer HP (1982) The influence of exogeneous factors such as maintenance and nutrition on the course and results of animal experiments. In: Bartosek I et al. (eds) Animals in toxicological research. Raven, New York, pp 13–32
4. Gillissen GJ (1982) Influence of cephalosporins on humoral immune response. In: Adam D, Hahn H, Opferkuch W (eds) The influence of antibiotics on the host-parasite relationship II. Springer, Berlin Heidelberg New York, pp 5–11
5. Gillissen G (1985) Antimicrobial chemotherapy in immunocompromised host. Cancer Treat Symp 1:37

6. Hauser W, Remington J (1982) Effect of antibiotics on the immune response. Am J Med 72:711
7. Hotzel D (1967) Contribution of the intestinal microflora to the nutrition of the host. Vitam Horm 24:115
8. Karch H, Goroncy-Bermes P, Opferkuch W, Kroll HP, O'Brien A (1985) Subinhibitory concentrations of antibiotics modulate amount of Shiga-like toxin produced by *Escherichia coli.* In: Adam D, Hahn H, Opferkuch W (eds) The influence of antibiotics on the host-parasite relationship II. Springer, Berlin Heidelberg New York, pp 239–245
9. Kollmorgen M, Longley R (1982) Dietary fat stimulates tumor growth and inhibits immune responses. 1st conference modulation and mediation of cancer by vitamins, Tucson, 1982
10. Limbert M, Bartlett RR, Dickneite G, Klesel N, Schorlemmer HU, Seibert G, Winkler I, Schrinner E (1984) Cefodizime, an aminothiazolyl cephalosporin. J Antibiot (Tokyo) 37:1719
11. Marx JL (1982) The immune system "belongs in the body". Pervasive anatomical and biochemical links between the immune and nervous systems help explain how mood might influence disease susceptibility. Science 227:1190
12. McCord JM, Fridovich I (1969) Superoxide dismutase. An enzymatic function for erythrocuprein (hemocuprein). J Biol Chem 244:6049
13. Milatovic D (1983) Antibiotics and phagocytosis. Eur J Microbiol 2:414
14. Mishell BB, Shiggi SM (1980) Selected methods in cellular immunology. WH Freeman, San Francisco
15. Monjau AA, Collector MI (1977) Stress induced modulation of the immune response. Science 196:307
16. Pawelzik M, Schumann U, Wiemer C (1985) The effect of sublethal concentrations of antibiotics on the host-parasite relationship. Zbl Bakt Hyg [A] Suppl 13:165
17. Opferkuch W, Pawelzik M (1986) Der Einfluß von Antibiotika auf die Keim-Phagozyten-Interaktion. FAC 5-3:431
18. Opferkuch W, Büscher KH, Leying H, Pawelzik M, Suerbaum S (1987a) The influence of subinhibitory concentrations of antibiotics on the bacterial surface with respect to host defense mechanisms. In: Szentivanyi A, Friedman H, Gillissen G (eds) Antibiosis and host immunity. Plenum New York, pp 15–25
19. Opferkuch W, Büscher KH, Leying H, Klimetzek V (1987b) Interaction of *Escherichia coli* and macrophages: alteration by treatment of bacteria with β-lactam antibiotics. Zbl Bakt Hyg [A] 266:116–126
20. Pawelzik M, Opferkuch W (1986) The influence of antibiotics on the host-parasite relationship. Clin Immunol Newsletter 7:81
21. Roszkowski K, Ko HL, Roszkowski W, Jeljaszewicz J, Pulverer G (1985) Effect of some antimicrobial antibiotics on sarcoma L-1 tumor growth in mice. Zbl Bakt Hyg [A] Suppl 13:199
22. Roszkowski W, Ko HL, Roszkowski K, Jeljaszewicz J, Pulverer G (1985) Effect of selected antibiotics on the cellular and humoral immune response in mice. Zbl Bakt Hyg [A] Suppl 13:59
23. Roszkowski W, Ko HL, Roszkowski K, Jeljaszewicz J, Pulverer G (1985) Antibiotics and immunomodulation: effects of cefotaxime, amikacin, mezlocillin, piperacillin and clindamycin. Med Microbiol Immunol (Berl) 173:279
24. Roszkowski W, Ko HL, Roszkowski K, Ciborowski P, Jeljaszewicz J, Pulverer G (1986) Effects of ciprofloxacin on the humoral and cellular immune responses in Balb/c mice. Zbl Bakt Hyg [A] 262:396
25. Suerbaum S, Leying H, Kroll HP, Gmeiner J, Opferkuch W (1987) Influences of β-lactam antibiotics and ciprofloxacin on the cell envelope of *Escherichia coli.* Antimicrob Agents Chemother 31:1106
26. Van der Waaij D (1969) Similarities between germfree mice and mice with an antibiotic decontaminated tract. In: Miraud EA, Bach N (eds) Germ-free biology, Plenum, New York, p 181
27. Van der Waaij D, Heidt PJ (1977) Intestinal bacterial ecology in relation to immunological factors and other defense mechanisms. In: Hambraens L, Hansen LA, McFarland H (eds) Food and immunology. Almquist and Wiskell, Stockholm, p 183

Influence of Ciprofloxacin Treatment In Vivo on Cell-Mediated Immunity to *Listeria monocytogenes*

S. Ehlers and H. Hahn

Introduction

The new quinolone derivative, ciprofloxacin, has been claimed to be an efficient chemotherapeutic drug in infections with the intracellular bacterium *Listeria monocytogenes* [1]. Recently, however, it was shown in an in vitro assay that high concentrations of ciprofloxacin irreversibly inhibit *Listeria*-specific T-cell proliferation [2].

To determine the in vivo relevance of this finding we examined various parameters of cell-mediated immunity generated during experimental *Listeria* infections in mice subjected to different protocols of antibiotic treatment.

Materials and Methods

Two experimental series were performed:

I. Groups A–D: B6D2F1 female mice were i.v. infected with 1×10^3 viable *L. monocytogenes* and treated i.v. with antibiotics for three consecutive days. Bacterial growth in the spleen was followed against time. Delayed-type hypersensitivity (DTH) reaction was elicited on day 6 and reinfection was performed with 1×10^5 *L. monocytogenes* i.v. on day 14. For adoptive transfer of protection, 1.5 ml proteose peptone was injected i.p. on day 7, peritoneal exudate cells harvested on day 10, and peritoneal equivalents or pooled cells infused into naive recipients together with a challenge dose of 5×10^4 *L. monocytogenes.*

II. Groups E, F, G: Mice were i.v. infected with 8.5×10^3 *L. monocytogenes* and treated i.p. with antibiotics for 5 days. DTH was elicited on day 6, and reinfection was performed with 1×10^5 *L. monocytogenes* i.v. on day 21. For adoptive transfer of protection, single cell suspensions of spleens harvested from treated donors on day 7 were prepared and either one for two splenic equivalents or 3×10^8 pooled spleen cells were infused into naive recipients together with a challenge dose of 5×10^4 *L. monocytogenes*. Controls received spleen cells of nonimmune, untreated donors.

Department of Medical Microbiology, Freie Universität Berlin 45, Hindenburgdamm 27, 1000 Berlin 45, Federal Republic of Germany

The Influence of Antibiotics on the Host-Parasite Relationship III
Edited by G. Gillissen, W. Opferkuch, G. Peters, and G. Pulverer

Antibiotic Treatment. Sodium ampicillin and ciprofloxacin ampoules (10 mg/ml) were kindly provided by Bayer AG, Wuppertal, FRG, and diluted to the appropriate doses in phosphate-buffered saline (PBS). Group A received 2 × 2 mg ciprofloxacin daily, group B 2 × 1 mg ciprofloxacin daily, group C 2 × 4 mg ampicillin daily, and group C PBS only, 0.4 ml twice daily. Injections were performed in a lateral tail vein in a volume of 0.4 ml at 12-h intervals starting in a lateral tail vein in a volume of 0.4 ml at 12-h intervals starting 6 h after the primary infection, a total number of six therapeutic injections being administered. In the second set of experiments, intraperitoneal treatments were carried out with the following doses: group E received 2 × 3 mg ampicillin daily, group F was given 2 × 1.5 mg ciprofloxacin daily, and group G received 2 × 0.5 ml PBS daily as a volume control. Treatment was continued for 5 days at 12-h intervals starting 6 h after the primary infection with 8.5×10^3 *L. monocytogenes.*

Results and Discussion

Influence of Antibiotic Treatment on the Primary Infection

The course of the primary infection during antibiotic treatment with ciprofloxacin and ampicillin is depicted in Fig. 1. Although the dosages used in these experiments were high (2 × 1 mg ciprofloxacin daily, representing an approximate 20-fold maximum dose calculated on a per kilogram body weight recommended dose for the i.v. therapeutic use in humans [3]), none of the treatment groups were entirely cleared of their bacterial load by antibiotic treatment alone, once again emphasizing the supreme importance of the host's own imune response to effectively counteract infection [4]. Moreover, there was a strong rebound of replicating bacteria after treatment was stopped after the first 3 days or, in fact, even after 5 days, reinforcing the rationale for prolonged treatment procedures in *Listeria* infections [5]. It is, however, intriguing to note that, when a high inoculum dose was used, ciprofloxacin was significantly less effective than the standard treatment with ampicillin (Fig. 1 b).

Influence of Antibiotic Treatment on the Development of DTH to Listeria Antigen (sAg)

The DTH response on day 7 for all groups is shown in Fig. 2. Treatment with ampicillin and ciprofloxacin 2 × 1 mg resulted in a significant reduction of the DTH response to sAg which in the high-dose ciprofloxacin treatment group came close to its complete abrogation (Fig. 2 a). With a higher inoculum dose, however, even a prolonged course of treatment with 1.5 mg ciprofloxacin did not severely compromise the DTH reaction of treated animals. In contrast, an efficient therapy with 2 × 3 mg ampicillin i.p. over 5 days significantly reduced this reaction (Fig. 2 b).

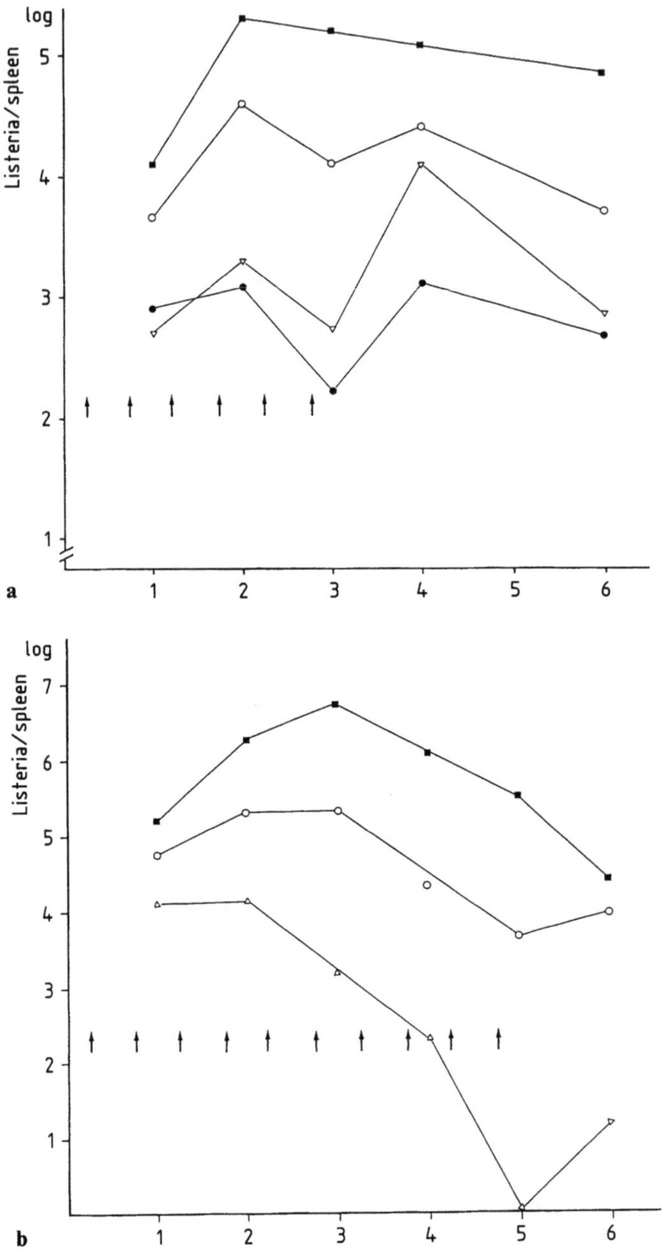

Fig. 1. a Course of primary infection (inoculum 1×10^3 *L. monocytogenes*) during treatment with: ■, D PBS only; ○, B 2×1 mg ciprofloxacin/day i.v.; ▽, C 2×4 mg ampicillin/day i.v.; ●, A 2×2 mg ciprofloxacin/day i.v. *Arrows* indicate the time of antibiotic administration. Means of five mice per time point. **b** Course of primary infection (inoculum 8.5×10^3 *L. monocytogenes*) during treatment with: ■, G PBS only; ○, F 2×1.5 mg ciprofloxacin/day i.p.; △, E 2×3 mg ampicillin/day i.p. *Arrows* indicate the time of antibiotic administration. Means of five mice per time point

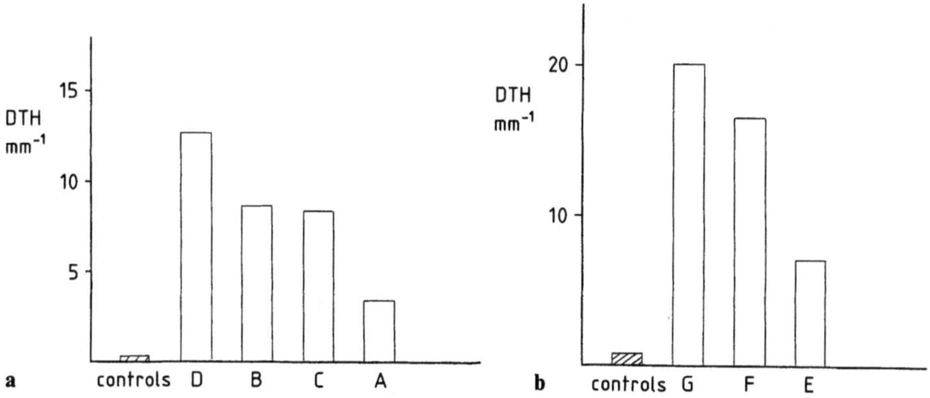

Fig. 2. a Delayed-type hypersensitivity on day 7 after primary infection with 1×10^3 *L. monocytogenes* 3-day treatment course. *A*, 2 × 2 mg ciprofloxacin/day i.v.; *B*, 2 × 1 mg ciprofloxacin/day i.v.; *C*, 2 × 4 mg ampicillin/day i.v.; *D*, PBS only. Means of five mice per group. **b** Delayed-type hypersensitivity on day 7 after primary infection with 8.5×10^3 *L. monocytogenes*; 5-day treatment course. *E*, 2 × 3 mg ampicillin day/i.p.; *F*, 2 × 1.5 mg ciprofloxacin day/i.p.; *G*, PBS only. Means of five mice per group

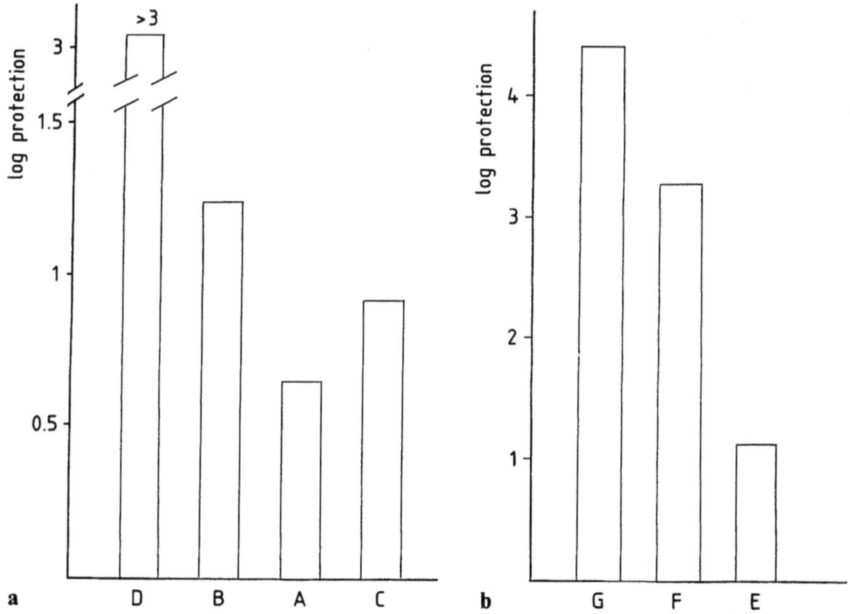

Fig. 3. a Protection during reinfection with 1×10^5 *L. monocytogenes* after a 3-day treatment course of primary infection (inoculum 1×10^3 *L. monocytogenes*) with: *D*, PBS only; *B*, 2 × 1 mg ciprofloxacin/day i.v.; *A*, 2 × 2 mg ciprofloxacin/day i.v.; *C*, 2 × 4 mg ampicillin/day i.v. Means of five mice per group. **b** Protection during reinfection with 1×10^5 *L. monocytogenes* after a 5-day treatment course of primary infection (inoculum 8.5×10^3 *L. monocytogenes* with: *G*, PBS only; *F*, 2 × 1.5 mg ciprofloxacin/day i.p.; *E*, 2 × 3 mg ampicillin/day i.p. Means of five mice per group

Effect of Antibiotic Treatment on the Generation of the Anti-Listeria Response

As Evidenced During Reinfection (Fig. 3a, b). A significant reduction in the level of protection was observed in all the treatment groups with an obvious relationship to the amount of replicating bacteria that had been present during the primary infection.

As Evidenced by Adoptive Cell Transfer. When one or two peritoneal exudate equivalents obtained from treated mice were transferred into recipient mice, there was no evidence of adoptive protection (data not shown). In an attempt to clarify the reason for this, we counted the number of cells that could be washed out from the peritoneal cavities of the animals in each treatment group. The data are given in Table 1, showing that treatment had substantially lowered the number of cells capable of entering the exudate. We therefore adjusted the number of cells transferred into each recipient to 1.5×10^7 and 2.4×10^7 in order to compare the functional capacity of the cells to confer protection. Although the level of adoptive protection was very low throughout the experiments, there was only a nonsignificant difference between the various treatment groups, thus pointing to a functional equivalence of the cells transferred (Fig. 4a). When spleen cells of treated donors were transferred, the same picture emerged (Fig. 4b): the control group exhibited a high amount of protection, reflecting an efficient T-cell reponse to a heavy and persistent primary infection. The ciprofloxacin-treated group showed less protection on a per spleen basis; yet when cell numbers were adjusted, no difference could be found in the protective capacities of treated and untreated immune spleens. Ampicillin-treated donors had mounted only a marginal degree of protective immunity as reflected by the low number of spleen cells (Table 1). When cell numbers were adjusted, transferred protection could be significantly enhanced, pointing to a quantitative rather than a qualitative deficiency of donor T-cells. The cumulative data of the experiments presented here are entirely consistent with the established dogma [6–8] that it is the level and length of replication of viable bacteria during the primary infection that ultimately determine the pro-

Table 1. Numbers of cells washed out from the peritoneal cavities

Peritoneal exudate cells	
Treatment group	Cells washed out per animal
A. 2 × 2 mg ciprofloxacin/day i.v.	3.44×10^6
B. 2 × 1 mg ciprofloxacin/day i.v.	6.15×10^6
C. 2 × 4 mg ampicillin/day i.v.	5.07×10^6
D. 2 × 0.4 ml PBS i.v.	15.80×10^6
Spleen cells	
Treatment group	Spleen cells per animal
E. 2 × 3 mg ampicillin/day i.p.	8.70×10^7
F. 2 × 1.5 mg ciprofloxacin/day i.p.	1.10×10^8
G. 2 × 0.5 ml PBS/day i.p.	1.24×10^8
– No treatment	6.94×10^7

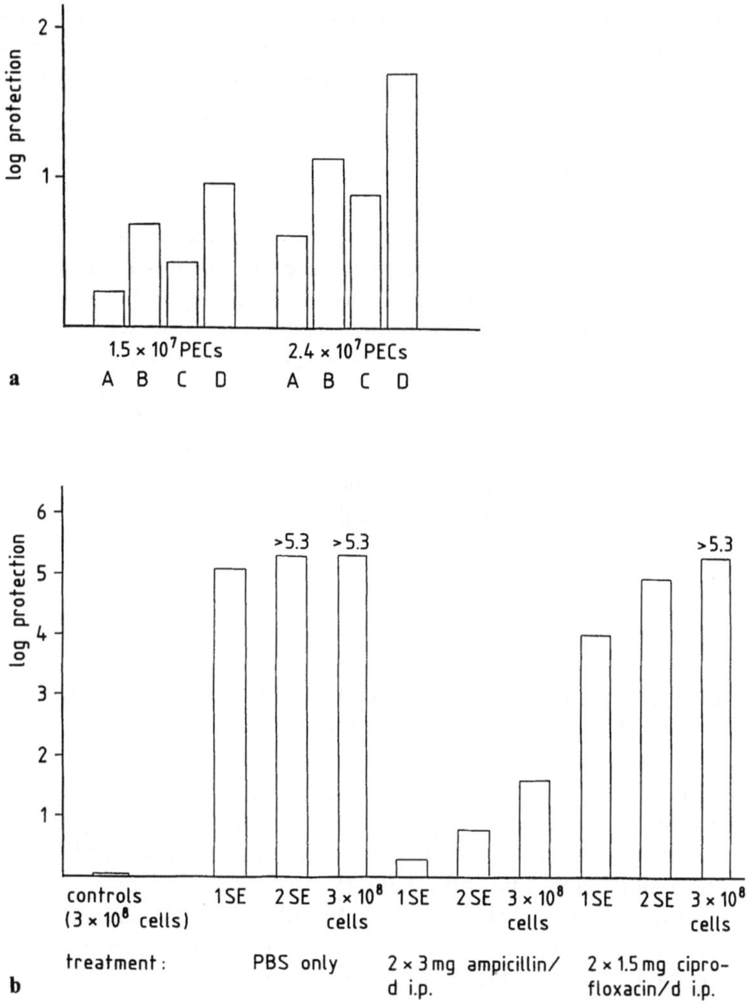

Fig. 4. a Adoptive immunity by transfer of adjusted numbers of peritoneal exudate cells (PECs) of treated donors (primary infection: 1×10^3 *L. monocytogenes*); 3-day treatment course with: *A*, 2×2 mg ciprofloxacin/day i.v.; *B*, 2×1 mg ciprofloxacin/day i.v.; *C*, 2×4 mg ampicillin/day i.v.; *D*, PBS only. Challenge dose: 5×10^4 *L. monocytogenes*. Means of five mice per group. **b** Adoptive immunity by transfer of splenic equivalents (SEs) or 3×10^8 splenocytes of treated donors (primary infection: 8.5×10^3 *L. monocytogenes*); 5-day treatment course. Challenge dose: 5×10^4 *L. monocytogenes*. Means of five mice per group

tective capacity acquired by the animal. Thus, whenever the number of cells transferred was adjusted to equal amounts, no differences between the recipient groups could be detected, pointing to numerical deficiency, yet functional equivalence of, protective cells generated in the treated infection.

Nonetheless, we cannot formally dismiss the hypothesis that an additional antiproliferative effect of ciprofloxacin may also exist in vivo. In fact, during most of the infection, the number of bacterial counts in treatment group B was only about 1 log unit lower than in the control group, yet the amount of protective immunity generated was about equal to that built up by group C (ampicillin), which at least during the first 3 days of infection had significantly lower numbers of bacteria in the spleen. However, the finding that during rebound *Listeria* numbers approached about the same level in both groups might resolve this apparent contradiction.

Since the prolonged treatment course afforded the advantage of reducing the rebound after cessation of treatment, the interfering effect of the latter seen during the first experimental series was virtually negligible and the distinction between the groups became even more clear cut. Thus, when spleen cells were adjusted numerically on transfer, no difference on the amount of protective capacity of the transferred cells could be observed when compared with the control group. In fact, any reduction of immune potency observed throughout the experiments could always be most easily explained by the reduction of the bacterial load by ciprofloxacin when given during the primary infection. In summary, ciprofloxacin seems to have no immunomodulatory effect in vivo.

Summary

The intravenous and intraperitoneal administration of ciprofloxacin in high doses (2×1 mg/day up to 2×2 mg/day can reduce the bacterial load of mice experimentally infected with the intracellular bacterium *Listeria monocytogenes*.

The T-cell response generated during the treated infection is affected in much the same way as it is during antibiotic treatment with ampicillin, i.e., the protective immunity established directly correlates with the number of bacteria present during an extended period during the primary infection.

Although an additional antiproliferative effect of ciprofloxacin on expanding T-cells as evidenced in in vitro experiments cannot be excluded, our data in summary favor the view that in vivo this effect is at most of minor importance.

Acknowledgment. We thank D. Oberbeck-Müller for preparing the figures.

References

1. Hof H, Zinn U, Ströder J (1985) Die Wirkung von Chinolinderivaten auf Listerien. ZAC 3:115
2. Hahn H, Wos B, Sperling U (1985) Influence of Ciprofloxacin on specific interactions of *Listeria*-specific T cells with antigen in vitro. In: Adam D, Hahn H, Opferkuch W (eds) The influence of antibiotics on the host-parasite relationship II. Springer, Berlin Heidelberg New York, p 96
3. Bassaris HP, Chrysanthopoulos C, Skoutelis A, Politi-Makrypoulia V (1986) Treatment of pneumonias with ciprofloxacin. In: Neu HC, Weuta H (eds) 1st international ciprofloxacin workshop. Excerpta Medica, p 241

4. Hof H, Emmerling P, Seeliger HPR (1981) Murine model for therapy of listeriosis in the compromised host. Chemotherapy 27:214
5. Nieman RE, Lorber B (1980) *Listeria* in adults: a changing pattern. Report of 8 cases and review of the literature. Rev Infect Dis 2:207
6. North RJ, Berche PA, Newborg MF (1981) Immunologic consequences of antibiotic-induced abridgement of bacterial infection: effect on generation and loss of protective T cells and level of immunologic memory. J Immunol 127(1):342
7. Emmerling P, Hof H, Finger H (1978) Resistance to infection with *Listeria monocytogenes* in normal and thymusless mice treated with ampicillin. Zbl Bakt Hyg I Abt Orig A 240:339
8. North RJ (1973) The mediators of anti-*Listeria* immunity as an enlarged population of short-lived, replicating T-cells. Kinetics of their production. J Exp Med 138:342

Enzymatic Conversion of [^{3}H]Clindamycin by the Human Neutrophil *

L. AMARAL and V. LORIAN

Introduction

Human neutrophils have been shown to concentrate radioactively labeled clindamycin approximately 12-fold compared with its concentration in the medium [1]. This concentrating effect was shown in this study to be dependent upon cellular energy at 37 °C. The amount of radioactively labeled clindamycin associated with formalin-fixed neutrophils was about twice the concentration of the medium and was interpreted by the authors to represent the binding of the antibiotic to the surface of the neutrophils.

The concentration of an antibiotic within a human phagocyte is of obvious interest with the possibility that after the phagocytosis of bacteria the penetration of the antibiotics into the cell allows the extension of antibiotic activity on the ingested bacteria. However, in order that this takes place the antimicrobial activity within the phagocyte, by necessity, must remain similar to its extracellular activity. Furthermore, inasmuch as the neutrophil (phagocyte) contains a large number of hydrolytic enzymes, the penetration of the antibiotic into the phagocyte may be rapidly followed by its degradation, and its antimicrobial activity may be lessened to the degree that it is ineffective. In this study, we investigated the molecular integrity of [^{3}H]clindamycin after its penetration into the human neutrophil.

Materials and Methods

Human neutrophils were purified by gradient centrifugation in dextran. Purified human neutrophils were cultured in TC 199 medium at various temperatures for varying periods in the presence of increasing concentrations of [^{3}H]clindamycin (specific activity 1.8 μCi/mm, New England Nuclear Corporation) generously provided by UpJohn Company, Kalamazoo, Michigan. At the end of the incubation period the neutrophils were centrifuged at 4000 g for 1 min and the supernate quickly removed. The insides of the culture tubes were wiped with cotton swabs in order to remove as much extracellular [^{3}H]clindamycin as possible. Examination of the duplicate set of cultures containing [^{14}C]inulin did not indicate a sig-

* Supported by a grant from the UpJohn Company, Kalamazoo, Michigan, USA
Department of Pathology and Department of Epidemiology, Infection Control and Bronx-Lebanon Hospital Center. Bronx, NY 10456

The Influence of Antibiotics on the Host-Parasite Relationship III
Edited by G. Gillissen, W. Opferkuch, G. Peters, and G. Pulverer

nificant contamination of [^{3}H]clindamycin present extracellularly when compared with the amount associated with the pellet (less than 0.8%). [^{3}H]clindamycin was extracted from the pelleted neutrophils with reagent-grade chloroform. The chloroform phase was removed and concentrated to 10 μl and applied to salica thin-layer plates. Chromatography was conducted with a mixture of acetone, water, and ethyl acetate (8: 1 : 5 vol/vol) for 30 min at 26 °C. The chromatographic plates were dried and incubated with Kodak X-ray film for various periods at −70 °C, developed, and scanned with the aid of a Beckman computer-assisted densitometer.

Results

The chloroform extract obtained from pelleted neutrophils incubated at 37 °C for various intervals yielded two autoradiographic bands in the developed X-ray film that overlaid the chromatographic plate. Comparison of the relative mobilities of these two bands to that separately exhibited by clindamycin and its metabolites indicated that the faster-moving band was [^{3}H]clindamycin and that the slower-moving band was demethyl clindamycin. Densitometric evaluation of the corresponding optical densities of these two respective autoradiographic bands, summarized in Table 1, indicated that, whereas the amount of [^{3}H]clindamycin remained constant, the amount of [^{3}H]demethyl clindamycin increased with incubation time. Parallel cultures conducted at 4 °C exhibited only one band that corresponded to [^{3}H]clindamycin. The optical density of this band remained essentially constant throughout the incubation period, and at a level below that exhibited at 37 °C.

Neutrophils incubated for 30 min at 37 °C with the same amount of [^{3}H]clindamycin but with additional increasing separate amounts of either nonradioactive clindamycin or nonradioactive demethyl clindamycin yielded the results presented in Table 2. The separate additions of either form of clindamycin at increasing concentrations resulted in comparable reductions of both autoradiographic bands. This reduction in the intensity of the bands was equally pronounced with addition of demethyl clindamycin. The presence of inhibitors of glycolysis in the

Table 1. Relative amounts of [^{3}H] clindamycin and [^{3}H] demethyl clindamycin extracted from human neutrophils incubated with 35 μg [^{3}H] clindamycin at 4 °C and 37 °C for varying periods

	Time (min)				
	5	15	30	60	120
4 °C					
[^{3}H] Clindamycin band	0.175	0.180	0.165	0.180	0.180
[^{3}H] Demethyl clindamycin band	0.000	0.000	0.000	0.000	0.000
37 °C					
[^{3}H] Clindamycin band	0.185	0.155	0.170	0.180	0.175
[^{3}H] Demethyl clindamycin band	0.235	0.495	0.530	0.505	0.525

Figures are optical densities of the autoradiographic band.

Table 2. Effects of measuring concentrations of either clindamycin or demethyl clindamycin on the relative amount of [^{3}H] clindamycin and [^{3}H] demethyl clindamycin extracted from human neutrophils incubated for 30 min with 25 μg [^{3}H] clindamycin at 37 °C

	Optical density of	
	[^{3}H] Clindamycin band	[^{3}H] Demethyl clindamycin band
25 μg [^{3}H] clindamycin	0.195	0.585
Plus 25 μg clindamycin	0.050	0.185
Plus 50 μg clindamycin	0.000	0.000
Plus 25 μg demethyl clindamycin	0.065	0.155
Plus 50 μg demethyl clindamycin	0.000	0.000

Table 3. Effect of glycolytic inhibitions on the optical density of [^{3}H] clindamycin and [^{3}H] demethyl clindamycin bands, neutrophils, and culture condition identical to those employed in the experiment described in Table 2

	Optical density of	
	[^{3}H] Clindamycin band	[^{3}H] Demethyl clindamycin band
Control	0.200	0.595
Iodoacetic acid 10^{-5} M	0.190	0.000
$HgCl_2$ 10^{-5} M	0.205	0.000
Dinitrophenylbenzene 10^{-5} M	0.190	0.000

culture medium yielded the results presented in Table 3. From the data presented it is clear that whereas the clindamycin band remains essentially equal to that of the control, the presence of these glycolytic inhibitors at the concentrations employed prevented the formation of the demethyl clindamycin band.

Discussion

The incubation of human neutrophils in the presence of [^{3}H]clindamycin results in the conversion of the antibiotic into demethyl clindamycin. The formed demethyl clindamycin increases with time. Culture conditions that reduce or obviate the production of cellular energy reduce or negate this conversion, hence favoring the existence of an enzyme involved in the conversion of clindamycin to the demethyl form. The autoradiographic band corresponding to [^{3}H]clindamycin was not severely affected regardless of term of incubation, temperature, or presence of glycolytic inhibitors. These results suggest a binding to the surfaces of the neutrophil. Because this band can be reduced in intensity by increasing concentrations of nonradioactive clindamycin, the binding of clindamycin to specific "surface receptors" is probable. Furthermore, inasmuch as increasing concentrations of demethyl clindamycin also reduce the optical density of the band, demethyl clindamycin may also bind to these same receptors.

The antimicrobial activity of demethyl clindamycin on sensitive strains of *Staphylococcus aureus* was examined and found to be approximately 10% higher than that obtained with identical concentrations of clindamycin (data not presented). Consequently, the enzymatic conversion of clindamycin by the human neutrophil, supposedly after its binding to a surface receptor and subsequent penetration into the cell, does not negatively affect its antimicrobial properties on *S. aureus*. The concentration of demethyl clindamycin many times over that concentration in the medium, coupled with its retained antimicrobial activity, would lead one to suspect that *S. aureus* phygocytosed in the presence of demethyl clindamycin by human neutrophils would result in increased killing. Unfortunately, this is not the case. This leads one to suspect that the concentrated drug remains compartmentalized and separate from the phygocytosed organism.

Although no real advantages are afforded by the concentration of demethyl clindamycin by the human neutrophil with respect to enhanced killing activity, the portion of the molecule that binds to the surface receptor of the neutrophil is of obvious importance for the design of antileukemic drugs with target specificity for the leukemic neutrophil.

Summary

Human neutrophils, when incubated in medium containing [^{3}H]clindamycin, convert the molecule into [^{3}H]demethyl clindamycin in increasing amounts with time. The conversion is temperature dependent and inhibited by the presence of inhibitors of glycolytic energy.

Reference

1. Hand WL, King-Thompson NL, Steinberg TH (1983) Interactions of antibiotics and phagocytes. J Antimicrob Chemother 12 [Suppl C]:1

Antibiotic Modulation of Host Defense

B. P. OVERBEEK and J. VERHOEF

Introduction

Infection is a major cause of morbidity and mortality in man. Many gram-negative bacteria are sensitive to the bacteriolytic activity of serum alone. When bacteria are not lysed by serum, as is common for gram-positive microorganisms, they usually become opsonized and subsequently phagocytized by phagocytic cells and rapidly killed. Optimal phagocytosis requires the participation of opsonins, including serum complement and immunoglobulin (Ig). Although opsonization with complement is primarily mediated through activation of complement via IgG at the bacterial cell surface, these factors may also become fixed to microorganisms without the participation of antibody. Receptors on polymorphonuclear leukocytes (PMNs) with specificity for C3b and C3bi (the activated third complement components) and for the Fc fragment of the antibody molecule have been described, and evidence suggests that these receptors play a major role in phagocytosis of staphylococci opsonized in normal serum.

Severalantimicrobial agents have been shown to interfere directly with the phagocytic process, by influencing the chemotactic, phagocytic, or bactericidal activity of the phagocytic cells. Modulation of the phagocytic process by antibiotics has been extensively reviewed elsewhere [4]. Recently, however, it has been shown that antibiotics may also indirectly influence the phagocytic process: some bacteria become more susceptible to phagocytosis after exposure to certain antibiotics.

In this paper we describe the results of experiments designed to study the effect of subinhibitory concentrations of antibiotics on phagocytosis of staphylococci and *Escherichia coli*.

Materials and Methods

Bacteria

Staphylococcus aureus Cowan I; *S. aureus* Cowan I NG, a protein A-deficient mutant of *S. aureus* Cowan I; *S. aureus* Wood 46; *S. aureus* HSmR; and three clinical isolates were studied. *E. coli* strains O1; O1:K1; O7; O7:K1; O8; O8:K43; O78K80; O111; and its Rc mutant *E. coli* J5 were used.

Department of Clinical Microbiology and Laboratory for Infectious Diseases, University Hospital, Postbus 80125, 3508 TC Utrecht, The Netherlands

The Influence of Antibiotics on the Host-Parasite Relationship III
Edited by G. Gillissen, W. Opferkuch, G. Peters, and G. Pulverer

Labeling

The strains were grown overnight at 37 °C in Mueller-Hinton broth (MHB, Difco Laboratories, Detroit, Michigan, United States), containing 5 μCi [^{3}H]thymidine/ml in *E. coli* studies, in the presence or absence of one-fourth or one-half of the minimal inhibitory concentration (MIC) of antibiotic.

Phagocytosis and Killing Assay

The uptake of radiolabeled bacteria by PMNs was measured by the method of Verhoef et al. [9]. In brief: radiolabeled bacteria were opsonized in different concentrations of serum for various periods. Equal amounts of preopsonized bacteria (5×10^7/ml) and PMNs (5×10^6/ml) were incubated in a 37 °C shaking water bath. At indicated times phagocytosis was stopped by the addition of ice-cold phosphate-buffered saline. The percentage of bacteria taken up by PMNs at each time interval was calculated from the uptake of radioactivity by the phagocytes and the total added radioactivity. Radioactivity was determined by liquid scintillation counting (Philips, Almelo, The Netherlands).

Colony-forming units, representing the viable leukocyte-associated bacterial population after 12 min phagocytosis, were determined as described by Veringa [11].

Quantification of Cell Wall Protein A

A modification of the method of Peterson et al. [6], described by Veringa, was used [10]. The amount of protein A was determined quantitatively by indirect hemagglutination with sheep red blood cells (SRPCs), previously sensitized with a subagglutinating dose of IgG antibody to SRBCs.

Effect on the Outer Membrane of E.coli

The effect on the outer membrane (OM) was studied in ELISA, SDS-gel electrophoresis, and immunoblot experiments [5].

Results

Effects on Gram-positive Bacteria

Phagocytosis. When *S. aureus* Cowan I, a protein A rich strain, was grown in subinhibitory concentrations of clindamycin and subsequently opsonized for 1, 5, or 10 min in 1% normal human serum, these bacteria were phagocytized much more efficiently than opsonized control bacteria not grown with clindamycin [10]. This effect is dose dependent. After 12 min of incubation with PMNs, 22% of the con-

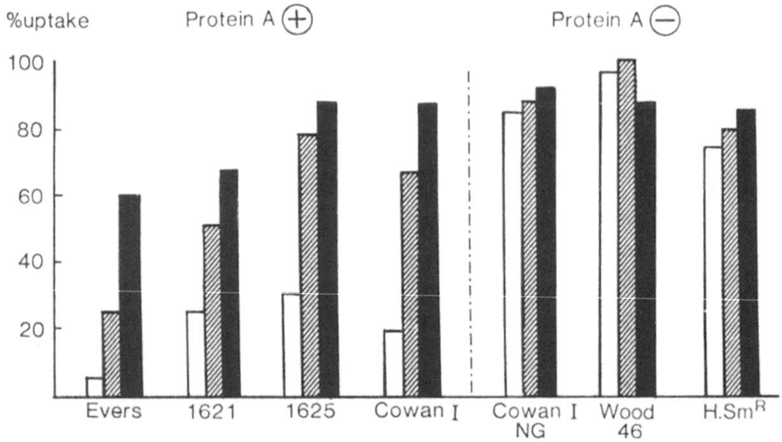

Fig. 1. Influence of clindamycin (▨, 0.25 × MiC; ■, 0.5 × MIC) on uptake of protein A-rich and protein A-poor *S. aureus* strains (□, control bacteria). Bacteria were opsonized in 1% normal serum for 1 min

trol bacteria were taken up, compared with 68% (0.25 × MIC) and 88% (0.5 × MIC) of the clindamycin-treated bacteria (Fig. 1).

No enhancement of uptake by PMNs was observed with clindamycin-treated *S. aureus* Cowan I NG, a protein A deficient mutant of *S. aureus* Cowan I.

Comparable results were observed after opsonization with agammaglobulinemic serum, heated antiserum, or C3-deficient serum. Clindamycin-treated *S. aureus* was also better killed by PMNs than control bacteria [11].

Effect of Clindamycin on Cell Wall Protein A. Table 1 shows that there is a dose-dependent reduction of cell wall protein A in protein A rich *S. aureus* strains when these strains were grown in the presence of subinhibitory concentrations of clindamycin.

Table 1. Reduction of the amount of protein A by clindamycin in protein A-rich *S. aureus* strains [10]

Strain	Amount of protein A (μg/10^9 bacteria)		
	Control	0.25 × MIC clindamycin	0.5 × MIC clindamycin
Staphylococcus aureus Ev.	5	0.16	ND
Staphylococcus aureus 1621	1.25	0.32	ND
Staphylococcus aureus 1625	20	0.16	0.16
Staphylococcus aureus Cowan I	20	1.25	0.32

ND, not done. Minimal detectable amount of protein A: 0.16 μg/10^9 bacteria.

Effects of Antibiotics on Gram-negative Bacteria

Phagocytosis. When normal human serum was used as opsonic source, all five unencapsulated strains of *E. coli* except for *E. coli* 0111 were phagocytized more readily than the four encapsulated *E. coli* strains [12]. Overnight incubation with subinhibitory concentrations of carumonam and azthreonam, two monocyclic beta-lactam antibiotics, resulted in an enhanced uptake of *E. coli* 0111 and the four encapsulated strains. Experiments with heat-inactivated serum showed that this effect was complement dependent (data not shown).

Influence of Monobactams on the Outer Membrane of Gram-negative Bacteria. Incubation of *E. coli* 0111 in subinhibitory concentrations of monobactam antibiotics increases its reactivity with antiserum to its rough mutant *E. coli* J5. This enhancement appeared to be due to an increased binding of antibodies directed to the core glycolipid and/or cell wall antigens, due to a relative loss of *O*-polysaccharide [5] (Figs. 2, 3).

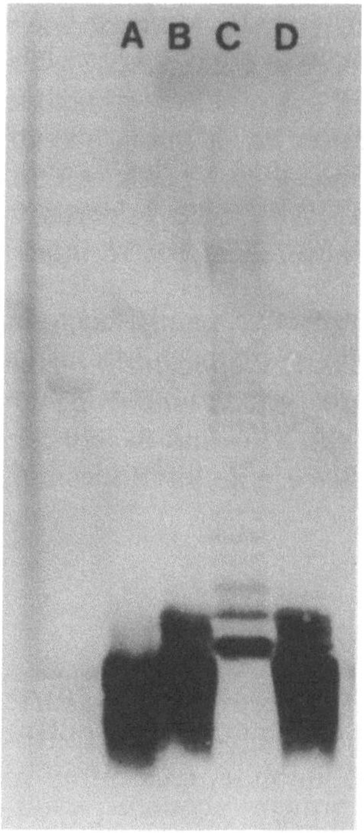

Fig. 2. SDS-polyacrylamide gel electrophoresis of proteinase K-treated cell walls of *E. coli* 0111 and J5. *Lane A*, *E. coli* J5, *Lane B*, monobactam-treated *E. coli* J5; *Lane C*, *E. coli* 0111; *Lane D*, monobactam-treated *E. coli* 0111

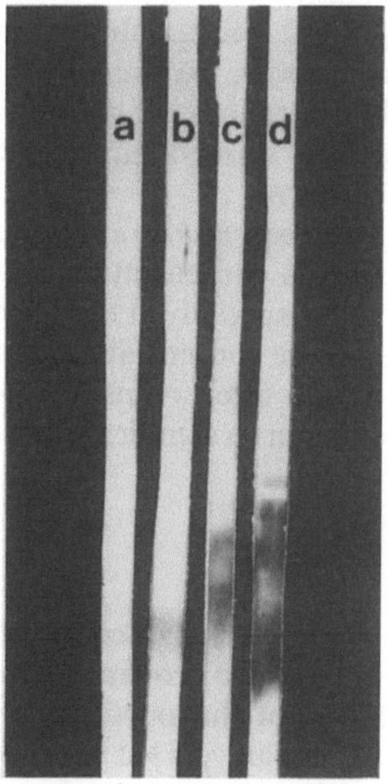

Fig. 3. Lipopolysaccharide-immunoblotting with a mouse monoclonal antibody against *E. coli* J5 core glycolipid. *Lanes A, B*, *E. coli* 0111; *Lanes C, D*, *E. coli* 0111, grown in a subinhibitory concentration of monobactam antibiotic

Discussion

Opsonization, which is an important process in the host defense system against invaded bacteria, can be impaired by bacterial structures. Protein A, a component of the cell wall of *S. aureus*, impairs opsonization by serum complement and by antibodies [7]. Because clindamycin at subinhibitory concentration decreases the amount of protein A in the cell wall of staphylococci, it is possible that this effect on protein A is the reason why clindamycin enhances uptake of these bacteria by PMNs.

In *E. coli* capsular polysaccharide has been shown to be a major virulence factor [3, 8]. Incubation of *E. coli* with monobactam antibiotics reduces the amount of K-antigen. This may then lead to increased opsonization and subsequent phagocytosis.

Monobactam antibiotics also have an effect on the *O*-polysaccharide side chain of lipopolysaccharides. On SDS gels, *O*-antigens were reduced dramatically when wild-type strains were exposed to these antibiotics. The *O*-polysaccharide of *E. coli* can serve as a shield. It can protect the bacteria against binding of antibodies to the core region [2, 7]. Antibodies directed to this core region have been shown to be cross-reactive with other gram-negative bacteria [1]. Also, a protective effect of this kind of antibodies on mortality has been demonstrated in humans and in animal studies in the case of septicemia by gram-negative bacteria [13, 14]. Because the amount of *O*-polysaccharide is reduced by the monobactam antibiotics, exposure to these antibiotics results in an increased binding of antibodies to the core glycolipid and/or the bacterial cell wall. Antibodies to core glycolipid showed enhanced cross-reactivity when bacteria were exposed to monobactams.

In conclusion, antibacterial agents may not only be effective against bacteria when a concentration above the MIC is reached, but in low concentrations as well. Especially at the site of infection (e.g., abscesses), where it commonly occurs that the concentration of antibacterial agents is below the MIC and the concentration of opsonins is significantly lower than in serum, certain antibiotics may still exert a significant effect.

Summary

The rates of uptake and intracellular killing of *S. aureus* were shown to be correlated to the protein A content of the cells: Strains with a high protein A content were not phagocytized as well. Strains incubated in subinhibitory concentrations of clindamycin led to dose-dependent reduction in their protein A content, resulting in enhanced uptake and killing. Comparable results were obtained after opsonization with agammaglobulinemic serum, heated antiserum, or C3-deficient serum. Protein A-deficient mutants were not affected by clindamycin pretreatment.

Two monocyclic, β-lactam antibiotics, carumonam and azthreonam, seem to influence the phagocytosis of gram-negative bacteria. Incubation of encapsulated *E. coli* in subinhibitory concentrations of the two monobactams enhances phagocytosis. This enhancement appears to be due to a selective loss of O-polysaccharide side chains of the lipopolysaccharide. Furthermore, an increase in the binding of antibodies directed to the core glycolipid could be demonstrated using rough mutant antiserum.

Thus, subinhibitory concentrations of clindamycin influenced the protein A content of *S. aureus* and subinhibitory concentrations of monobactams influenced the outer membrane of gram-negative bacteria, both resulting in a lower resistance to host defense mechanisms.

References

1. De Jongh-Leuvenink J, Bouter AS, Marcelis JH, Schellekens J, Verhoef J (1986) Cross-reactivity of monoclonal antibodies against lipopolysaccharides of gram-negative bacteria. Eur J Clin Microbiol 5:148–151
2. Gigliotti F, Shenep JL (1983) Failure of monoclonal antibodies to the core glycolipid to bind intact smooth strains of *Escherichia coli*. J Infect Dis 151:1005–1011
3. Horwitz MA, Silverstein SC (1980) Influence of the *Escherichia coli* capsule on complement fixation and on phagocytosis and killing by human phagocytosis. J Clin Invest 65:82–94
4. Milatovic D (1983) Antibiotics and phagocytosis. Eur J Clin Microbiol 2:414–425
5. Overbeek BP, Schellekens JFP, Lippe W, Dekker BAT, Verhoef J (1987) Carumonam enhances reactivity of *Escherichia coli* with mono- and polyclonal antisera to rough mutant *Escherichia coli* J5. J Clin Microbiol 25:1009–1013
6. Peterson PK, Verhoef J, Sabath LD, Quie PG (1977) Effect of protein A on staphylococcal opsonization. Infect Immun 15:706–746
7. Van der Ley P, Kuipers O, Tommassen J, Lugtenberg B (1986) *O*-Antigenic chains of lipopolysaccharide prevent binding of antibody molecules to an outer membrane pore protein in *Enterobacteriaceae*. Microb Pathogenesis 1:43–49
8. Van Dijk WC, Verbrugh HA, van der Tol ME, Peters R, Verhoef J (1979) Role of *Escherichia coli* K capsular antigens during complement activation, C fixation and opsonization. Infect Immun 25:603–609
9. Verhoef J, Peterson PK, Quie P (1977) Kinetics of staphylococcal opsonization, attachment, ingestion and killing by human polymorphonuclear leukocytes: a quantitative assay using [^{3}H]-thymidine labeled bacteria. J Immunol Methods 14:303–313
10. Veringa EM, Verhoef J (1986) Influence of subinhibitory concentrations of clindamycin on opsonophagocytosis of *Staphylococcus aureus:* a protein A dependent process. Antimicrob Agents Chemother 30:796–797
11. Veringa EM, Verhoef J (1987) Clindamycin at subinhibitory concentrations enhances antibody and complement dependent phagocytosis by human polymorphonuclear leukocytes of *Staphylococcus aureus*. Chemotherapy 33:243–249
12. Veringa E, Box A, Rozenberg-Arska M, Vernoef J (1988) Monobactam antibiotics in subinhibitory concentrations enhance opsonophagocytosis and serum bacteriolysis in certain *Escherichia coli* strains. Drugs Exp Clin Res 14:1–8
13. Ziegler EJ, Douglas H, Sherman JE, Davis CE, Braude AI (1973) Treatment of *E. coli* and *Klebsiella* bacteremia in agranulocytic animals with antiserum to an UDP-Gal epimerase-deficient mutant. J Immunol 111:433–438
14. Ziegler EJ, McCutchan JA, Fierer J, Glauser MP, Sadoff JC, Douglas H, Braude AI (1982) Treatment of gram-negative bacteremia and shock with human antiserum to a mutant *Escherichia coli*. N Engl J Med 307:1225–1230

In Vitro and Ex Vivo Effect of Cefodizime on Phagocytosis

A. Fietta, C. Bersani, T. Santagada, F.M. Grassi, and G. Gialdroni-Grassi

Among the newer cephalosporins, cefodizime, an α-methoxy-imino-2-thiazolyl derivative, has been reported to display direct and indirect effect on some components of the host defense system against infection [3–7]. The aim of our research was to study the in vitro and ex vivo direct effect of cefodizime on human mononuclear and polymorphonuclear phagocytes in order to better understand the mechanism of its immunomodulating properties.

Random migration, chemotaxis, phagocytosis frequency and index, nitroblue tetrazolium (NBT) reduction, and microbicidal activity were investigated according to the methods described by Gialdroni Grassi et al. [1]. Briefly, locomotion was assessed in modified Boyden chambers, with and without endotoxin-activated human serum as chemoattractant; phagocytosis and NBT reduction were performed using plastic-adherent phagocytes; microbicidal activity against *Candida albicans* was measured microbiologically. Tests were performed in the presence of cefodizime concentrations ranging from 1 to 200 μg/ml. Phagocytes and particles used as phagocytic challenge (i.e., zymosan or heat-killed *C. albicans*) were separately pretreated with the same drug concentrations and carefully washed before the assays in order to remove extracellular and non-cell-bound drug. Cefodizime at concentrations ranging from 1 to 200 μg/ml did not influence in vitro random migration, chemotaxis, NBT reduction frequency to formazan deposits, and microbicidal activity against *C. albicans* (data not shown). On the contrary the antibiotic seemed to modulate phagocytosis frequency and index. Experiments performed by leaving the antibiotic in the test system during the phagocytosis assay demonstrated that cefodizime did not influence phagocytosis when serum-opsonized particles (i.e., zymosan or heat-killed *C. albicans*) were used as phagocytic challenge (data not shown). A significant dose-related increase of both frequency and index of phagocytosis was shown when nonopsonized particles were used as phagocytic challenge (Tables 1, 2).

Phagocytes and zymosan particles were separately incubated with cefodizime for 30 min and then carefully washed before the assay in order to remove extracellular and non-cell-bound drug. Phagocytes again showed increased phagocytic activity for nonopsonized zymosan. This enhancing effect was shown at cefodizime concentrations equal or superior to 50 μg/ml. On the other hand zymosan pretreated with cefodizime seemed better recognized and ingested by both phagocytic cells than untreated particles. In this case the effect was significant at lower concentrations of the antibiotic (from 25 μg/ml).

Department of Chemotherapy, University of Pavia, Via Taramelli 5,27100 Pavia, Italy

The Influence of Antibiotics on the Host-Parasite Relationship III
Edited by G. Gillissen, W. Opferkuch, G. Peters, and G. Pulverer

Table 1. In vitro effect of cefodizime on nonspecific phagocystosis by adherent human neutrophils

	Concentrations (μg/ml)			
	25	50	100	200
Phagocytosis frequency				
A (%)	114.5*	131.2**	134.5**	134.5**
B (%)	103.8	115.4*	132.2**	131.0*
C (%)	117.5	137.0	142.5**	150.3**
Phagocytosis index				
A (%)	108.4	131.3**	136.1**	174.7**
B (%)	106.1	120.7*	136.6*	158.5**
C (%)	103.6	120.7*	156.1**	170.7**

Results, obtained from ten experiments using cells from different healthy volunteers, are expressed as percentages of phagocytosis indexes for cefodizime-treated/untreated cells and particles, assumed as 100%. Statistical significance of $P<0.05$ (*) and $P<0.01$ (**) (Student's *t*-test) is shown. A, in presence of cefodizime concentrations; B, monocytes treated for 30 min with cefodizime and carefully washed before the assay; C, zymosan treated for 30 min with the antibiotic and carefully washed before the assay.

Table 2. In vitro effect of cefodizime on nonspecific phagocystosis by adherent human monocytes

	Concentrations (μg/ml)			
	25	50	100	200
Phagocytosis frequency				
A (%)	132.4**	145.2**	154.8**	158.3**
B (%)	134.2	161.5*	178.8**	181.8**
C (%)	165.7**	191.6**	199.2**	220.8**
Phagocytosis index				
A (%)	136.4	154.1**	192.9**	227.0**
B (%)	139.3*	160.6*	191.8*	226.2*
C (%)	173.2**	201.2**	208.5**	237.8**

Symbols as in Table 1.

The effect of cefodizime on phagocyte functions was investigated following its administration to seven healthy volunteers. Subjects were treated intravenously at a daily dose of 4 g for 6 days. Neutrophil and monocyte functions were examined before and 12 h after the end of treatment. In agreement with the results obtained in vitro, the administration of this molecule produced a significant improvement of phagocytosis frequency and index of both neutrophils and monocytes when nonopsonized zymosan was used as phagocytic challenge (Fig. 1).

Our data indicated that cefodizime modulated in vitro and ex vivo nonspecific phagocytosis of adherent human phagocytes. The antibiotic probably did not penetrate either phagocytes or other mammalian cells [6], but only bound to their surfaces. The lack of effect on specific phagocytosis suggested that the antibiotic

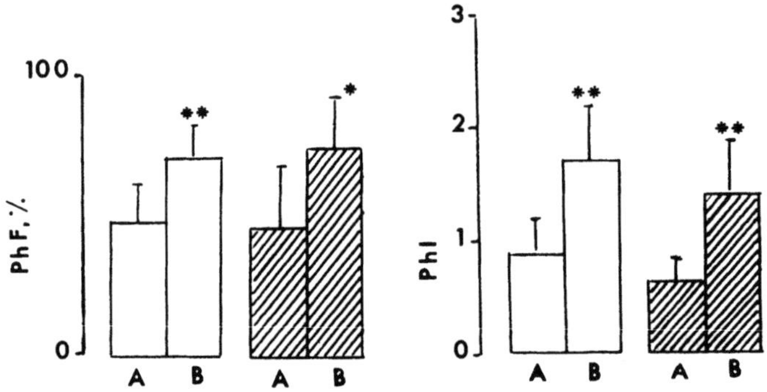

Fig. 1. Ex vivo effect of cefodizime on nonspecific phagocytosis frequency (*PhF*) and index (*PhI*) by monocytes (□) and neutrophils ( ). Results represent the mean values ±SD obtained from seven healthy subjects treated for 6 days with 4 g i.v. cefodizime. Nonopsonized zymosan was used as phagocytic challenge. *A*, before drug administration; *B*, 12 h after the end of the treatment; $*P<0.05$; $**P<0.01$ as estimated by Student's *t*-test

did not interact with surface serum receptors of phagocytic cells and opsonized particles.

The enhancing effect on nonspecific phagocytosis was shown not only when the drug was present during the assay but also when phagocytic cells or zymosanor heat-killed *C. albicans* were pretreated with the antibiotic, carefully removed before the assay. This dual effect suggested that the drug could bind some surface components of both types of cells, such as sugar residues of the phagocyte plasma membrane and carbohydrates or sugar-binding proteins of yeast cell surface [2]. Through an interaction in this process, cefodizime could provide an increased number of bridging moieties, amplifying the ingestion process.

Summary

The activity of cefodizime, a recent α-methoxy-imino-2-thiazolyl cephalosporin derivative, on phagocytic functions was tested in vitro and ex vivo. In vitro, at concentrations ranging from 1 to 200 μg/ml, it did not influence random migration, chemotaxis, nitroblue tetrazolium reduction, or microbicidal activity of neutrophils and monocytes. It did not affect phagocytosis when serum-opsonized particles were used as phagocytic challenge, while a significant increase of both frequency and index of phagocytosis was shown when nonopsonized zymosan or heat-killed *Candida albicans* were used as phagocytic challenge.

The effect of cefodizime on phagocytosis was evaluated following its administration of seven healthy volunteers (4 g daily i.v. for 6 days). Neutrophil and monocyte functions were tested before and 12 h after the end of treatment. A significant enhancement of phagocytosis frequency and index of both neutrophils and monocytes was observed when nonopsonized zymosan was used as phagocytic challenge.

References

1. Gialdroni Grassi G, Fietta A, Sacchi F, De Rose V (1984) Influence of ceftriaxone on natural defense systems. Am J Med 77 [Suppl 4 C]:37–41
2. Godman R, Bar-Shavit Z (1982) Phagocytosis – modes of particle recognition and stimulation by natural peptides. In: Karnovsky ML, Bolis L (eds) Phagocytosis past and future. Academic, New York, pp 259–285
3. Labro MT, Babin-Chevaye C, Hakim J (1986) Effects of cefotaxime and cefodizime on human granulocyte functions in vitro. J Antimicrob Chemother 18:233–237
4. Labro MT, Amit N, Babin-Chevaye C, Hakin J (1987) Cefodizime (HR 221) potentiation of human neutrophil oxygen-independent bactericidal activity. J Antimicrob Chemother 19:331–341
5. Leyhausen G, Seibert G, Maidhof A, Muller WEG (1984) Differential stimulation of lymphocyte cell growth in vitro by cephalosporins. Antimicrob Agents Chemother 26:752–756
6. Nagayama A, Nomura S, Taen H (1986) Enhanced killing of cefodizime (HR 221) treated *Escherichia coli* by macrophages and leukocytes. In: Marget W, Lang W, Gabler-Sandberger E (eds) Proc IXth international congress of infectious and parasitic diseases, vol II. Bacterial infections, antibacterial chemotherapy, addendum. MMV Medizin, Munich, pp 26–28
7. Yokota T, Nozawa R, Suzuki E, Arai K (1986) Synergy of antibacterial activity between cefodizime (THR 221) and the serum complement, and mouse polymorphonuclear leukocytes (PMNs) and/or macrophages (MO) In: Marget W, Lang W, Gabler-Sandberger E (eds) Proc. IXth international congress of infectious and parasitic diseases, vol II. Bacterial infections, antibacterial chemotherapy, addendum. MMV Medizin, Munich, pp 29–30

Antibacterial Substance(s) from *Hypericum perforatum*: Influence on Phagocytosis of *Escherichia coli* by Human Neutrophils *

E. LINGAAS [1] and T. MIDTVEDT [2]

Introduction

The presence of antibacterial substances in the plant genus *Hypericum* has been known for more than 40 years. In 1943, Osborn [10] demonstrated that extracts of a number of *Hypericum* species were active against *Staphylococcus aureus* but inactive against *Escherichia coli.* In the case of *Hypericum perforatum* (St. John's Wort), Neuwald and Hagenstrøm [9] found the petroleum ether and acetone extracts of the flowering herb and the dry fruits to be active against *S. aureus* but not against *Salmonella typhi* and *E. coli.* Gaind and Ganjoo [5] confirmed their results and obtained evidence of the presence of two compounds exhibiting activity against a number of gram-positive organisms. Such extracts have been used as food preservatives [7], and also to treat infections [6]. One of the active principles of *Hypericum,* designated hyperforin, was isolated and characterized in 1971 [6]. Recently, its structure and stereochemistry has been revised by Brondz et al. [1, 2].

Polymorphonuclear neutrophils are important contributors to host defense reactions in bacterial infections. Inadequate host defense may result in serious infections, as sometimes seen in immunocompromised hosts. In such patients infections should not only be treated with traditional chemotherapy but, ideally, with antimicrobial drugs stimulating host defense reactions, such as phagocytosis. In the present report, the influence of an extract of *H. perforatum* on the in vitro phagocytosis of *E. coli* by human polymorphonuclear neutrophils (PMNs) has been studied.

Materials and Methods

Neutrophils. Blood from healthy donors was separated according to the technique of Bøyum [3] and the PMNs recovered were washed in Krebs Ringer phosphate buffer enriched with 10 m*M* glucose (KRG). A quantity of 2.5×10^6 cells/ml was added to Leighton tubes (16×125 mm, Bellco, United States) and incubated in KRG in a horizontal position at 37 °C for 60 min. By that time, a monolayer of neutrophils with approximately 5000 cells/mm^2 had been established.

* This work was supported by grants from Legatet til Henrik Homans Minde, and from Det Kongelige Sosialdepartements stipendier til farmaceutiske studender.

[1] Kaptein W. Wilhelmsen og frues Bakteriologisk Institutt, Rikshospitalet, University of Oslo, 0027 Oslo 1, Norway
[2] Department of Medical Microbial Ecology, Karolinska Institutet, Stockholm, Sweden

The Influence of Antibiotics on the Host-Parasite Relationship III
Edited by G. Gillissen, W. Opferkuch, G. Peters, and G. Pulverer

Bacteria. A suspension of radiolabeled *E. coli* O:86, B:7, strain X-7, was prepared as described earlier [8]. The bacteria were opsonized either with 10% autologous serum or with rabbit anti *E. coli* IgG.

Phagocytosis. The uptake was started by adding 1-ml aliquots of the suspensions of nonopsonized or opsonized *E. coli* to the PMN monolayers, and stopped after 30 min by washing with cold KRG. For the study of release of bacterial breakdown products from the PMNs, the cells were washed with prewarmed KRG (37 °C) and incubated for another 60 min at 37 °C with 10% serum.

Hypericum perforatum Extract. An extract from dried leaf material of *Hypericum perforatum* purchased from Norsk Medisinal depot, Oslo, Norway, was kindly provided in a resin-like form by Ilia Brondz, Institute for Chemistry, University of Oslo. The extraction procedure has previously been described [6]. A stock solution of 50 mg/ml was stored at 4 °C in 96% ethanol, sheltered from light. Immediately before use, the solution was diluted with KRG to a final concentration of 1, 10, or 100 μg/ml. The extract, bacteria, opsonins, and neutrophils were combined in the following four ways:

1. The bacteria were preincubated with the extract for 30 min, washed and submitted to phagocytosis in the absence of extract.
2. The PMNs were preincubated for 30 min before the start of phagocytosis, which took place in the absence of extract.
3. Both PMNs and *E. coli* were preincubated with the extract, after which the uptake took place in its presence.
4. Same as [3], but the PMNs were also exposed to extract for 60 min after uptake had been finished.

Quantitation of Uptake and Release. Cell protein and radioactivity was measured as described earlier [8]. Uptake of *E. coli* by the PMNs was expressed as counts per milligram cell protein per minute and the release was expressed as percentage radioactivity released from the PMNs during the first 60 min after uptake had been finished.

Results

Influence of Opsonization on Phagocytosis. When phagocytosis took place in the presence of 10% autologous serum, the uptake of *E. coli* increased by a factor of 23.0 ± 3.0 (mean $\pm$ SD, $n=41$), compared with the uptake of nonopsonized bacteria. Correspondingly, opsonization by anti *E. coli* IgG resulted in an enhancement of the uptake by 35.8 ± 15.7 (mean $\pm$ SD, $n=35$).

Preincubation of E.coli by (Extract) Hypericum perforatum. The uptake of pretreated *E. coli* is outlined in Table 1. With nonopsonized bacteria, a significant stimulation of uptake was observed at 100 μg/ml, whereas the uptake of serum-opsonized and IgG-opsonized *E. coli* was inhibited at 10–100 μg/ml of the extract.

Table 1. Uptake of *E. coli* by human PMNs after preincubation of bacteria with an extract from *H. perforatum*[a, b]

Extract concentration (μg/ml)	*E. coli*		
	Nonopsonized	Serum-opsonized	IgG-opsonized
1	107.2 ± 13.0	103.2 ± 3.2	91.5 ± 6.7
10	102.4 ± 13.8	94.4 ± 4.9	86.0 ± 4.9*
100	178.8 ± 17.7***	80.0 ± 4.8**	74.8 ± 4.3***

[a] All values are means ± SEM as percentages of controls.
[b] Compared with controls: * $P<0.05$; ** $P<0.01$; *** $P<0.001$ (Student's *t*-test).

Table 2. Uptake of *E. coli* by human PMNs after preincubation of the neutrophils with an extract from *H. perforatum*[a, b]

Extract concentration (μg/ml)	*E. coli*		
	Nonopsonized	Serum-opsonized	IgG-opsonized
1	107.8 ± 6.5	102.1 ± 3.0	105.3 ± 5.6
10	107.7 ± 3.8	97.6 ± 5.3	79.2 ± 9.1*
100	619.4 ± 39.9***	75.9 ± 9.1*	102.0 ± 22.5

[a] All values are means ± SEM as percentages of controls.
[b] Compared with controls: * $P<0.05$; ** $P<0.01$; *** $P<0.001$ (Student's *t*-test).

Preincubation of the Neutrophils. After preincubation of the neutrophils, but not the bacteria, a similar pattern was seen (Table 2). However, the uptake of nonopsonized *E. coli* was more efficiently stimulated at 100 μg/ml after preincubation of the neutrophils than after preincubation of the bacteria. Regarding serum-opsonized bacteria, the inhibiting effect was of the same magnitude as that seen after preincubation of the bacteria. On the other hand, after neutrophil preincubation with the extract, the inhibiting effect on the uptake of IgG-opsonized bacteria was less pronounced than after preincubation of the bacteria. Only a slight but significant inhibition was seen at 10 μg/ml.

Preincubation of the Neutrophils and Bacteria and Uptake in the Presence of the Extract. Table 3 shows that preincubation of the neutrophils for 30 min and of the bacteria for 5 min followed by uptake in the presence of the extract resulted in even more pronounced effects. With 100 μg/ml, the uptake of nonopsonized *E. coli* increased almost 50-fold and the uptake of IgG-opsonized *E. coli* more than 3-fold. The uptake of serum-opsonized bacteria, however, was reduced by approximately 40% at 100 μg/ml.

Release of Bacterial Breakdown Products from the Neutrophils. Table 4 shows the elimination of radiolabeled bacterial breakdown products from the neutrophils during the 1st h of the postingestion phase. When the neutrophils and bacteria were pretreated with the extract, and uptake and elimination took place in its

Table 3. Uptake of *E. coli* by human PMNs in the presence of an extract from *H. perforatum* and after preincubation of neutrophils and bacteria with the extract[a, b]

Extract concentration (μg/ml)	*E. coli*		
	Nonopsonized	Serum-opsonized	IgG-opsonized
1	143.1± 7.9***	97.8±6.6	119.5± 7.9*
10	512.9± 50.6***	93.8±3.1	90.3+ 6.1*
100	4839.8±379.4***	61.1±3.3***	352.2±43.0***

[a] All values are means±SEM as percentages of controls.
[b] Compared with controls: * $P<0.05$; ** $P<0.01$; *** $P<0.001$ (Student's *t*-test).

Table 4. Release of bacterial breakdown products from human PMNs in the presence of 10 μg/ml of an extract from *H. perforatum* after uptake of *E. coli*[a, b]

Extract concentration (μg/ml)	*E. coli*		
	Nonopsonized	Serum-opsonized	IgG-opsonized
0	50.0±3.9	47.2±4.2	48.0±3.9
10 μg/ml	56.7±5.0	51.9±2.9	63.6±4.1*

[a] All values are percentage radioactivity released during the first 60 min after cessation of uptake, expressed as means±SEM.
[b] Compared with controls: * $P<0.05$; ** $P<0.01$; *** $P<0.001$ (Student's *t*-test).

presence (10 μg/ml), the elimination of nonopsonized *E. coli* proceeded normally, while the elimination of IgG-opsonized bacteria was stimulated.

Discussion

During recent years it has become clear that, despite the availability of a large number of potent broad-spectrum antimicrobial agents, we are still unable to cure many infections, particularly in immunocompromised patients. In these patients defective host defense often results in serious microbial infections. In addition to traditional chemotherapy, immunocompromised patients would benefit from agents that stimulate host defense reactions, such as phagocyte functions, through the development of so-called immunomodulating drugs. The search for such agents has also included substances derived from plants. As shown by Delaveau et al. [4], intraperitoneal phagocytosis of *E. coli* in mice was simulated by a large number of plant extracts. They also tested *Hypericum vulgare L.* (*H. perforatum* L.), but found it to be inactive. However, they used a different extraction procedure than that used for the present study. We found that substance(s) extracted from *H. perforatum* markedly enhanced phagocytosis of nonopsonized *E. coli.* The "drug" seemed to bind firmly to both bacteria and neutrophils as preincubation followed by washing in both cases enhanced subsequent phagocytosis in its absence. However, the most pronounced stimulation of phagocytosis was seen when the extract was present during the uptake phase. In this case, at 100 μg/ml it promoted uptake approximately twice as efficiently as 10% serum and opsonization with IgG.

The binding to the bacteria obviously interfered to some extent with the binding of IgG. However, binding to the neutrophil seemed to affect the Fc-receptor only marginally. When the extract was present at high concentration during uptake of IgG-opsonized bacteria, the slight inhibiting influence on the binding to the neutrophil Fc-receptor was therefore outweighed by the phagocytosis-promoting effect of the extract per se. The extract therefore seemed to act like an opsonin by itself.

The experiments with serum-opsonized *E. coli* demonstrated that the substance(s) interferes with opsonins other than IgG. This was particularly evident from the experiments where the extract was present during phagocytosis (Table 3). In contrast to the stimulating effect seen on the uptake of IgG-opsonized *E. coli* in this setting, the inhibitory effect of the extract was potentiated compared with the effect of preincubation of bacteria or neutrophils alone.

In spite of the inhibitory effect on the uptake of serum-opsonized *E. coli*, intracellular degradation of the bacteria in the neutrophils was not inhibited. On the contrary, with IgG-opsonized bacteria the breakdown of ingested bacteria proceeded more efficiently in the presence of the extract.

The present in vitro observations on the effect of substance(s) from *H. perforatum* on phagocytosis by neutrophils have not yet been confirmed in vivo. Whether this agent also promotes phagocytosis in vivo should be examined. If it does, it may become a valuable drug for treating infections, particularly in immunocompromised patients, in spite of its rather narrow antibacterial spectrum.

Summary

Hyperforin is an antibacterial agent extracted and purified from the plant *Hypericum perforatum* L. Its antibacterial spetrum includes a number of Gram-positive organisms, but it is inactive against Enterobacteriaceae. In the present study, an extract from *H. perforatum* was found to have a major influence on phagocytosis of *Escherichia coli* by human polymorphonuclear neutrophils in vitro.

The most striking effect was seen on the uptake of nonopsonized bacteria, which was stimulated up to 50-fold at 100 μg/ml. The uptake of IgG-opsonized bacteria was also stimulated at 100 μg/ml, but the extract inhibited IgG opsonization per se. On the other hand, the uptake of serum-opsonized *E. coli* was inhibited by approximately 40% at this concentration. The substance(s) in the extract seemed to bind to both neutrophils and *E. coli*.

In spite of the inhibitory effect on the uptake of serum-opsonized *E. coli*, intracellular degradation of the bacteria in the neutrophils was not inhibited. On the contrary, with IgG-opsonized bacteria the breakdown of ingested bacteria proceeded more efficiently in the presence of the extract of *H. perforatum*.

Acknowledgments. The authors gratefully acknowledge the technical assistance of Olaug Bjertnæs, David Bradfield, and Ingrid Fagerheim.

References

1. Brondz I, Greibrokk T, Groth PA, Aasen AJ (1982) The relative stereochemistry of hyperforin – an antibiotic from *Hypercium perforatum* L. Tetrahedron Lett 23:1299–1300
2. Brondz I, Greibrokk T, Groth P, Aasen AJ (1983) The absolute configuration of hyperforin, an antibiotic from *Hypericum perforatum L.*, based on the crystal structure determination of its *p*-bromobenzoate ester. Acta Chem Scand Ser A 37:263–265
3. Bøym A (1968) Isolation of leukocytes from human blood. Further observations. Methylcellulose, dextran and Ficoll as erythrocyte aggregating agents. Scand J Clin Lab Invest 21 [Suppl 97]:31–50
4. Delaveau P, Lallouette P, Tessier AM (1980) Stimulation of the phagocytic activity of the r.e.s. by plant extracts. Planta Med 40:49–54
5. Gaind KN, Ganjoo TN (1959) Antibacterial principle of *Hypericum perforatum* Linn. Indian J Physiol Pharmacol 21:172–175
6. Gurevich AT, Dobrynin VN, Kolosov MN, Poravko SA, Ryabova ID, Chernov BK, Derbentzeva NA, Aizenman BE, Garagulya AD (1971) Antibiotik hyperforin iz *Hypericum perforatum* L. Antibiotiki 16:510–513
7. Jensen LB, Miller WA (1951) Antibiotic from St. John's wort as a food preservative. Chem Abstr 45:7724
8. Lingaas E, Midtvedt T (1985) Dissociated effect of amphotericin B and desoxycholate on phagocytosis of *Escherichia coli* by human polymorphonuclear neutrophils. Drugs Exp Clin Res 11:747–754
9. Neuwald F, Hagenstrøm U (1954) Untersuchungen über die antibakterielle Wirkung von *Hypericum perforatum* L. Arch Pharm (Weinheim) 287:439–441
10. Osborn EM (1943) On the occurrence of antibacterial substances in green plants. Br J Exp Med 24:227–231

Influence of the Tetrachlorodecaoxygen Anion Complex on Phagocytosis of Peripheral Human Polymorphonuclear Cells in Chemiluminescence Assays

G. GILLISSEN and H. OSTENDORP

Introduction

Topically, the tetrachlorodecaoxygen anion complex (TCDO) has a therapeutic effect in wound healing [2, 9] with an increase of pO_2 in the capillary blood [3] and systematically in experimental infections [1]. It constitutes a negatively charged complex of chlorine and oxygen $(Cl_4O_{10})n$, $MW_{n=1}=301.8$. Incubation with hemoproteins leads to complex degradation and the appearance of oxygen water in chloride [4], whereby toxic oxygen species are not formed [8]. Heme-activated TCDO was described to be bactericidal for a number of microbial species [6, 7], to enhance phagocytosis by resident peritoneal macrophages of mice [7], and to stimulate humoral and cellular immunity [1]. TCDO enhanced the phagocytosis-dependent chemiluminescence (CL) of polymorphonuclear cells (PMNs) only in whole blood in the presence of peroxidase but not using isolated cells [6].

It was, therefore, of interest to investigate the conditions which influence the TCDO effect on phagocytosis-dependent CL with special reference to a modulating effect of lymphocytes.

Material and Methods

Tetrachlorodecaoxygen anion complex (Oxochemie, Heidelberg (FRG) was available in an isotonic water solution of 15.5 mmol/liter. It was diluted with saline immediately before use.

Chemiluminescence Assay

For all assays the Biocounter M2000 (Lumac, Schaesberg, The Netherlands) adapted to a temperature of 37 °C and Lumanol™-100/3 M (purified 3-aminophthalhydracid, 10^{-3} *M* in NaOH, pH 12.0, diluted before use 1:10 with phosphate-buffered saline (PBS, pH 7.2) were used.

The mixture for assays, always to a volume of 0.8 ml, was composed of 5×10^5 PMNs or 5×10^5 lymphocytes or both cells together suspended in 0.1 ml Hank's

Department of Medical Microbiology, Medical Faculty, Pauwelsstraße, 5100 Aachen, Federal Republic of Germany

The Influence of Antibiotics on the Host-Parasite Relationship III
Edited by G. Gillissen, W. Opferkuch, G. Peters, and G. Pulverer

balanced salt solution 199 without phenol red (Flow Lab, UK), with 10% autologous serum, TCDO in concentrations of 0.04 or 0.16 µmol/0.1 ml (PBS alone for controls), opsonized *Candida* with 5×10^6 cells/0.1 ml PBS, 0.1 ml Lumanol, and 0.4 ml Hank's solution without serum. Preincubation of human cells without or with subsequent washing was performed together with TCDO for 30 min at 37 °C in an atmosphere of 5% CO_2. Cell activity was measured over 75 min and the maximum relative light units (RLUmax) was taken for comparison.

Isolation of Human PMNs and Lymphocytes

Human blood was taken with 100 IU heparin/ml (Heparin-Na 5000, Braun, Melsungen, FRG) and centrifuged at 200 g for 15 min. The buffycoat cells were resuspended in centrifuged (20 min at 750 g) platelet-free plasma. After sedimentation of erythrocytes for 30 min at 37 °C (inclined position), PMNs and lymphocytes were separated by superposing cell suspensions on Ficoll medium, density 1.077 (Seromed, Biochrom KG, Berlin, FRG) and centrifugation (15 min at 1000 g). PMNs and lymphocytes with a purity of 95%–98% and 98%–100% respectively were adapted to a density of 5×10^6 cells/ml in Hank's 199 medium with 10% autologous serum after washing.

Opsonization of Candida

Candida albicans ATCC 10231 of an 18-h culture in glucose-containing broth was adapted after washing to 5×10^7 cells/ml PBS. Two volumes were incubated with 1 volume of autologous serum for 30 min at 37 °C, washed and readapted to 5×10^7 cells/ml PBS.

Results

Tetrachlorodecaoxygen anion complex in both concentrations of 0.04 and 0.16 µmol/0.1 ml did not modulate the activity of PMNs in chemiluminescence assays induced by opsonized *Candida* cells if the ingredients of the test system were given together at the same time and measured immediately thereafter. This was independent of whether autologous lymphocytes were additionally present or not (Fig. 1, upper). Under the same experimental conditions, lymphocytes alone, i.e., without the phagocytic PMNs, also showed a certain reactivity with small values of 350–950 RLUmax compared with 2000–4000 RLUmax observed with PMNs. This reactivity of lymphocytes was reduced in the presence of TCDO (Fig. 1, upper).

Preincubation of PMN cells with TCDO for 30 min at 37 °C before the addition of opsonized *Candida* but without subsequent washing resulted in a considerable increase of reactivity of over 120% in the case of the higher TCDO concentration (Fig. 1, lower). The presence of lymphocytes under otherwise identically experimental conditions reduced this effect to a certain extent, but not completely. In both cases, the smaller TCDO concentration had no effect.

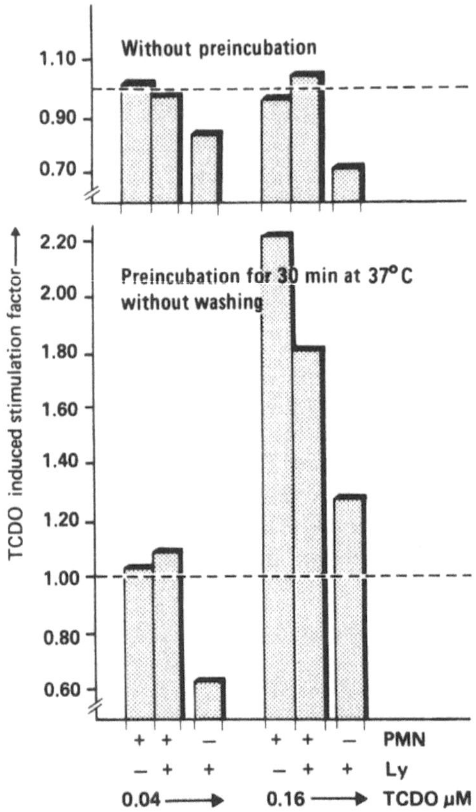

Fig. 1. Effect of TCDO on peripheral human PMNs alone or together with lymphocytes relative to controls without TCDO. TCDO concentration in µmol/0.1 ml PBS. Pretreatment of cells by incubation of equal parts of cell suspensions and TCDO solutions before the addition of opsonized *Candida*

Preincubation of lymphocytes alone with TCDO but without subsequent washing before the addition of *Candida* resulted in an increased reactivity in the case of the higher TCDO concentration but in a decrease by the smaller one. Also in this case, preincubation changed the reactivity.

In further experiments, cells were washed after the preincubation with TCDO and before the addition of opsonized *Candida*. In this way, an attempt was made to obtain information about the TCDO effect on different leukocyte classes and their interactions. As shown in Fig. 2, TCDO-pretreated PMNs showed an increased reactivity upon the addition of opsonized *Candida* which was most pronounced with the lower concentration. The addition of lymphocytes pretreated with small concentrations of TCDO to preincubated normal PMNs had no effect when compared with controls using not TCDO-treated, but preincubated lymphocytes. In the case of higher TDCO concentrations for pretreating lymphocytes, there was an increased reactivity, though smaller than without lymphocytes. This result was by and large reproducible (Fig. 2). Pretreatment of lympho-

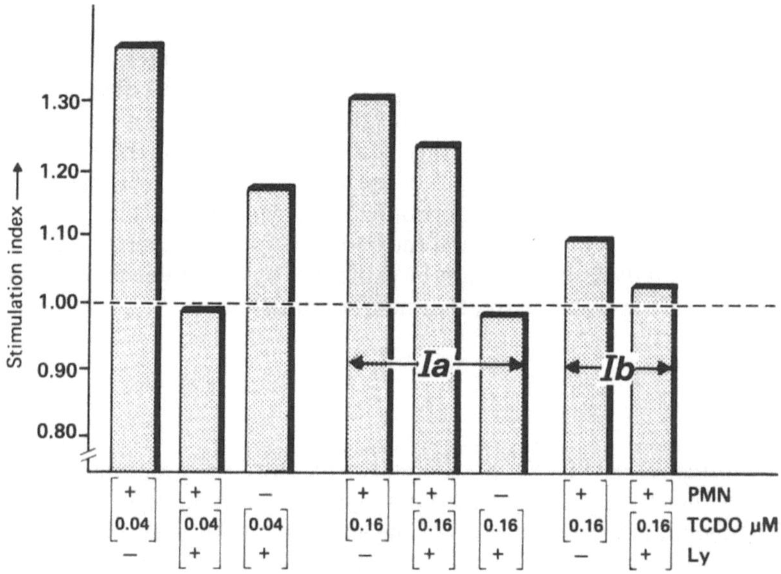

Fig. 2. Influence of TCDO pretreatment of cells and subsequent washing before the addition of opsonized *Candida* on their further activity in chemiluminescence assays in comparison with values in the absence of TCDO. TCDO concentration in µmol/0.1 ml PBS. [], preincubation; *Ia, Ib*, assays on different days

cytes alone with TCDO in smaller concentrations and subsequent washing resulted in a stimulation whereas the higher concentration was not effective.

Discussion

The activation of PMNs by phagocytosis evaluated in chemiluminescence assays is not modulated by the presence of TCDO. This corresponds to the observation by others, who have shown that no activation could be observed with isolated PMNs even in the presence of biocatalysts [6]. In contrast, phagocytosis-induced activity of PMNs is considerably increased if they are pretreated by incubation with TCDO before the addition of opsonized *Candida*. This happens, though hemoproteins, i.e., activators [4], as catalysts have not been added to the assay system.

The TCDO effect by preincubation with phagocytes may be regarded as a delayed onset of stimulation possibly due to liberation of cellular catalase activity or to the time necessary for penetration of TCDO into the cells. As shown with the higher TCDO concentration, the presence of lymphocytes reduced the stimulatory TCDO effect.

Washing of pretreated PMNs did not abolish the TCDO effect on phagocytosis-induced cell activation; smaller TCDO concentrations were even enhancing under these conditions. Here again, the addition of TCDO-pretreated lymphocytes relative to not treated but only preincubated ones resulted in reduced chemiluminescence values (Fig. 2). This was more pronounced if pretreatment and testing of lymphocytes alone gave higher values, leading to the suggestion that TCDO affects different lymphocyte classes differently depending possibly on various conditions such as concentration or time of contact with feedback impulses on PMN activity. In this context, it must also be considered whether TCDO treatment induces a shift of the $T_h/T_{c/s}$ cell ratio, with immunological consequences. These assays are in progress and will be published later.

Lymphocytes by themselves showed a distinct increase in reactivity after contact with *Candida,* which might be explained by an influence on adrenergic receptors [5] as shown also with other microorganisms.

Summary

The influence of TCDO in different concentrations on human PMN cells alone or together with autologous lymphocytes was examined in phagocytosis-dependent chemiluminescence assays. The experiments showed that TCDO had no influence at room temperature as already described. This was independent of whether lymphocytes were additionally present or not. Preincubation of PMNs with TCDO, however, increased their reactivity considerably, which was also demonstrable if pretreated cells were washed before the addition of opsonized *Candida.* Autologous lymphocytes exhibited a modulating effect in this test system whether they were pretreated simultaneously with PMNs and TCDO or separately with this substance and subsequently added to not pretreated PMNs before the phagocytosis assay. These results indicate a direct influence of TCDO on human PMNs concerning their phagocytic reactivity in chemiluminescence assays as well as on lymphocytes with a possibly differential sensitivity of lymphocyte classes.

References

1. Gillissen G, Kühne FW, Breuer-Werle M, Melzer B, Ostendorp H (1986) Increased resistance towards two systemic experimental infections by tetrachlorodecaoxygen anion complex. Drug Res 36(II):1778–1782
2. Hinz J, Hautzinger H, Stahl KW (1986) Rationale for and results from a randomised, double-blind trial of tetrachlorodecaoxygen anion complex in wound healing. The Lancet I:825–828
3. Hinz J, Kühne FW, Schöning v G, Sell G, Seebach v B, Seebach v A (1985) Behandlung chronisch therapieresistenter Wunden mit dem biokatalytisch aktivierbaren Sauerstoffträger Tetrachlorodecaoxid. Med Welt 36:210–215
4. Hollfelder K (1984) Hämaktivierte antimikrobielle Eigenschaften des Sauerstoffträgers Tetrachlorodecaoxid (TCDO). Diplomarbeit, Institut für Mikrobiologie der Techn Univ München, p 1–94
5. Szentivanyi A, Middleton JrE, Williams JE, Friedman H (1983) Effect of microbial agents on the immune network and associated pharmacological reactivities. In: Middleton JrE, Reed CE, Ellis EF (eds) Allergy: principles and practice, vol 1. Mosby, St. Louis, USA
6. Ullmann U, Kühne FW (1985) In vitro investigations on the antibacterial action and the influence on phagocytic chemiluminescence of tetrachlorodecaoxide – a new non-metallic oxygen complex. Infection 13 [Suppl 2]:236–240

7. Woerly G, Lombard Y, Stahl KW, Poindron Ph (1986) Capacity of tetrachlorodecaoxygen anion complex and bacterial lipopolysaccharide to accelerate phagocytosis of subcultured normal mouse resident macrophages. Abstract, Internat. Congress on the biological and clinical aspects of phagocytic function. Pavia, Italy
8. Youngman RJ, Wagner GR, Kühne FW, Elstner EF (1985) Biochemical oxygen activation as the basis for the physiological action of tetrachlorodecaoxide (TCDO) Z Naturforschung 40 c:409–414
9. Zenker W, Thiede A, Dommes M, Ullmann U (1986) Die Wirksamkeit von Tetrachlorodecaoxid (TCDO) zur Behandlung komplizierter Wundheilungsstörungen. Chirurg 57:334–339

Influence of RO 236240 on Human Polymorphonuclear Leukocytes In Vitro *

P. van der Auwera and M. Husson

Introduction

RO 236240 is a new trifluoroquinolone with very high in vitro activity against gram-negative and gram-positive bacteria particularly against methicillin-resistant *Staphylococcus aureus*. Since staphylococci may behave like intracellular pathogens [1, 2], we have studied the influence of RO 236240 on the functions of polymorphonuclear leukocytes (PMNLs) with a special interest for the intracellular killing.

Materials and Methods

Strains. Two strains of *S. aureus* were studied: 42 D is a strain susceptible to oxacillin [minimal inhibitory concentration (MIC), 0.8 mg/liter] and MAT is a strain resistant to oxacillin (MIC, > 50 mg/liter).

Neutrophils. Neutrophils were obtained from the peripheral blood of healthy volunteers. Blood was collected on ACD (Acetate, Citric acid, Dextrose; Gibco, Ghent, Belgium). Sedimentation in dextran for 1 h was allowed, followed by separation of the leukocyte-rich supernatant on Ficoll-Hypaque (Pharmacia). After lysis of residual erythrocytes by hypotonic shock, the cells were resuspended in Hank's balanced salt solution (HBSS) (Gibco) and stored on ice until used. Counting and the viability test (trypan blue exclusion) were performed before each experiment.

Chemotaxis. Chemotaxis was studied using an agarose gel technique described by Nelson et al. [3], and PMNLs were preincubated for 30 min with 10 mg/liter RO 236240 in HBSS, the agar gel containing the same concentration. The stimulus was opsonized zymosan. Each test was done ten times. Chemotactic and random migration were measured and averaged from the ten plates. Results were expressed as the differential chemotactic migration in millimeters.

---

* This study was supported by a grant from Produits Roche sa, Brussels, Belgium.
Service de Médecine et Laboratoire d'Investigation Clinique H. J. Tagnon, Institut Jules Bordet, Centre des Tumeurs de l'Université Libre de Bruxelles, rue Héger-Bordet 1, 1000 Brussels, Belgium

The Influence of Antibiotics on the Host-Parasite Relationship III
Edited by G. Gillissen, W. Opferkuch, G. Peters, and G. Pulverer

Superoxide Production. Neutrophils were suspended at concentration of 1.5×10^6 cells/ml and were preincubated for 60 min with or without antibiotics at 37 °C in a shaking water bath. Superoxide production was then determined by a fixed-time assay according to Babior and Cohen [4], with horse heart cytochrome C (Sigma type III) (30 mg/ml) and PMA (phorbol myristate acetate, Sigma) as the stimulus. Results were expressed as a percentage of the control activity obtained in the absence of any antibiotic. The PMNLs from three different donors were tested.

Radioisotopic Phagocytosis. The radioisotopic method using heat-killed bacteria was used [5]. Polymorphonuclear neutrophils (PMNs) were incubated for 15 min with the antibiotic prior to the test. Phagocytosis was allowed in the presence of the antibiotic in 10% fresh serum. Each concentration was tested in duplicate using PMNs prepared from three different volunteers.

Intracellular Killing. This was studied according to Leijh et al. [6].

Effect of Pretreating the Inoculum. The strains were grown for 1 h at 37 °C in MIC and MIC/4 concentrations of RO 236240, were washed twice, and were centrifuged for 5 min at high speed in a Hawksley Microfuge. Fifty microliters of the inoculum [2×10^7 colony-forming units (CFUs/ml] was incubated with 0.4 ml PMNLs at 6×10^6 cells/ml and 0.1 ml fresh human serum, in a shaking water bath. The number of surviving bacteria at 0, 1, 2, and 4 h was assessed by duplicate 10- µl samplings of the mixtures, subjected to osmotic lysis of leukocytes in ice-cold distilled water for 20 min. Various dilutions were done in distilled water and plated on Mueller-Hinton agar. After overnight incubation, colonies were counted and recorded as the mean CFUs/ml from at least six different counts. Results were compared with those for bacteria not preexposed to antibiotic. Unopsonized inoculum pretreated with Ro 236240 was also tested, as well as inoculum opsonized with heat-inactivated serum (56 °C).

Effect of Adding RO 236240 at the Time of Phagocytosis. RO 236240 at MIC and MIC/4 concentrations was added to PMNLs at the same time as the opsonized inoculum.

Effect of Adding RO 236240 After Phagocytosis. After 2 min of phagocytosis, the PMNLs were incubated in the presence of the antibiotic at MIC and MIC/4.

Intracellular Concentration of RO 236240. A sensitive bioassay was developed in small petri plates (5 cm in diameter) using Antibiotic Medium No 2 (Oxoid) as the medium and *Klebsiella pneumoniae* IJB87/1 as the test organism. The calibration curve ranged from 0.2 to 8 mg/liter. The PMNLs were incubated for 1 h with RO 236240 (5 and 10 mg/liter). Rifampin (2, 5, 10 mg/liter) was tested as a control antibiotic. After incubation, the PMNLs were rapidly washed at 4 °C and centrifuged in antibiotic-free HBSS for 2 min. This procedure has been showed to minimize extracellular contamination without losing intracellular antibiotic significantly [7]. The pellet was sonicated, an aliquot tested for protein content by Lowry's method, and the remainder assayed microbiologically, each test being done in triplicate. The intracellular concentration was calculated assuming that 1 mg protein corresponded to 5 µl intracellular fluid [8].

Results

Chemotaxis. RO 236240 at 10 mg/liter and not significantly influence the directed migration nor the random migration in agar. The control differential migration ($n=10$) was 0.61 mm (SD=0.087 mm). After 30 min preincubation of PMNLs with 10 mg/liter RO 236240, the differential migration ($n=10$) was 0.80 mm (SD=0.10 mm).

Superoxide Production. The mean superoxide production of PMNLs preincubated for 60 min with 10 mg/liter RO 236240 (range, 1.88–1.95 n$M/10^6$ cells per minute) was 98.1% (SD=4.5%, $n=3$) of the superoxide production by untreated control PMNLs (range, 1.86–2.07 n$M/10^6$ cells per minute).

Phagocytosis. The mean absolute uptakes of radiolabeled *S. aureus* by untreated control PMNLs obtained from three different volunteers were 31% of the initial inoculum (range, 26%–36%) for the strain 42 D and 32% (range, 18%–42%) for the strain MAT. Phagocytosis, in the presence of RO 236240, was 101% (SD= 6.7%) of the control for the strain 42 D and 104.8% (SD=3.2%) for the strain MAT.

Intracellular Killing. Polymorphonuclear leukocyte killing ability and viability were not affected by pretreatment with RO 236240 10 mg/liter for 1 h before phagocytosis. During incubation with the bacteria the viability (trypan blue exclusion) was >95% at time 0, >95% at 1 h, 94%–97% at 2 h, and 90%–96% after 24 h.

Effect of Pretreating the Inoculum. Pretreating the two strains with MIC or MIC/4 concentrations of RO 236240 had no significant influence on intracellular killing (not shown). Pretreatment of the inoculum with RO 236240 did not affect the opsonization requirement, since no killing was observed after opsonization with heat-inactivated serum or no opsonization.

Effect or Adding RO 236240 at the Time of Phagocytosis. Table 1 shows that RO 236240 had no influence on the intracellular killing of the strain MAT. However, the strain 42 D was significantly better killed in the presence of MIC or MIC/4 concentrations of RO 236240.

Effect of RO 236240 on Phagocytosed Microorganisms. Table 2 shows that RO 236240 at MIC and MIC/4 concentrations did not improve the intracellular killing of strain MAT. However, RO 236240 at the MIC concentration tested was able to prevent the regrowth of intracellular bacteria which occurred after 24 h of incubation. At this time the PMNL viability was 95%–99% for the PMNLs with bacteria without antibiotics, and 85%–98% when they were incubated with bacteria and antibiotics.

Table 1. Intraphagocytic killing of two strains of *S. aureus*. Polymorphonuclear leukocytes were incubated with MIC and MIC/4 concentrations of RO 236240 from the beginning of phagocytosis and for 24 h

	Incubation conditions	Viable counts (10^4 cfus/ml) after			
		0 h	1 h	2 h	24 h
Strain 42 D (oxacillin-susceptible)					
Controls	HBSS	171	188	418	1012
	RO 236240 0.1 mg/liter	175	187	371	1062
	RO 236240 0.4 mg/liter	178	167	301	1100
PMNLs	HBSS	142	31	15	690
	RO 236240 0.1 mg/liter	180	14	6	23
	RO 236240 0.4 mg/liter	163	14	6	42
Strain MAT (oxacillin-resistant)					
Controls	HBSS	250	320	440	2730
	RO 236240 0.1 mg/liter	288	360	380	3300
	RO 236240 0.4 mg/liter	285	310	407	3500
PMLs	HBSS	382	89	18	176
	RO 236240 0.1 mg/liter	297	114	26	99
	RO 236240 0.4 mg/liter	264	112	23	287

Table 2. Intraphagocytic killing of two strains of *S. aureus*. The PMNLs were incubated with MIC and MIC/4 concentrations of RO 236240, which was added after 2 min of phagocytosis and removal of extracellular staphylococci

Incubation conditions	Viable counts (10^3 CFUs/ml) after				Viability
	0 h	1 h	2 h	24 h	(%)
Strain 42 D (oxacillin-susceptible)					
HBSS	124	10	9	3250	95
RO 236240 0.1 mg/liter	130	10	8	386	95
RO 236240 0.4 mg/liter	124	6	12	10	95
Strain MAT (oxacillin-resistant)					
HBSS	214	18	15	2510	99
RO 236240 0.1 mg/liter	196	27	12	2427	98
RO 236240 0.4 mg/liter	186	17	18	2230	97

Intracellular Concentration of RO 236240. The between-assay variability of the RO 236240 bioassay was 8.4% ($n=5$) (4 mg/liter) and that of the rifampin assay was 4.7% ($n=5$) (1.25 mg/liter). The ratio between the intra- and extracellular concentration was about 2 for RO 236240 and about 5 for rifampin.

Discussion and Conclusion

RO 236240 is a new fluorinated quinolone with a very high in vitro activity. We were not able to identify any negative interaction between RO 236240 and the functions of PMNL tested, although, at concentrations below expected serum concentrations, RO 236240 improved the killing of internalized *S. aureus* 42 D. We found an intracellular penetration of rifampin (I/E ratio of 4.3–5.4) which was very similar to that reported by Hand and King-Thompson [9]. The penetration of RO 236240 was high in PMNLs, being twice as high as the extracellular concentration. Furthermore, the intracellular drug appeared to remain bioactive in the lysosomes since one of the strain was significantly better killed in the presence of extracellular RO 236240 than in its absence. In conclusion, RO 236240 did not decrease any of the PMNL functions tested; on some occasions RO 236240 was able to improve intracellular killing. The clinical significance of these results remains to be assessed in susceptible patients with impairement of PMNL functions.

Summary

The influence of RO 236240, a new trifluoroquinolone with high in vitro activity against gram-positive bacteria on the functions of polymorphonuclear leukocytes, was studied using two strains of *Staphylococcus aureus,* one susceptible and one resistant to oxacillin. RO 236240 (10 mg/liter) had no influence on superoxide generation stimulated by phorbol myristate acetate, neither on phagocytosis of opsonized *S. aureus,* nor on chemotaxis in agar using opsonized zymosan as the stimulus. RO 236240 (MIC and MIC/4) did not modify the intracellular killing of the two strains when they were preincubated. However, in aerobic conditions, RO 236240 was able to prevent the overgrowth of phagocytosed *S. aureus* 42D after 24 h of incubation. Using a microbiological assay, RO 236240 intracellular concentration was twice as high as the extracellular concentration.

References

1. Mandell GL (1975) Interaction of intraleukocytic bacteria and antibiotics. J Clin Invest 55:561–566
2. Rogers DE, Tompsett R (1952) The survival of staphylococci within human leucocytes. J Exp Med 95:209–230
3. Nelson RD, Quie PG, Simmons RL (1975) Chemotaxis under agarose: a new and simple method for measuring chemotaxis and spontaneous migration of human polymorphonuclear leukocytes and monocytes. J Immunol 115:1650–1656
4. Babior BM, Cohen HJ (1981) In: Cline MJ (ed) Leukocyte function. Methods in hematology 3. Churchill Livingstone, London, pp 1–38
5. Metcalf JA, Gallin JI, Nauseef WM, Root RK (1986) Laboratory manual of neutrophil function. Raven, New York, 1–191
6. Leijh PCJ, van den Barselaar MT, Dubbeldeman-Rempt I, van Furth R (1980) Kinetics of intracellular killing of *Staphylococcus aureus* and *Escherichia coli* by human granulocytes. Eur J Immunol 10:750–757
7. Renard C, Vanderhaeghe HJ, Claes PJ, Zenebergh A, Tulkens PM (1987) Influence of conversion of penicillin G into a basic derivative on its accumulation and subcellular localization in cultured macrophages. Antimicrob Agents Chemother 31:410–416
8. Steinman RM, Brodie SE, Cohn ZA (1976) Membrane flow during pinocytosis. A stereological analysis. J Cell Biol 68:665–687
9. Hand WL, King-Thompson NL (1986) Contrasts between phagocyte antibiotic uptake and subsequent intracellular bactericidal activity. Antimicrob Agents Chemother 29:135–140

Interactions Among Subinhibitory Antibiotics, Aerobic Gram-negative Rods, and Human Polymorphonuclear Neutrophils

L. A. MANDELL and M. AFNAN

Introduction

In the treatment of bacterial infection with antibiotics, drug levels in tissues at the site of infection may be below the minimal inhibitory concentration (MIC) for the infecting organism [1, 2]. Exposure of bacteria to sub-MIC antibacterial drugs can result in alterations in bacterial morphology [3–5] and proliferation [6, 7] as well as changes in sensitivity of the organisms to serum [8, 9].

Despite the fact that adequately functioning phagocytes play a major role in recovery from acute bacterial infection, relatively little is known about effects of sub-MIC antibiotics on interactions between phagocytes and bacteria.

The present studies were done to investigate how sub-MIC antibiotics affect such interactions. Our initial hypothesis was that drugs acting on the bacterial cell wall (e.g., beta-lactams such as ticarcillin) would be more likely to result in alterations in phagocytosis than would drugs acting at a ribosomal level (e.g., aminoglycosides such as tobramycin). Studies of ingestion and killing of drug-treated and control organisms by polymorphonuclear neutrophils (PMNs) were done and investigations of possible mechanisms were carried out.

Materials and Methods

Microorganisms and Radioactive Labeling

The method of radioactive labeling and the techniques used for measurement of phagocytosis and killing were those of Verbrugh and Verhoef [10, 11]. A modified form of this method has been reported by us previously [12]. A serum-resistant strain of *Escherichia coli* O18 : K1 : H7 was used and serum resistance was tested prior to and following exposure of the *E. coli* to sub-MIC concentrations of the test antibiotics [13]. The organisms were maintained on blood agar at 4 °C. For the studies, one colony was transferred to Mueller-Hinton broth (Difco, Detroit, United States) for 5 h at 37 °C, then 0.1 ml was subcultured into 1.0 ml Mueller-Hinton broth containing 0.005 mCi thymidine-methyl-^{3}H (specific activity, 5 Ci/mmol; Amersham, Bucks, UK) for radiolabeling and to place the bacteria in the logarithmic phase of growth. Organisms were grown for 18 h at 37 °C then 0.1 ml

McMaster Medical Unit, Henderson General Hospital, 711, Concession Street, Hamilton, Ontario, Canada L8V 1C3

The Influence of Antibiotics on the Host-Parasite Relationship III
Edited by G. Gillissen, W. Opferkuch, G. Peters, and G. Pulverer

was transferred to a fresh tube of Mueller-Hinton broth (1 ml) for 1 h. The bacteria were then washed with phosphate-buffered saline (PBS) (GIBCO, Grand Island, NY), pH 7.4, and adjusted to a final concentration of 5.0×10^8 colony-forming units (CFUs)/ml using a standard turbidimetric technique [14]. The MIC of the test drugs was determined using a broth dilution technique [15].

Preparation of PMNs and PMN Extracts

Thirty milliliters of blood from healthy volunteers on no medication were drawn into heparinized 50-ml plastic syringes (10 units heparin/ml blood). Fifteen milliliters of 6% dextran 70 (Fluka, Buchs, Switzerland) was added and the red blood cells were allowed to settle for 1 h.

The PMN-rich supernatant was separated and centrifuged at 160 g for 10 min. The resulting cell pellet was washed in 0.87% ammonium chloride to lyse the red cells, the PMNs were resuspended in Hank's balanced salt solution (HBSS), and total and differential cell counts were obtained. Following this, PMNs were adjusted to a final concentration of 0.25×10^8 cells/ml.

For experiments involving cytochalasin-B (cyto-B), the PMNs were preincubated with 5 µg/ml of the compound for 10 min at 37 °C before bacteria were added.

Crude leukocyte extracts were prepared by sonicating the PMNs for 15 min in 1.0 *M* NaCl, 0.05 *M* Na_2HPO_4, pH 7.4. The cellular debris was then removed by centrifugation at 3000 g for 30 min at 4 °C [16].

Pretreatment of E.coli with Sub-MIC Antibiotics

Stock solutions of the test antibiotics (ticarcillin, 852; tobramycin, 918 µg active substance/mg respectively) were prepared using distilled water as a diluent and were stored at −70 °C.

The bacterial suspension was divided into 1.0-ml aliquots in plastic tubes (12 × 75 mm Falcon, Oxnard, California, United States) to which was added either 1.0-ml sterile PBS (control group) or 1.0 ml antibiotic preparation (final concentrations $^1/_2$, $^1/_8$, $^1/_{32}$ MIC). The antibiotic-bacterial mixtures were incubated at 37 °C for 90 min. Bacteria were then removed by centrifugation at 2000 g for 15 min and washed with PBS.

Opsonization

Normal human serum from seven healthy donors was pooled and stored at −70 °C. To each of the bacterial pellets, 2.0 ml 10% serum was added for 30 min at 37 °C. Following this, the tubes were centrifuged at 2000 g for 15 min and the bacterial pellets were then resuspended in 2.0 ml HBSS. When necessary, serum was decomplemented by heating to 56 °C for 30 min.

Phagocytosis and Killing Assays

Polymorphonuclear neutrophils and control and drug-treated *E. coli* were incubated for predetermined times. The reactions were then stopped and the PMNs were separated from the bacteria by differential centrifugation. The principle of the phagocytic and killing assays depends upon the determination of counts per minute (CPM) and CFUs respectively associated with the PMNs at a particular time and the CPM and CFU associated with the bacteria at the beginning of the experiment (time zero).

Total Colony-Forming Units and Radioactivity

0.1 ml HBSS was added to 0.1-ml suspensions of opsonized bacteria followed immediately by the addition of 0.8 ml ice-cold PBS (time zero). Samples were taken for colony counts and the tubes were then centrifuged at 2000 g for 15 min. The bacterial pellet was left overnight, then 6.0 ml scintillation liquid [toluene containing PPO, POPOP (Amersham), and 20% Triton X-100 (Amersham)] were added and CPM were determined using a liquid scintillation counter (Beckman LS3133T).

Colony-Forming Units at Specific Times (3, 10, 20 Min)

0.1 ml of the PMN suspension was added to 0.1-ml suspensions of opsonized bacteria. For all experiments, the bacteria: PMN ratio was 10:1. At each of three predetermined times (3, 10, and 20 min), appropriate tubes were removed and placed in an ice bath, and 1.0 ml ice-cold PBS was added to each tube. The tubes were spun at 160 g × 5 min at 4 °C and the PMNs resuspended in PBS. Samples were taken from the tubes and the PMNs were lysed with distilled water. Serial dilutions were then prepared for pour plate colony counts.

Polymorphonuclear Neutrophil Associated Radioactivity at Specific Times

After samples were taken from the various tubes for determination of CFUs, the tubes were spun at 160 g for 5 min at 4 °C. The PMN pellet was left overnight, the PMNs were solubilized in 6.0 ml scintillation liquid, and CPM were determined.

The following formulas were used to calculate the results. The percentage of the total bacterial population that was leukocyte associated at a given sampling time (percentage uptake) was calculated using formula 1:

1. Percentage uptake at measured time

$$= \frac{\text{CPM in leukocyte pellet at measured time}}{\text{CPM in total bacterial pellet (time zero)}} \times 100$$

2. Percentage CFUs in leukocyte pellet at measured time

$$= \frac{\text{CUFs in leukocyte pellet at measured time}}{\text{CFUs at time zero}} \times 100$$

The leukocyte-associated bacterial population that was viable at 3, 10., and 20 min incubation was calculated according to formula 3:

3. Percentage viable leukocyte-associated bacteria at measured time

$$= \frac{\text{Percentage CFUs in leukocyte pellet at measured time}}{\text{Percentage uptake at measured time}} \times 100$$

where the numerator and denominator were derived from formulas 2 and 1 respectively. Percentage bacteria killed = 100% − % viable.

Statistical Analysis

Initial testing of the phagocytic and bactericidal assays showed minimal "within" and "between" experiment error. Accordingly, experiments were done in duplicate on any given day and repeated on three separate occasions.

Comparisons of means at specific time points were done using two-way analysis of variance. Direct comparisons of two means were done using paired *t*-tests. *P* values of less than 0.05 were considered statistically significant.

Results

Effects of Pretreatment with Sub-MIC Antibiotic on Killing of E.coli by PMNs

The overall means and their standard errors for killing of antibiotic-pretreated and control *E. coli* are shown in Table 1. Statistically significant differences in killing were noted at 3 and 10 min with both drugs, with the maximal potentiating effects seen at 3 min.

Table 1. Effects of sub-MIC antibiotic on killing of *E. coli* by PMNs

Time (min)	% killed ½ MIC (SEM)	⅛ MIC (SEM)	1/32 MIC (SEM)	Control (SEM)	*P*
Ticarcillin					
3	46.5 (6.68)	29 (7.48)	24 (6.95)	32 (6.68)	0.025
10	57 (5.35)	53 (3.74)	34 (5.08)	51 (6.68)	0.001
20	64 (5.08)	50 (7.48)	51 (5.08)	59 (4.54)	NS
Tobramycin					
3	50 (10.6)	38 (11)	17 (8.3)	23 (7.7)	0.02
10	74 (4.6)	66 (3.1)	50 (8.1)	65 (4.5)	0.043
20	63 (12)	52 (11.3)	40 (11.7)	58 (9.6)	NS

NS = $P > 0.05$.

Table 2. Effects of sub-MIC antibiotic on phagocytosis of *E. coli*

Time	% Uptake				
(min)	$^1/_2$ MIC (SEM)	$^1/_8$ MIC (SEM)	$^1/_{32}$ MIC (SEM)	Control (SEM)	*P*
Ticarcillin					
3	42 (6.41)	35 (6.15)	36 (6.95)	39 (7.48)	NS
10	44 (5.88)	42 (5.08)	34 (4.81)	49 (6.95)	NS
20	52 (5.08)	39 (4.54)	47 (6.68)	51 (7.22)	0.005
Tobramycin					
3	50 (6.4)	39 (3.9)	34 (5.2)	37 (6.2)	NS
10	55 (6.7)	45 (6.8)	42 (6.2)	38 (3.25)	NS
20	47 (4.3)	48 (9.1)	43 (8.6)	32 (4.3)	NS

NS = $P > 0.05$.

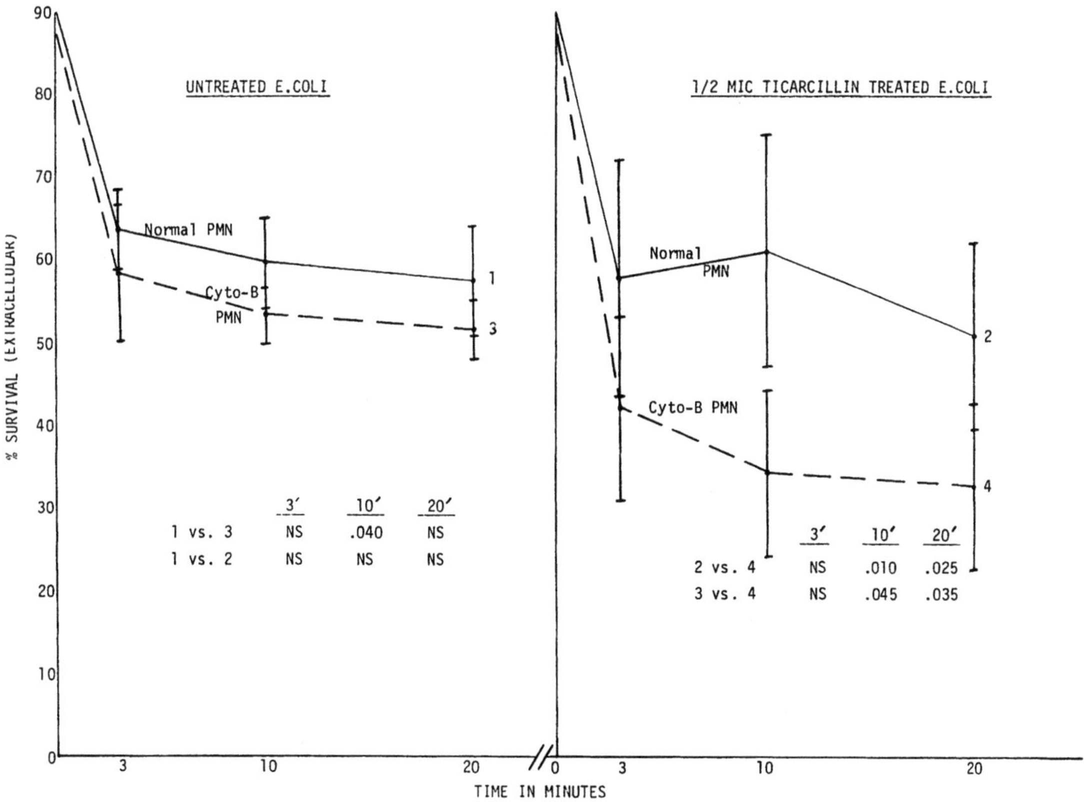

Fig. 1. Effect on *E. coli* of pretreatment with ½ MIC ticarcillin

Effects of pretreatment with Sub-MIC Antibiotic on Phagocytosis of E. coli by PMNs

The overall means and their standard errors for uptake of antibiotic-pretreated and control *E. coli* are shown in Table 2. For ticarcillin, no statistically significant differences were seen at 3 min or 10 min. At 20 min, there was a significant overall difference ($P<0.005$) across the four groups. This difference, however, appeared to be due to some suppression of uptake of *E. coli* by $^1/_8$ and $^1/_{32}$ MIC ticarcillin.

With tobramycin there was no statistically significant enhancement or suppression of uptake of antibiotic-treated compared with control *E. coli* at any of the three times.

Studies with Cyto-B-Treated PMNs: Effects of Drug Pretreatment on Killing of E.coli

To investigate possible mechanisms of increased susceptibility to killing by PMNs of sub-MIC antibiotic-treated *E. coli*, studies with cyto-B-treated PMNs were

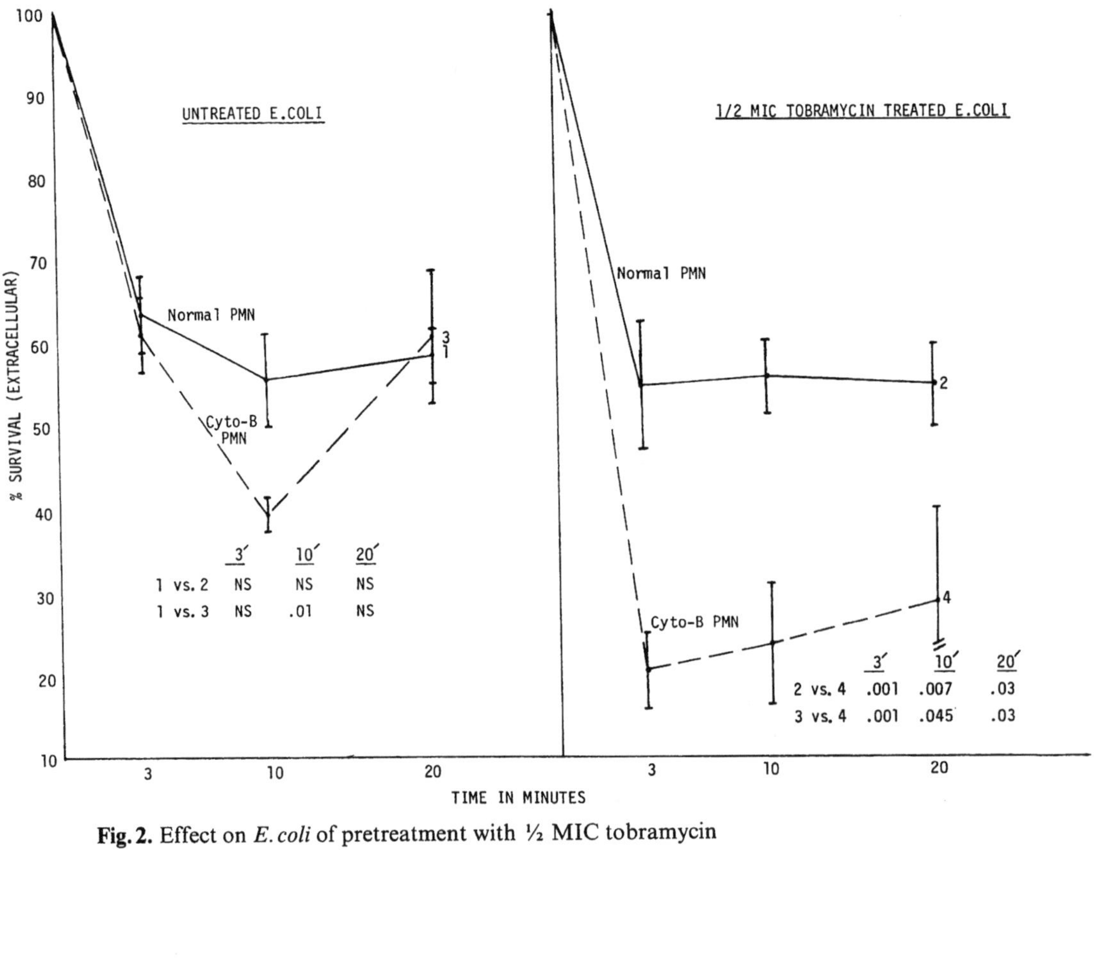

Fig. 2. Effect on *E. coli* of pretreatment with ½ MIC tobramycin

done. Addition of cyto-B to PMNs converts the phagocytic cells into secretory cells. Because of this effect, extracellular as opposed to intracellular killing of control and antibiotic-treated organisms was measured. The data for these experiments are shown in Fig. 1. Curves 1 and 2 represent percentage extracellular survival of control and ½ MIC ticarcillin-treated *E. coli* respectively when incubated with normal PMNs. No statistically significant differences were found between the two curves at 3, 10, or 20 min.

Curves 3 and 4 show percentage extracellular survival of the bacteria when cyto-B-treated PMNs were used with control and ½ MIC ticarcillin-treated *E. coli* respectively. The percentage reduction in extracellular survival of the drug-treated bacteria was significantly greater than that of the control *E. coli*, indicating greater killing of these organisms by the cyto-B PMNs.

Figure 2 shows the results for experiments done with *E. coli* exposed to ½ MIC tobramycin. The results are similar to those for ticarcillin except that the disparity between extracellular survival of tobramycin-treated *E. coli* incubated with cyto-B-treated PMNs and normal PMNs appears to be even greater than that shown in Fig. 1 for ticarcillin.

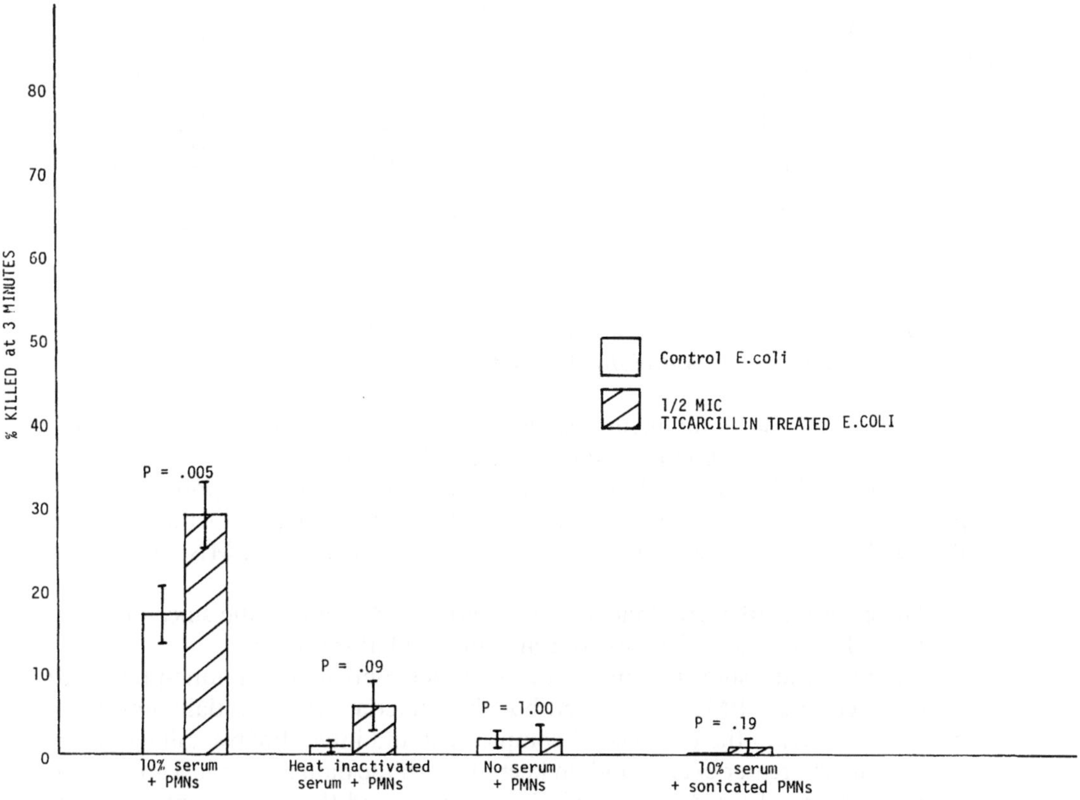

Fig. 3. Role of opsonizing serum in bacterial killing by intact PMNs

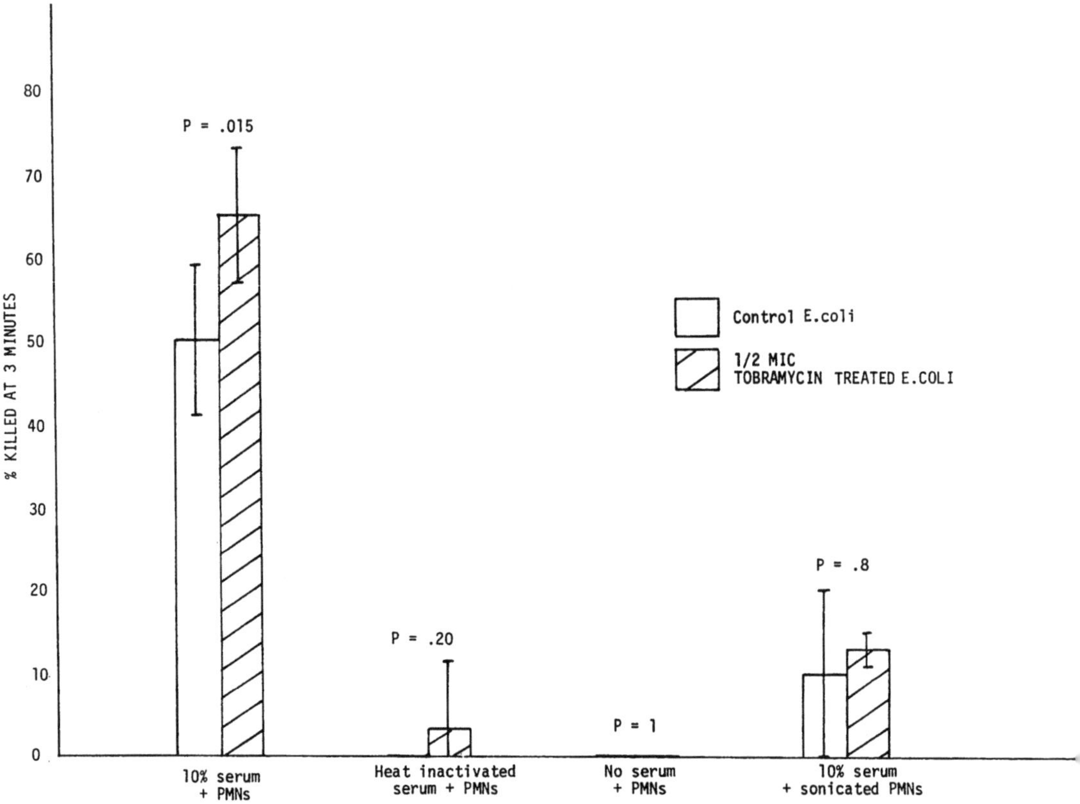

Fig. 4. Role of opsonizing serum in bacterial killing by intact PMNs

Requirements for Opsonins in the Presence of Intact PMNs for Enhanced Killing of Antibiotic-Treated Bacteria

To determine these requirements, experiments were carried out in which complement, was present or absent and PMNs were intact or sonicated. Control, ½ MIC ticarcillin, and ½ MIC tobramycin-pretreated *E. coli* were exposed to 10% pooled human serum, heat-inactivated serum, or PBS prior to incubation with PMNs. In one experiment, 10% pooled serum was used but PMNs were sonicated.

The experiments were done at 3 min with ½ MIC antibiotic since maximal killing had been noted with this concentration and at this time.

Figures 3 and 4 show minimal killing of either control or antibiotic-pretreated *E. coli* when intact PMNs were used but the bacteria were essentially not opsonized. However, in the presence of complement and intact PMNs, killing occurred to a much greater extent, and, in keeping with the data shown in Table 1, significantly more of the drug-treated *E. coli* were killed than were control organisms.

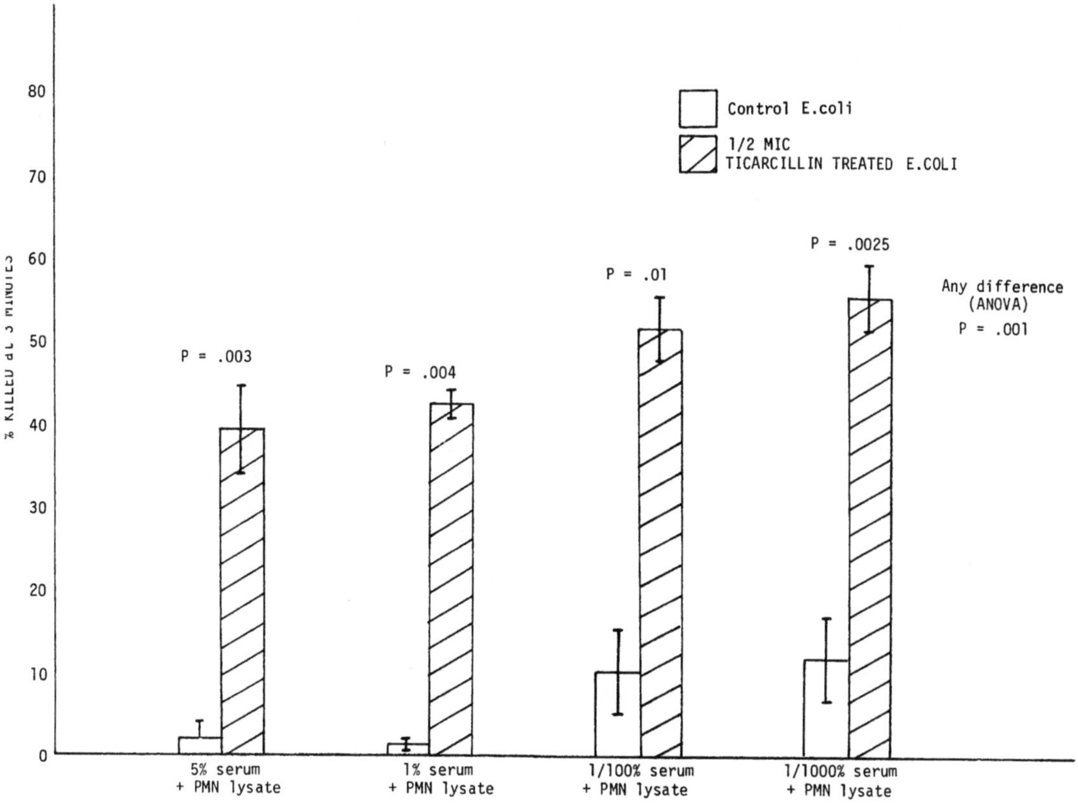

Fig. 5. Killing by PMN lysates in the presence of decreasing serum concentrations

When PMNs were sonicated, little killing of control or antibiotic-treated bacteria was seen. To determine whether this was related to inhibition of lysate killing by serum, the following experiments were done.

Studies of Bacterial Killing by PMN Lysates

Experiments were done in which control and ½ MIC ticarcillin-pretreated *E. coli* were exposed to increasing dilutions of serum (5%, 1%, 1/100%, 1/1000%) and were then washed and incubated with PMN lysates.

As more dilute serum was used, a statistically significant increase in killing of antibiotic-treated *E. coli* was seen (Fig. 5). Statistical analysis also showed significant differences between ½ MIC drug-treated *E. coli* and control *E. coli*, with the former being killed much more readily.

Discussion

Our initial hypothesis was that any increase in killing of antibiotic-treated organisms would simply be a reflection of enhanced uptake. We also felt that such results would more likely be seen with cell wall active drugs such as ticarcillin than with drugs acting at a subcellular locus such as tobramycin.

As shown in "Results," both ticarcillin and tobramycin treatment of *E. coli* resulted in increased killing of the organisms. This result, however, was independent of any increases in ingestion of the organisms by the PMNs.

In order to minimize possible confounding effects and to allow us to distinguish between the effects of antibiotics on bacteria rather than on PMNs, the test organisms were pretreated with antibiotic and washed prior to their incubation with PMNs.

The fungal metabolite cyto-B allows binding of opsonized bacteria to PMNs but impairs their ingestion. It essentially converts the neutrophils from phagocytic cells into secretory cells, allowing one to measure extracellularly processes which normally occur within the cell [17]. Pretreatment with either ticarcillin or tobramycin made the *E. coli* more susceptible than the untreated organisms to extracellular killing by the cyto-B-treated PMNs.

In the presence of intact PMNs, opsonization of the bacteria was necessary for enhanced killing to occur. This suggests that intimate contact probably mediated via opsonin receptors plays a role. The finding that PMN lysates did not kill opsonized *E. coli* suggested a possible inhibitory effect by the serum adherent to the bacteria.

Subsequent experiments showing killing by PMN lysates of control and drug-treated *E. coli* exposed to increasingly dilute serum suggested that in fact such inhibition was taking place.

Despite having different mechanisms of action, sub-MIC ticarcillin and tobramycin may be able to elicit structural or functional changes in the capsular, outer membrane or peptidoglycan layers of the bacteria. Such changes may render the organisms more susceptible to the bactericidal mechanisms of PMNs.

Summary

Sub-MIC antibiotic-treated *E. coli* is more susceptible to killing by intact PMNs and PMN lysates than control *E. coli*.

With intact PMNs:
- Enhanced killing of drug-treated bacteria is independent of any increases in ingestion of organisms.
- Enhanced killing of drug-treated bacteria persists in the presence of cyto-B-treated PMNs.
- Opsonizing serum is necessary in the presence of intact PMNs.

With PMN lysates:
- ½ MIC ticarcillin-treated *E. coli* is more susceptible to killing by lysates than control *E. coli*.
- Prior incubation of the bacteria in 10% serum inhibits this killing.

References

1. Yourtee EL, Root RK (1982) Antibiotic-neutrophil interactions in microbial killing. In: Gallin JI, Fauci AS (eds) Advances of host defense mechanisms, vol 1. Raven, New York, p 187
2. Zak O, Kradolfer F (1979) Effects of subminimal inhibitory concentrations of antibiotics in experimental infections. Rev Infect Dis 1:862–879
3. Lorian V, Sabath LD (1972) Penicillins and cephalosporins: differences in morphologic effects on *Proteus mirabilis*. J Infect Dis 125:560–564
4. Perkins RL, Miller MA (1973) Scanning electron microscopy of morphological alterations in *Proteus mirabilis* induced by cephalosporins and semisynthetic penicillins. Can J Microbiol 19:251–255
5. Lorian V, Atkinson B (1975) Abnormal forms of bacteria produced by anibiotics. Am J Clin Pathol 64:678–688
6. Lorian V (1975) Some effects of subinhibitory concentrations of penicillins on the structure and division of staphylococci. Antimicrob Agents Chemother 7:864–870
7. Shah PM, Heetderks G, Stille W (1976) Activity of amikacin at sub-inhibitory levels. J Antimicrob Chemother 2:97–100
8. Adam D (1971) Studies on the influence of host defence mechanisms on the antimicrobial effect of chemotherapeutic agents. I. The influence of serum constituents on the in vitro effect of gentamicin and polymyxin. Int J Clin Pharmacol Ther Toxicol 4:175–182
9. Lorian V, Atkinson B (1978) Effects of serum on gram-positive cocci grown in the presence of penicillin. J Infect Dis 138:865–871
10. Verbrugh HA, Peters R, Peterson PK, Verhoef J (1978) Phagocytosis and intracellular killing of staphylococci by polymorphonuclear and mononuclear leukocytes. J Clin Pathol 31:539–545
11. Verhoef J, Peterson PK, Sabath LD, Quie PG (1977b) Kinetics of staphylococcal opsonization, attachment, ingestion and killing by human polymorphonuclear leukocytes: a quantitative assay using (^{3}H) – thymidine labelled bacteria. J Immunol Methods 14:303–311
12. Mandell LA (1985) Interactions between human polymorphonuclear neutrophils and ampicillin treated *E. coli*. In: Adam D, Hahn H, Opferkuch W (eds) The influence of antibiotics on the host-parasite relationship – II. Springer, Berlin Heidelberg New York, pp 166–178
13. Taylor PW, Roberts HP et al. (1972) Evaluation of a technique for the estimation of serum bactericidal activity against gram-negative organisms. Medical Lab Technol 29:272–279
14. McFarland J (1907) Nephelometer: an instrument for estimating the numbers of bacteria in suspensions used for calculating the opsonic index and for vaccines. JAMA 49:1176–1178
15. Washington JA, Barry AL (1974) Dilution test procedures. In: Lenaette EH, Spaulding EH, Truant JP (eds) Manual of clinical microbiology, 2nd edn. American Society for Microbiology, Washington DC, p 410
16. Weitz JI, Landman SL, Crowley KA, Birken S, Morgan FJ (1986) Development of an assay for in vivo human neutrophil elastase activity. J Clin Invest 78:155–162
17. Goldstein IM (1984) Neutrophil degranulation. In: Snyderman R (ed) Contemporary topics in immunology, vol 14. Regulation of leukocyte function. Plenum, New York, pp 189–219

Effects of Glycopeptide and Lipopeptide Antibiotics on Granulocyte Function In Vitro

F. SCHUMACHER-PERDREAU [1], E. SCHELL-FREDERICK [2], G. PETERS [1], and G. PULVERER [1]

Introduction

Vancomycin and the newly developed teicoplanin are glycopeptide antibiotics with high activity against gram-positive bacteria, especially staphylococci and streptococci [8]. LY 146032 is a new cyclic polypeptide antibiotic containing a fatty acid moiety [3]. Similar to vancomycin and teicoplanin, the new cyclic lipopeptide demonstrates excellent activity against a broad range of gram-positive bacteria including methicillin-resistant strains of *S. aureus* and *S. epidermidis* [9].

There are several case reports in the literature of vancomycin-associated neutropenia without bone marrow depression following prolonged administration of the antibiotic [1, 5, 6, 11, 12]. Failure of teicoplanin therapy indicated by increasing or persisting fever and signs of infections, associated with a progressive decrease of white blood cells, was also observed during a clinical trial with this antibiotic in our institution (R. Stuttmann, G. Peters, personal communication). The decrease in white blood cells (WBCs) with teicoplanin therapy was striking. After stopping therapy and changing to another antistaphylococcal drug, normalization of body temperature as well as a rise in WBCs was observed with resolution of the infection. Teicoplanin appeared to affect leukocyte homeostasis in vivo. Bone marrow taken from a patient revealed no signs of marrow depression but a marked left-shift in the granulocyte cell lines, suggesting that granulocytes are the affected leukocyte population and teicoplanin may act peripherally.

These observations led us to examine granulocyte function in vitro in the presence of these peptide antibiotics. The effects of teicoplanin, vancomycin, and LY 146032 on luminol-enhanced chemiluminescence and on the release of granule enzymes were investigated. The possible cytotoxicity of these antibiotics was also evaluated.

[1] Institute of Hygiene, University of Köln, Goldenfelsstr. 19–21, 5000 Köln 41, Federal Republic of Germany

[2] Department of Medicine I, University of Köln, Joseph-Stelzmann-Str. 9, 5000 Köln 41, Federal Republic of Germany

The Influence of Antibiotics on the Host-Parasite Relationship III
Edited by G. Gillissen, W. Opferkuch, G. Peters, and G. Pulverer

Material and Methods

Bacteria

Staphylococcus aureus SG 511-Jena was used. The bacteria were grown overnight at 37 °C in Mueller-Hinton broth (Difco Lab., Detroit, USA) and washed three times in saline before use.

Antibiotics

Teicoplanin (Le Petit, Milan, Italy), vancomycin and LY 146032 (Eli Lilly, Indianapolis, United States) were used in this study. The antibiotics were diluted in MEM (Gibco) for chemiluminescence study.

Leukocyte Preparation

Thirty-five milliliters of blood from healthy volunteers on no medication (age range 23–60 years) were drawn by venipuncture using preservative-free heparin (10 units/ml). Fifteen milliliters of 6% dextran T 70 (Pharmacia Fine Chemicals AB, Uppsala, Sweden) were added. The red blood cells were allowed to settle for 45 min at 37 °C. The neutrophil-rich supernatant was separated and centrifuged at 160 × g for 10 min. Residual red blood cells were removed by hypotonic lysis. The neutrophils were washed in Hanks's balanced salt solution (HBSS), resuspended in MEM (free of phenol red), supplemented with 10% heat-inactivated fetal calf serum, and adjusted to a final concentration of 5×10^6/ml. For the measurement of the release of β-glucuronidase and lysozyme, Ficoll-urographin-purified granulocytes were used [4].

The neutrophils were preincubated with the antibiotics teicoplanin, vancomycin, and LY 146032 at concentrations 50–150 µg/ml for 30 min at 37 °C. Neutrophils from the same donor incubated without antibiotics were used as a control.

Opsonization

Zymosan (Sigma) was suspended in phosphate-buffered saline (PBS) at a concentration of 20 mg/ml. The zymosan suspension was washed twice in PBS, suspended in normal pooled human serum (1 : 6 diluted) for 30 min at 37 °C, and washed again twice before being resuspended to the same concentration in MEM. The same procedure was followed to opsonize the bacteria adjusted to a concentration of 10^9 colony-forming units(CFUs)/ml.

Chemiluminescence Assay

Measurement of the luminol-dependent chemiluminescence was performed according to Easmon et al. [2]. Briefly: 5×10^6 neutrophils in 0.25 ml MEM supplemented with heat-inactivated fetal calf serum were added to luminol (Sigma, 10^{-9} molar). The system was activated by the addition of *N*-formyl-methionyl-leucyl-phenylalanine (FMLP, 10^{-8} molar), serum-opsonized zymosan (2 mg zymosan), or serum-opsonized *Staphylococcus aureus* SG 511-Jena (10^8 CFUs). The time trace of chemiluminescence was recorded in millivolts using a LKB-Wallace-1251 luminometer.

Lactate Dehydrogenase, Beta-glucuronidase, Lysozyme

The polymorphonuclear neutrophil (PMN) samples (1.0×10^7/ml) were preincubated in the presence or absence of antibiotic for 30 min at 37 °C. The cells were then centrifuged, resuspended in fresh medium containing the appropriate stimulus and the same concentration of antibiotic, and further incubated for 30 min at 37 °C. Enzymes were measured in aliquots of cell-free supernatants according to Klebanoff and Clark [7]. At least three PMN samples from three different donors were investigated.

Cytotoxicity

Release of indium from prelabeled and twice-washed mixed leukocytes was measured as previously described [10].

Results

Opsonized *S. aureus* SG 511, opsonized zymosan, and the soluble stimulus FMLP induced a significant chemiluminescence response in PMNs from all 25 samples (12 donors), the amplitude being donor dependent. The peak was obtained after about 150 s for FMLP and 12 min for the particles. The stimulation of PMNs exposed to the antibiotics vancomycin, teicoplanin, and LY 146032 revealed different patterns of reactivity.

Vancomycin. (Sixteen out of 25 PMN preparations incubated in the presence of 50, 100, and 200 μg/ml vancomycin showed no difference in the amount of chemiluminescence in comparison with the controls. The dose of antibiotic did not influence either the amplitude or the time trace of chemiluminescence emitted. Seven PMN samples showed a slight decrease compared with the mV output of control cells (Fig. 1), and two samples taken from the same donor at 2-month intervals showed a drastic decrease in chemiluminescence following vancomycin pretreatment. For each donor parallel results were obtained with the three stimuli used.

Teicoplanin. Four out of 25 samples showed chemiluminescence similar to that of the control. Twenty-one samples showed a dose-dependent reduction in the amplitude of chemiluminescence (Fig. 2). A similar decrease in chemilumi-

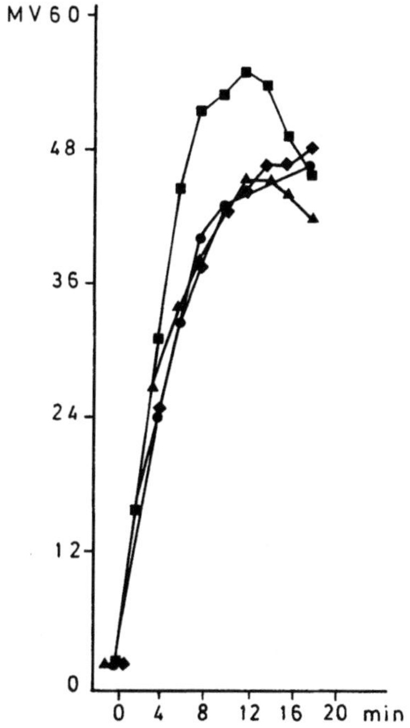

Fig. 1. Time trace of chemiluminescence of human PMNs pretreated with vancomycin (50 μg/ml ●, 100 μg/ml ▲, 200 μg/ml ◆) after stimulation with opsonized *S. aureus* SG 511-Jena (control: ■), mv = millivolt

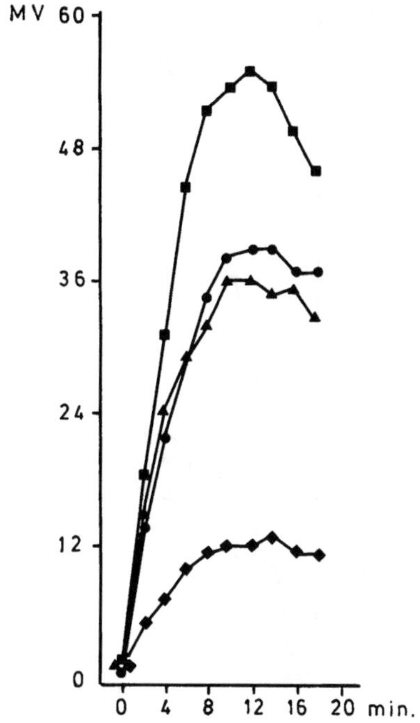

Fig. 2. Time trace of chemiluminescence of human PMNs pretreated with teicoplanin (50 μg/ml ●, 100 μg/ml ▲, 200 μg/ml ◆) after stimulation with opsonized *S. aureus* SG 511-Jena (control: ■)

nescence was measured using FMLP. If the leukocytes were washed twice following preincubation with teicoplanin before chemiluminescence measurement, the inhibitory effect was largely reversed. Teicoplanin did not have a light-quenching effect. FMLP-stimulated chemiluminescence was not inhibited if teicoplanin was added to the system immediately after FMLP and immediately before measurement. In addition, if the complete system in a small tube was measured in a larger tube containing teicoplanin up to 1000 μg/ml, no quenching was observed.

LY 146032. The response of PMNs pretreated with the lipopeptide LY 146032 varied depending on the stimulus used. With opsonized zymosan or *S. aureus,* PMNs pretreated with LY 146032 generated more chemiluminescence than control cells (five PMN samples from five different donors). As illustrated by the results from one donor (Fig. 3), this stimulation was most striking after preincubation with 200 μg/ml of the drug. In contrast, with FMLP an inhibition of chemiluminescence was observed after drug pretreatment (14 PMN samples from 8 different donors). The extent of the inhibitory effect was dependent both on the concentration of the antibiotic and on the donor.

None of the antibiotics investigated in concentrations up to 500 μg/ml demonstrated a cytotoxic effect on mixed leukocytes or isolated granulocytes. Trypan

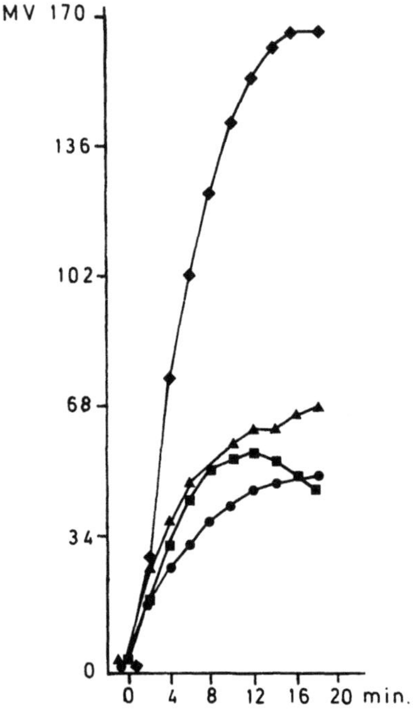

Fig. 3. Time trace of chemiluminescence of human PMNs pretreated with LY 146032 (50 μg/ml ●, 100 μg/ml ▲, 200 μg/ml ◆) after stimulation with opsonized *S. aureus* SG 511-Jena (control: ■)

Table 1. Lactate dehydrogenase release (units/liter) by human PMNs pretreated with glycopeptide or lipid antibiotics

PMNs	50.0
PMNs + teicoplanin (200 μg/ml)	49.1
PMNs + teicoplanin (500 μg/ml)	44.5
PMNs + vancomycin (200 μg/ml)	50.3
PMNs + vancomycin (500 μg/ml)	50.1
PMNs + LY 146032 (200 μg/ml)	46.7
PMNs + LY 146023 (500 μg/ml)	46.3

blue exclusion was greater than 92% in all cell preparations. There was no increase in the release of the cytoplasmic enzyme lactate-dehydrogenase when granulocytes were incubated with antibiotic for 30 min at 37 °C (Table 1). Cells in the presence of antibiotics incubated for a further 30 min after addition of cytochalasin B (5 μg/ml) and FMLP (1×10^{-7} molar) did not show a higher lactate dehydrogenase (LDH) release than control cells. Indium-prelabeled leukocytes did not release increased label during a 30-min incubation with the drug.

The effect of 250 μg/ml teicoplanin, vancomycin, and LY 146032 on basal and stimulated granule enzyme release was investigated. Lysozyme release was suppressed in teicoplanin-pretreated cells (Table 2). No influence of vancomycin or LY 146032 was noted. Similar results were found for beta-glucuronidase release

Table 2. Lysozyme release by human PMNs pretreated with glycopeptide or lipopeptide antibiotics

	Δ *E*/min	%
PMNs	0.06	
PMNs+FMLP	0.65	100
PMNs+teicoplanin (250 μg/ml)	0.05	
PMNs+FMLP	0.37	56
PMNs+vancomycin (250 μg/ml)	0.05	
PMNs+FMLP	0.62	95
PMNs+LY 146032 (250 μg/ml)	0.05	
PMNs+FMLP	0.65	100

Table 3. Beta-glucuronidase release (percentage maximum) by human PMNs pretreated with glycopeptide or lipopeptide antibiotics

PMNs	2.0		4.8
PMNs+FMLP	28.7	+ zymosan (1 mg/ml)	19.2
PMNs+teicoplanin (250 μg/ml)	1.4		4.6
PMNs+FMLP	15.7	+ zymosan	15.0
PMNs+vancomycin (250 μg/ml)	2.1		5.0
PMNs+FMLP	29.2	+ zymosan	20.3
PMNs+LY 146032	–		5.0
PMNs+FMLP	–	+ zymosan	20.5

–, not tested.

(Table 3). Teicoplanin again inhibited the enzyme release from FMLP or zymosan-stimulated PMNs.

Discussion

Polymorphonuclear neutrophils stimulated in vitro with soluble or corpuscular stimuli emit light. Oxygen metabolites and radicals, e.g., superoxide anion and singlet oxygen, are thought to be responsible for this reaction.

The chemiluminescence response in PMNs pretreated with antibiotics is highly dependent on the drug itself, the concentration of the drug, and the blood donor. Teicoplanin and to a considerably less extent vancomycin suppress luminol-enhanced chemiluminescence in granulocytes triggered in vitro with FMLP and opsonized zymosan or bacteria in a high number of apparently healthy donors. After preincubation with LY 146032, particular stimuli generated an enhanced chemiluminescence response whereas the response by FMLP was depressed. Only teicoplanin was shown to affect granule enzyme release at the concentrations tested.

The antibiotics were not cytotoxic in these short-term experiments, as measured by trypan blue exclusion, LDH release, and indium-111 release, and by the reversibility of teicoplanin inhibition of chemiluminescence after washing the cells.

The in vitro results show clear but different effects of these glycopeptide and lipopeptide antibiotics on granulocyte function. The extent varies between donors. It is so far unclear whether these functional changes observed in vitro contribute to the neutropenia observed in occasional patients following glycopeptide therapy.

Summary

Teicoplanin is a new glycopeptide and LY 146032 a new lipopeptide antibiotic, both similar to vancomycin in antibacterial spectrum and activity. Several cases of neutropenia have been reported following prolonged vancomycin therapy and it appears also to be a possible side effect of teicoplanin therapy. This led us to investigate the effects of vancomycin, teicoplanin, and LY 146032 on luminol-enhanced chemiluminescence – stimulated with FMLP and opsonized zymosan and *S. aureus* – enzyme release, and indium-111 release of human PMNs. All these substances tested revealed no cytotoxic effect on PMNs. Vancomycin and teicoplanin showed a donor-dependent effect on PMN chemiluminescence, stimulated with FMLP, opsonized zymosan, and opsonized *S. aureus*. In most donors, teicoplanin inhibited PMN chemiluminescence to a significantly greater extent than vancomycin. LY 146032 inhibited FMLP-stimulated PMN chemiluminescence in all donors examined, but enhanced opsonized zymosan or opsonized *S. aureus*-stimulated chemiluminescence. Teicoplanin also inhibited the release of lysozyme, beta-glucuronidase, and lactate dehydrogenase in PMNs. The inhibitory effects on PMN function obtained in vitro may contribute to the neutropenia observed in occasional patients following glycopeptide therapy.

References

1. Borland CDR, Farras WE (1979) Reversible neutropenia from vancomycin. JAMA 242:2392–2393
2. Easmon CSF, Cole PJ, Williams AJ, Hastings M (1980) The measurement of opsonic and phagocytic function by luminol-dependent chemiluminescence. J Immunol Methods 41:67–71
3. Eliopoulos GMC, Thauvin B, Gerson RC, Moellering J (1985) In vitro activity and mechanism of action of A $21978C_1$, a novel cyclic lipopeptide antibiotic. Antimicrob Agents Chemother 27:357–362
4. Ferrante A, Thong YH (1980) Optimal conditions for simultaneous purification of mononuclear and polymorphonuclear leukocytes from human blood by the hypaque-ficoll-method. J Immunol Methods 36:109–117
5. Gopal V, Bisno AL, Silverblatt FJ (1976) Failure of vancomycin treatment in *Staphylococcus aureus* endocarditis. JAMA 236:1604–1606
6. Hook EW III, Johnson WD Jr (1978) Vancomycin therapy of bacterial endocarditis. Am J Med 65:411–415
7. Klebanoff SJ, Clark RA (1979) The neutrophil: function and clinical disorders. North-Holland, Amsterdam

8. Peters G, Pulverer G (1983) Antibacterial activity of teicomycin (MDL 507), a new glycopeptide antibiotic, in comparison to vancomycin. J Antimicrob Chemother 11:94–95
9. Peters G, Schumacher-Perdreau F, Pulverer G (1987) In vitro activity of the new peptolide antibiotic LY 146032 against staphylococci: a comparison with the glycopeptide antibiotics vancomycin and teicoplanin. Eur J Clin Microbiol 6:685
10. Schell-Frederick E, Frühling J, van der Auwera Ph, van Laethem Y, Klastersky J (1984) ^{111}Indium-oxine-labelled leucocytes in the diagnosis of localized infection in patients with neoplastic disease. Cancer 54:817–824
11. Weitzmann SA, Stossel TP, Desmond M (1978) Drug-induced immunological neutropenia. Lancet I:1068–1072
12. West BC (1981) Vancomycin-induced neutropenia. South Med J 74:1255–1256

Determination of Intracellular Antibacterial Activity of Antibiotics by Means of a Fluorochrome Microassay

W. Horn [1], R. Jantzen [1], and J. Lücke [2]

Introduction

Several antibiotics have been shown by use of radioactive labeling to accumulate in phagocytes. The most prominent representatives of this group are clindamycin and erythromycin, which can be concentrated by human [both normal and chronic granulomatous disease (CGD)] PMNs up to 40 times the extracellular concentration [5, 7]. The question as to whether the intracellular antibacterial activity of antibiotics parallels their intracellular concentration is more difficult to answer and has directly been addressed by a few studies only. For example, Silva et al. [9] incubated normal and CGD PMNs with 0.05 mg/liter clindamycin (MIC = 0.06 mg/liter) during, prior to, or after phagocytosis of *Staphylococcus aureus* and found no significant improvement of intracellular killing with both normal and CGD PMNs. This result contradicts the uptake studies. We therefore reevaluated the problem by using a fluorochrome microassay that allows simultaneous determination of uptake and killing of bacteria under the influence of subinhibitory concentrations of antibiotics. In order to test the intracellular activity of antibiotics it would be advantageous to employ either phagocytes with impaired killing function or microorganisms which survive intracellularly to a high degree. We tried both approaches: azide-treated or CGD PMNs were used for phagocytosis of staphylococci, thus establishing high intracellular survival rates due to defective granulocyte function; normal PMNs were used for phagocytosis of *Listeria,* which survived to 60% intracellularly without addition of antibiotics. Experiments with clindamycin-treated bacteria were also performed to determine the degree to which extracellular action of the antibiotic on bacteria influenced intracellular survival.

Materials and Methods

Eleven *S. aureus* strains isolated from patients and one *Listeria* strain were used for phagocytosis. Antibiotics tested were: clindamycin hydrochloride (Upjohn), vancomycin hydrochloride (Lilly), penicillin G (Grünenthal), erythromycin glucoheptonate (Schering), flucloxacillin, and gentamicin sulfate (both Beecham-Wülfing). All other materials and the basic method have previously been de-

[1] Medizinische Klinik III, University of Giessen, 6300 Giessen, Federal Republic of Germany
[2] Upjohn GmbH, Heppenheim, Federal Republic of Germany

The Influence of Antibiotics on the Host-Parasite Relationship III
Edited by G. Gillissen, W. Opferkuch, G. Peters, and G. Pulverer

scribed in detail [4]. Peripheral blood PMNs were sedimented onto glass slides, washed, and incubated with a bacterial suspension in a humid atmosphere at 37 °C. Thereafter the preparations were stained with acridin orange and dried. This procedure resulted in the fluorescence of intracellular bacteria only, with living bacteria fluorescing green and nonliving bacteria fluorescing red.

For the present study, this method was modified as follows: After an 18-h growth in Tryptic Soy Broth (TSB), stationary-phase bacteria were incubated with 10% of pooled human AB serum in Dulbecco's phosphate-buffered saline (DPBS) (staphylococci 1×10^8/ml, *Listeria* 3×10^7/ml) for 1 h at 37 °C for opsonization and in order to initiate growth. In the meantime, glass-adherent PMNs were incubated with antibiotics in DPBS for 30 min. The concentrations of antibiotics are given in "Results." Thereafter, antibiotics were added to aliquots of the bacterial suspensions to yield the same concentrations as in the respective solutions used fo preincubating the PMNs. The preincubation solutions were decanted and the bacterial suspensions immediately layered onto the cells. Where indicated, 1 m*M* sodium azide [6] was added to the *S. aureus* suspensions immediately before phagocytosis. Phagocytosis time was 45 min. One hundred and sixty PMNs on two slides were evaluated for each experiment. All other procedures were performed as described [4].

When the direct effect of ¼ MIC clindamycin on staphylococci was to be tested, an appropriate amount of clindamycin was added to the opsonization mixture after 15 min, and incubation was prolonged for another 45 min. This time was chosen to match phagocytosis time, i.e., the maximal period during which extracellular bacteria could be in contact with clindamycin before being phagocytized in the original experimental setting. Thereafter bacteria were washed twice, resuspended in opsonization medium without antibiotic, and added to untreated PMNs. The rest of the assay was performed as before.

Significances were determined by the *t*-test; results are given as mean values $\pm$ SD.

Results

Minimal inhibitory concentrations were determined in trypticase soy broth with 2×10^7/ml staphylococcal and 5×10^6/ml *Listeria* inoculum concentration. MICs of staphylococci – except for one clindamycin-resistant strain – were 0.08–0.16 mg/liter for clindamycin, 0.16–0.63 for flucloxacillin, 0.63–1.25 for gentamycin, and 1.25 for vancomycin. The MIC of the *Listeria* strain was 1.25 mg/liter for clindamycin and 0.16 for penicillin G and erythromycin.

Effect of Clindamycin on the Intracellular Survival of Staphylococci Phagocytized by Normal, Untreated PMNs. Clindamycin at concentrations of ½ or ⅛ MIC, added to PMNs as described in "Material and methods", did not influence the percentage of intracellularly surviving bacteria (17% $\pm$ 5.0%, ten strains, one to three experiments each). It did, however, increase the uptake of bacteria by roughly the same rate as did azide (about 30%). The latter phenomenon has previously been noted [4].

Effect of Clindamycin on the Intracellular Survival of Staphylococci Phagocytized by Azide-Treated PMNs. Addition of 1 m*M* sodium azide to the phagocytosis mixture increased the percentage of intracellularly surviving staphylococci from 17% ± 5.0% to 38% ± 5.3% in ten strains that were sensitive to clindamycin in vitro [6]. Clindamycin at a concentration of ¼ MIC, added as described in "Materials and methods," completely reversed the effect of azide in seven ("responder strains") of the ten sensitive strains (percentage of surviving bacteria, 14% ± 2.2%). The remaining three sensitive as well as the one resistant strain did not respond to clindamycin in this system.

With four of the responder strains, the effect of preincubating the staphylococci instead of PMNs with ¼ MIC clindamycin for 45 min (see "Materials and methods") was additionally tested: Table 1 shows that pretreatment of bacteria reduced intracellular survival by 40%, as compared with 100% when PMNs were pretreated.

Again, a slight enhancement of bacterial uptake by azide and clindamycin was noted (10 ± 1.1 bacteria/cell in untreated, 12 ± 1.5 in azide-treated, and 13 ± 1.9 in azide- plus clindamycin-treated PMNs).

Dose Response Curve. A responder strain that was also sensitive to all other antibiotics applied was chosen for a dose-response curve (Fig. 1). A slight improvement of intracellular killing was already observable at an extracellular clindamycin concentration of 1/32 MIC. At ¼ MIC, the effect of azide was fully balanced, as seen before. Gentamicin, vancomycin, and flucloxacillin, at concentrations of ¼ MIC, had no effect at all.

Test of the Method with PMNs of a CGD Patient. The reason why seven of the ten sensitive *S. aureus* strains did not respond to clindamycin in azide-treated PMNs is unclear. In order to circumvent treatment with azide and nevertheless

Table 1. Intracellular survival of staphylococci after treatment of PMNs or bacteria with ¼ MIC clindamycin

Treatment of		Strain number			
PMNs	Bacteria	7	8	9	10
–	–	18 ± 2.2	14 ± 3.0	13 ± 4.0	13 ± 2.0
A	–	32 ± 2.6	36 ± 3.4	43 ± 3.9	44 ± 2.6
A + C	–	14 ± 2.6	14 ± 1.2	14 ± 1.2	16 ± 1.3
–	–	16 ± 3.5	16 ± 3.6	13 ± 4.0	12 ± 2.6
–	C	21 ± 7.5	15 ± 2.6	12 ± 2.9	12 ± 3.0
A	–	35 ± 5.8	37 ± 4.5	40 ± 2.4	44 ± 4.5
A	C	31 ± 4.6	26 ± 2.7	29 ± 5.6	31 ± 5.1

Polymorphonuclear neutrophils or staphylococci were treated with ¼ MIC clindamycin as described in "Materials and Methods". Numbers denote the percentage of intracellularly surviving bacteria ± SD (n = three experiments for the upper part, four for the lower part of the table). A, 1 m*M* sodium azide; C, ¼ MIC clindamycin.

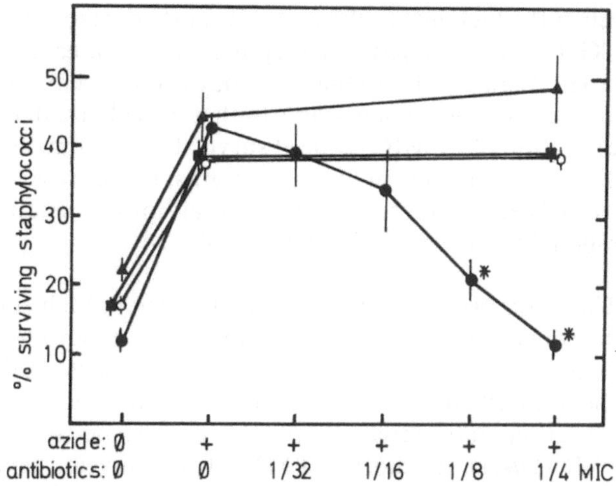

Fig. 1. Dependence of intracellular survival rate of *S. aureus* strain S2 phagocytized by azide-treated PMNs on extracellular concentrations of antibiotics. ●, clindamycin: ○, gentamicin: ▲, vancomicin: ■, flucloxacillin. Vertical lines = ±SE, $n = 3$; *, significant difference to zero value, as obtained with Student's t-test, $P < 0.001$

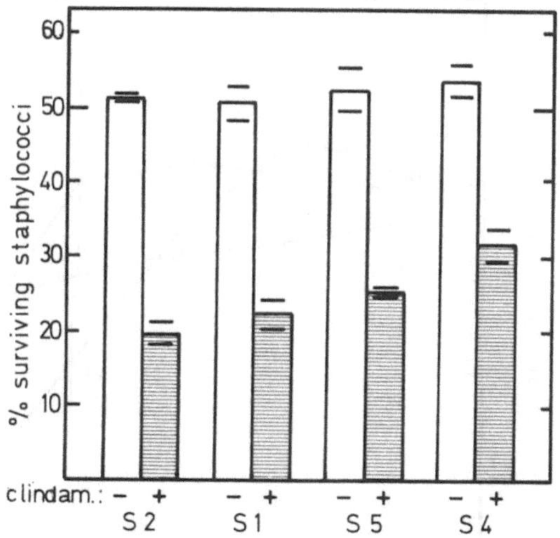

Fig. 2. Effect of 0.04 mg/liter clindamycin (= ¼ MIC) on intracellular survival of *S. aureus* strains phagocytized by CGD PMNs. S1, S2: responder strains; S4, S5: nonresponder strains. *Bars* represent the man value of two experiments, *horizontal lines* the individual experiments. The mean number of bacteria/PMN was 14.3 ± 0.44 (SE) without and 15.1 ± 1.43 with clindamycin

retain the high intracellular survival rate of staphylococci, PMNs of a child with CGD were employed. Two representatives of each group of staphylococci were tested. Figure 2 shows that, without clindamycin, the level of surviving intracellular bacteria was comparable to that in azide-treated cells. Clindamycin at a concentration of ¼ MIC reduced survival rates from 50% to 20–30% for all strains. Thus, all clindamycin-sensitive strains, in contrast to the experiment with azide-treated cells, behaved the same way, although a small difference seemed to persist, especially between strains S2 and S4.

Use of Listeria. A third approach to achieve high survival rates of phagocytized microorganisms without poisoning the phagocyte or employing PMNs with genetically defective killing function is to use bacteria that are naturally resistant to the intracellular killing mechanisms of the phagocyte. A well-known example of this group of bacteria is *Listeria.* A dose-response experiment was therefore done with *Listeria* and normal PMNs. Clindamycin, penicillin G, and erythromycin were applied at concentrations between ¹⁄₃₂ and ¼ MIC. Clindamycin reduced the intracellular survival rate significantly at concentrations of ⅛ and ¼ MIC. The effects of penicillin G and erythromycin in that concentration range were less pronounced and significant only for erythromycin at ¼ MIC (Fig. 3).

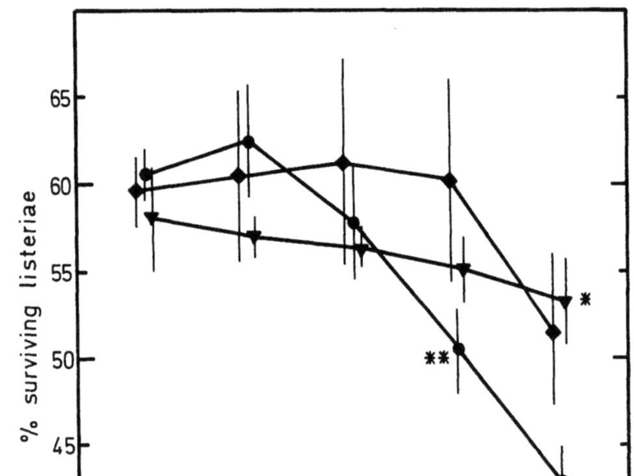

Fig. 3. Dependence of intracellular survival rate of a *Listeria* strain phagocytized by normal, native PMNs on extracellular concentrations of antibiotics. ●, clindamycin ($n=11$); ◆, penicillin G ($n=4$); ▼, erythromycin ($n=8$). *Vertical lines,* ±SE. Significant differences from zero value, as obtained with Student's *t*-test: *, $P<0.05$; **, $P<0.01$; ***, $P<0.001$

Discussion

The main purpose of this study was to investigate the problem of whether clindamycin is intracellularly as active as can be expected from its known accumulation in phagocytes. We also wanted to demonstrate the usefulness of the fluorochrome method for studies dealing with the interaction of bacteria, phagocytes, and antibiotics.

The method presented here measures the uptake and short-term (45-min) survival of bacteria phagocytized by PMNs that were incubated with subinhibitory concentrations of antibiotics 30 min before and during phagocytosis. Thirty minutes preincubation with clindamycin is sufficient to reach a plateau in intracellular accumulation [7, 5]. Presence of the antibiotic in the phagocytosis mixture at the same concentration as in the preincubation buffer is necessary since it reequilibrates rapidly with the extracellular medium [7]. In order to achieve a high basal survival rate, three approaches were made: azide-treated or CGD PMNs were employed with staphylococci, whereas native normal PMNs were used with *Listeria*.

Clindamycin at an extracellular concentration of ¼ MIC reduced survival of staphylococci in CGD PMNs from ca. 50% to 25%. Silva et al. [9] reported a mean reduction of surviving staphylococci in CGD PMNs from 90% to 82% after a 2-h incubation, with clindamycin at a concentration of 0.83 MIC in the test mixture. This difference in absolute numbers might be due to the different incubation times and to the fact that in the experiment of Silva et al. [9] cell-adherent bacteria contributed to the measurement of survival.

Clindamycin at an extracellular concentration of ¼ MIC reduced survival rates of *Listeria* in normal PMNs from 61% to 43%. A significant reduction to 50% was already observed with ⅛ MIC. This and the foregoing result are compatible with the hypothesis that clindamycin not only accumulates in PMNs but also retains its antibacterial activity. Erythromycin, which can also be concentrated intracellularly (e.g. [3]), only had a small effect at ⅛ MIC; penicillin G had none at ⅛ MIC. At ¼ MIC, both antibiotics reduced survival to ca. 53%.

Clindamycin at an extracellular concentration of ¼ MIC reduced survival of staphylococci in azide-treated PMNs from 38% to 14%, the level that pertains in native normal PMNs. This result, however, was only true for seven of ten clindamycin-sensitive strains ("responder strains"). The other sensitive strains as well as a resistant one did not respond to clindamycin under these conditions. The ten strains did not significantly differ in MICs, in uptake rates, in basal survival rates, or in the increase of survival after addition of azide. The divergence could also not be due to differences in the PMNs since various antibiotics were tested with PMNs of the same person, and vice versa. We did not attempt to resolve this problem in the present study.

Preincubation of staphylococci (responder strains) instead of PMNs with ¼ MIC clindamycin for 45 min reduced azide-induced enhanced intracellular survival by 40%, as compared with 100% when PMNs were pretreated with the antibiotic. These 40% would therefore be the maximal contribution of extracellular antibiotic to the overall effect of clindamycin in the latter system since phagocytosis time was also 45 min.

A dose-response experiment performed with a responder strain showed significant reductions of intracellular survival at ¼ and ⅛ MIC and a slight reduction even at $^1/_{16}$ MIC (Fig. 1), in accordance with the *Listeria* experiment (Fig. 3). Taken together, these two experiments demonstrate a good correlation between reported concentration ratios in PMNs (5–40 times the extracellular concentration, e.g., [7, 3, 5] and intracellular antibacterial activity. Gentamicin and penicillins, which are not concentrated by phagocytes [3], and vancomycin had no significant effect at ¼ MIC. This difference in intracellular antibacterial effectiveness between accumulated and not accumulated antibiotics has already been reported by Jacobs and Wilson [5], who, however, applied antibiotics at concentrations several times higher than MICs.

We observed a slight enhancement of ingestion of staphylococci by clindamycin, in agreement with other studies [8, 10]. These authors ascribe the phenomenon of antibiotic-induced enhancement of ingestion to an improved opsonization. In a fluorochrome phagocytosis assay similar to ours, Bassaris et al. [1] found that ingestion and killing rate of clindamycin-resistant (MIC > 64 mg/liter) *E. coli* was enhanced by preincubation of bacteria with 4 mg/liter clindamycin. These studies, in addition to the results presented here, demonstrate that the fluorochrome assay can also be useful if bacteria, instead of phagocytes, are preincubated with antibiotics, i.e., when the focus of interest is on the action of antibiotics on bacteria rather than on uptake of antibiotics by PMNs.

The failure of Easmon and Crane [2] to detect any enhancement by clindamycin – in contrast to rifampicin – of intracellular killing of staphylococci by normal PMNs, in spite of high basal survival rates, may be due to the fact that their phagocytosis mixture did not contain serum which stimulates intracellular killing. We, too, did not observe an effect of clindamycin on staphylococci phagocytized by normal PMNs. However, because of the low basal survival rate of staphylococci in our system, small differences induced by clindamycin may have remained undetected.

The main result of the present study is that subinhibitory concentrations of clindamycin in a serum-containing system very effectively reduced intracellular survival of staphylococci phagocytized by azide-treated or by CGD PMNs. This effect could primarily be ascribed to clindamycin accumulated in the PMNs. The function of normal PMNs was not further improved by subinhibitory concentrations of clindamycin.

Summary

Clindamycin has been shown to accumulate in phagocytes by a factor of 5–40 times the extracellular concentration. In the present study, the influence of subminimal inhibitory concentration (MIC) doses of clindamycin and other antibiotics was investigated by incubating glass-adherent human neutrophils prior to and during phagocytosis with antibiotics. Ingestion rate and intracellular survival of bacteria were assayed by a fluorochrome method using acridin orange. In neutrophils of a child with chronic granulomatous disease, an extracellular concentration of ¼ MIC clindamycin reduced survival of staphylococci from 50% to

25%. In normal neutrophils, the same concentration reduced survival of *Listeria* from 61% to 43%. In azide-treated (1 m*M*) normal neutrophils, seven of ten staphylococcal strains which were sensitive to clindamycin in vitro responded to intracellular clindamycin. In responder strains, ¼ MIC clindamycin completely reversed the increase of survival induced by azide. A dose-response curve showed a significant decrease of survival by ca. 50% at ⅛ MIC and a small effect even at 1/32 MIC. Other antibiotics were less or not effective. Preincubation of staphylococci instead of PMNs with ¼ MIC clindamycin diminished the azide-induced enhancement of survival by only 40%. We conclude that sub-MIC doses of clindamycin can enhance intracellular killing of sensitive bacteria, primarily by accumulation of clindamycin in the phagocytes.

Acknowledgments. We thank Dr. S. Bhakdi (Institute of Medical Microbiology) for staphylococcal strains isolated from patients and for the *Listeria* strain, and Dr. K. Bertram (formerly Children's Hospital) for blood of a child with CGD (both University of Giessen).

References

1. Bassaris HP, Lianou PE, Papavassiliou JT (1984) Interaction of subminimal inhibitory concentrations of clindamycin and *Escherichia coli:* effects on adhesion and polymorphonuclear leukocyte function. J Antimcrob Chemother 13:361–367
2. Easmon CSF, Crane JP (1984) Cellular uptake of clindamycin and lincomycin. Br J Exp Pathol 65:725–730
3. Hand WL, King-Thompson NL, Steinberg TH (1983) Interactions of antibiotics and phagocytes. J Antimicrob Chemother 12 [Suppl C]:1–11
4. Horn W, Hansmann C, Federlin K (1985) An improved fluorochrome microassay for the detection of living and non-living intracellular bacteria in human neutrophils. J Immunol Methods 83:233–240
5. Jacobs RF, Wilson CB (1983) Intracellular penetration and antimicrobial activity of antibiotics. J Antimcrob Chemother 12 [Suppl C]:13–20
6. Klebanoff SJ (1970) Myeloperoxidase: contribution to the microbicidal activity of intact leukocytes. Science 169:1095–1097
7. Klempner MS, Styrt B (1981) Clindamycin uptake by human neutrophils. J Infect Dis 144:472–479
8. Milatovic D (1982) Effect of subinhibitory antibiotic concentrations on the phagocytosis of *Staphylococcus aureus*. Eur J Clin Microbiol 1:97
9. Silva J Jr, Dembinski S, Schaberg (1983) Effects of subinhibitory antibiotics on bactericidal activity of chronic granulomatous disease granulocytes in vitro. J Antimicrob Chemother 12 [Suppl C]:21–27
10. Verhoef J, Milatovic D (1985) Influence of antibiotics on opsonization of staphylococci. In: Pulverer G, Jeljaszewicz J (eds) Chemotherapy and immunity. Zbl Bakt Hyg Suppl 13:115–120

Effect of New Antibacterial Agents on Intracellular Staphylococci and Mycobacteria

C. S. F. Easmon

Introduction

Intracellular bacteria are protected against most host defences and antibacterial agents. Antibiotics such as rifampicin and clindamycin are known to be taken up by cells and to be effective against intracellular bacteria [1, 2].

The purpose of this study was to examine the effect of new agents such as the 4-quinolones and new rifamycins and macrolides on the survival of either *Staphylococcus aureus* or *Mycobacterium* spp. within neutrophils and macrophages.

Materials and Methods

Bacteria

Staphylococcus aureus NCTC 6571 was used. The strains of *Mycobacterium fortuitum* and *M. chelonei* were kindly supplied by Mr. C. Collins, Public Health Laboratory, Dulwich, UK. Organisms were stored either at −70 °C or in liquid nitrogen. *S. aureus* was grown in Brain Heart Infusion Broth (Lab M) and on Columbia agar plates. Mycobacteria were grown in Middlebrook's 7H9 broth and on Columbia agar plates. For phagocytic experiments after growth in broth, organisms were washed twice and resuspended in tissue culture Medium 199 supplemented with 25 m*M* HEPES buffer pH 7.3 (Gibco).

Antibacterial Agents

Ciprofloxacin was supplied by Bayer, RO 236240 by Roche, difloxacin by Abbott, rifapentine and rifampicin by Lepetit and RU 28965 and erythromycin by Roussell.

Effect of Antibacterial Agents on Intracellular Survival

Bacteria were opsonized by incubation in 10% (v/v) pooled normal human serum for 15–30 min at 37 °C at a concentration of 5×10^6 colony-formingunits(CFUs)/

Department of Medical Microbiology, Wright-Fleming Institute, St. Mary's Hospital Medical School, London W2 1PG, United Kingdom

The Influence of Antibiotics on the Host-Parasite Relationship III
Edited by G. Gillissen, W. Opferkuch, G. Peters, and G. Pulverer

ml and washed twice. Neutrophils were separated from human venous blood by dextran sedimentation, hypotonic lysis and washing. Mouse peritoneal macrophages were collected by washing out the peritoneal cavity with 3–4 ml ice-cold 199 5 days after intraperitoneal injection of thioglycollate broth. Macrophages were suspended in 199 supplemented with 1% fetal calf serum at 1% gelatin.

Equal volumes of cells and bacteria were mixed in a ratio of 5 to 1 for 15 min to allow ingestion to occur. Cells were washed thoroughly to remove free bacteria and, where staphylococci were being used, further treated with lysostaphin. Cells from an aliquot of suspension were lysed by sonication in distilled water at the beginning of the experiment for viable bacterial counting. Varying concentrations of the antibacterial agent to be tested were added to the suspension and the cells further incubated for up to 6 h (neutrophils) or 20 h (macrophages). At intervals, further aliquots were taken and lysed for bacterial counting.

Results

Tables 1 and 2 show the effect of the macrolides erythromycin and RU 28965 on *S. aureus* in neutrophils and macrophages respectively. Neither agent had much

Table 1. Effect of pH on intracellular activity of erythromycin 28965 in human neutrophils

Antibiotic	pH	% Intracellular survival of *S. aureus* at	
		4 h	8 h
Control	7.4	23	16
Control	6.0	22	>100
Erythromycin	7.4	13	4
Erythromycin	6.0	13	2.5
28965	7.4	15	4.5
28965	6.0	12.5	1.4

Table 2. Effect of erythromycin (2.0 mg/litre), Ro 28965 (10 mg/litre) and rifampicin (0.1 mg/litre) on survival of *S. aureus* in macrophages

Antibiotic	pH	% Surviving *S. aureus* at		
		2 h	4 h	20 h
Control	7.3	68	60	OG
Control	6.0	81	69	OG
Erythromycin	7.3	52	41	20
Erythromycin	6.0	81	77	91
28965	7.3	56	39	10
28965	6.0	67	66	57
Rifampicin	7.3	14	3	< 0.01
Rifampicin	6.0	17	2	< 0.01

OG, overgrown.

Table 3. Effect of RO 236240 on survival of *S. aureus* 6571 within mouse peritoneal macrophages over 20 h

Ro 236240 concentration (mg/litre)	Initial inoculum	% Survival of intracellular *S. aureus* T 2	T 20
–	4 $\times 10^6$	58	40
5	4 $\times 10^6$	30	10
1	4 $\times 10^6$	33	11
–	3.7 $\times 10^6$	54	38
5	3.7 $\times 10^6$	26	10
1	3.7 $\times 10^6$	40	10
–	1.85 $\times 10^6$	54	124
5	1.85 $\times 10^6$	33	6.5
1	1.85 $\times 10^6$	49	12

Both 5 and 1 mg/litre produce significant reduction in intracellular staphylococcal survival at 20 h.

Table 4. Effect of Ro 236240 on survival of *S. aureus* 6571 in human neutrophils over 4 h

Ro 236240 concentration (mg/litre)	Initial inoculum	% Survival of intracellular *s. aureus* T 2	T 4
–	1.16 $\times 10^6$	38	33
5	1.16 $\times 10^6$	33	16
1	1.16 $\times 10^6$	30	18
–	1.4 $\times 10^6$	57	49
5	1.4 $\times 10^6$	58	26
1	1.4 $\times 10^6$	54	31
–	8 $\times 10^6$	33	29
5	8 $\times 10^6$	31	12.5
1	8 $\times 10^6$	25	24

The higher concentration reduces intracellular staphylococcal survival by 50% or more by 4 h.

effect after 4 h incubation, but both reduced *S. aureus* counts at 8 and 20 h respectively. Macrolides are slowly bactericidal and have little effect when short incubation periods are used. Reduction of pH to 6 had little effect with neutrophils but a marked effect on macrophages. This may be because of the longer incubation period. With the macrophages rifampicin at 0.1 mg/litre was included as a positive control.

The effects of rifampicin and rifapentine are compared in Table 5. With a sensitive *S. aureus* both antibiotics produced a rapid reduction of intracellular organisms. However, a 100-fold increase in extracellular concentrations of rifampicin and rifapentine had no effect on the intracellular survival of a resistant strain.

Table 5. Effect of rifampicin and rifapentine on sensitive and resistant *S. aureus* ingested by neutrophils

Extracellular antibiotic concentration (mg/litre)	*Staphylococcus aureus* sensitivity	% Surviving *S. aureus* at	
		1 h	2 h
0	S	25	24
0	R	73	64
Rifampicin (0.01)	S	2	1
Rifampicin (0.1)	R	73	60
Rifampicin (1.0)	R	78	67
Rifapentine (0.02)	S	1	1
Rifapentine (0.1)	R	67	62
Rifapentine (1.0)	R	84	71

S, sensitive; R, resistant.

Table 6. Effect of ciprofloxacin on survival of *S. aureus* and *M. fortuitum* in macrophages

Ciprofloxacin concentration	Test organisms	% Surviving bacteria at		
		2 h	4 h	20 h
0	*S. aureus*	74	69	OG
0.1	*S. aureus*	104	80	54
0.5	*S. aureus*	60	50	21
2.0	*S. aureus*	64	22	4
0	*M. fortuitum*	87	90	94
0.5	*M. fortuitum*	78	65	53
2.0	*M. fortuitum*	62	41	32

OG, overgrown.

Table 7. Effect of Ro 236240 on intracellular survival of *S. aureus*, *M. fortuitum* and *M. chelonei* in macrophages

Ro 236240 concentration (mg/litre)	Organism	% Survival at		
		2 h	20 h	48 h
0	*S. aureus*	63	OG	ND
0.5	*S. aureus*	71	5	ND
2.0	*S. aureus*	64	0.5	ND
0	*M. fortuitum*	115	650	924
0.5	*M. fortuitum*	84	90	110
2.0	*M. fortuitum*	79	15	0.05
0	*M. chelonei*	85	385	790
0.5	*M. chelonei*	101	323	820
2.0	*M. chelonei*	91	240	750

OG, overgrown; ND, not done.

The effect of ciprofloxacin and RO 236240 on *S. aureus* and on mycobacterial survival within cells is shown in Tables 6 and 7. Both 4-quinolones were active against the sensitive *S. aureus* and *M. fortuitum*. In contrast the quinolone-resistant *M. chelonei* was unaffected by RO 236240. Similar results have been found for difloxacin.

The new rifamycins, macrolides and 4-quinolones are all active against intracellular organisms. This is an important factor in treating diseases caused by genera as diverse as *Mycobacterium, Legionella, Salmonella* and *Chlamydia*.

Summary

Intracellular bacteria are protected against most host defenses and antibacterial agents. The purpose of this study was to examine the effect of new quinolones, rifamycins, and macrolides on the survival of either *Staphylococcus aureus* or *Mycobacterium* spp. within neutrophils and macrophages. The macrolides erythromycin and RU 28965 had a considerable effect on *S. aureus* in neutrophils and macrophages after longer incubation periods. Rifampicin and rifapentine had a significant effect on intracellular organisms of a sensitive *S. aureus*, but not of a resistant strain. The two quinolones ciprofloxacin and RO 236240 were both active against the sensitive *S. aureus* and *M. fortuitum*. However, the quinolone-resistant *M. chelonei* remained unaffected. The clinical implications of these results in treating diseases caused by intracellular organisms are discussed.

References

1. Easmon CSF (1979) The effect of antibiotics on the intracellular survival of *Staphylococcus aureus*. Br J Exp Pathol 60:24–28
2. Easmon CSF, Crane JP (1984) Comparative uptake of rifampicin and rifapentine (DL 473) by human neutrophils. J Antimicrob Chemother 13:585–591

Effects of Beta-Lactam Antibiotics on the Lymphocyte Responses In Vitro and in Animals

E. A. Chaperon and A. C. Stonnington

Introduction

The cephalosporin antibiotics continue to be further developed and are among the more popular agents for treating bacterial infections [14, 15]. It has been shown that certain cephalosporins, even in therapeutic concentrations, can suppress [^{3}H]-thymidine incorporation by human peripheral blood lymphocytes following stimulation with mitogens or specific antigens [4, 8, 10]. Potential clinical implications for such observations remain unclear, since there is no assurance that such in vitro phenomena are paralleled by in vivo events. Studies designed to evaluate immune responses in animals, after injection with cephalosporins, have produced somewhat conflicting results [3, 5, 13], but do support the hypothesis that these agents may have immunoregulatory activity.

The present study extends previous work with human lymphocytes to a mouse model, and supports the observations of others [3] in showing that cephalosporins in culture can suppress responses of mouse splenic lymphocytes in a pattern similar to that already seen with human lymphocytes. The effects of injecting cephalosporins into normal mice on lymphocyte mitogenic responses, plaque-forming cell responses to sheep erythrocytes, and delayed hypersensitivity footpad reactions to the same antigen are also examined.

Materials and Methods

Animals. Male C3H/HeJ and C3HeB/FeJ mice (Jackson Laboratories, Bar Harbor, ME, United States) were used to evaluate the effects of cephalosporins on in vitro lymphocyte responses and plaque-forming cell production following injection of the animals with sheep erythrocytes. Male Swiss Webster mice (Sasco, Omaha, NE, United States) were used to determine delayed hypersensitivity responses. All mice ranged in age from 6 to 8 weeks.

Antimicrobials. The cephalosporins were supplied in powdered form by the manufacturers. Cephalothin, cephalexin, cefamandole, and cefazolin were provided by Eli Lilly and Company; cefoxitin was obtained from Merk, Sharpe and Dohme; cephradine and cephapirin came from Smith, Kline, and French Laboratories.

Department of Medical Microbiology, Creighton University School of Medicine,
2500 California Street, Omaha, NE 68178-0213, USA

The Influence of Antibiotics on the Host-Parasite Relationship III
Edited by G. Gillissen, W. Opferkuch, G. Peters, and G. Pulverer

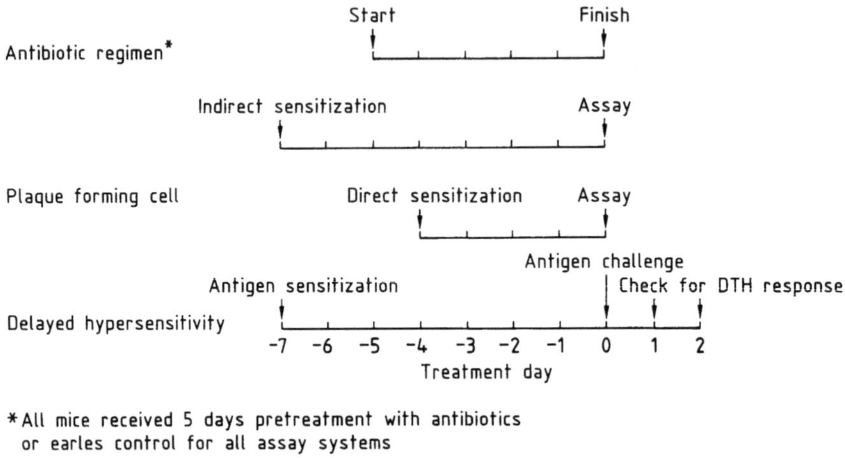

Fig. 1. Treatment schedule followed for evaluating the effect of pretreatment of mice with cephalosporins on lymphocyte responses to mitogens, PFC formation, and delayed hypersensitivity response. Mice received antibiotic (14 mg/kg body wt.) i.v. every 6 h for 5 days

Rifampin was obtained from Ciba-Geigy Corporation. Working solutions of all drugs were prepared in Earles balanced salt solution 10–30 min before use. The rifampin was dissolved in a small volume of methanol before dilution in saline.

Treatment of Mice. The animals were injected i.v. via tail vein every 6 h for 5 days (14 mg/kg body wt. in 0.5 ml). Controls received only diluent. There were four replicates per treatment group in each experiment. The same protocol was followed for all experiments (Fig. 1).

Determination of Antibiotic Serum Levels. The method of Bennett et al. [2] was followed. Log phase cultures of *Bacillus subtillis* (ATCC strain mic 10) in Mueller Hinton Broth (BBL) were adjusted to a #1 McFarland standard and swabbed in quadrant fashion on Kirby-Bauer plates. Blank sterile disks (BBL) were saturated with test sera or standards consisting of known concentrations of antibiotics in normal mouse serum. Zone diameters were measured after 18 h incubation at 37 °C, and unknown drug concentrations were determined from a standard curve of the appropriate standard.

Plaque-Forming Cells. A modification of the method of Jerne et al. [7] was used. On day 4 or 7 following i.p. immunization with 0.2 ml of a 20% suspension of washed sheep red cells (SRBCs) in Earles BSS, mice were killed, and splenic lymphocyte suspensions were prepared and tested for direct and indirect plaque-forming cells (PFCs).

Delayed-Type Hypersensitivity. The footpad swelling technique of Liew [9] as modified by McCarthy et al. [11] was employed. On day 7 following i.p. sensitization of mice with 0.2 ml of a suspension of washed SRBCs (10^8 cells/ml), pre-challenge thicknesses of both hind footpads were measured with a micrometer caliper. Left footpads were then injected with SRBCs (20 µl, 10^8 cells/ml), and right footpads were injected with buffer. Post challenge footpad thicknesses were measured at 24, 48, and 72 h.

Culture Conditions. Spleen cell cultures were performed using the method of Strong et al. [17]. Mice were killed by cervical dislocation, the spleens were removed aseptically, and the lymphocytes were teased with forceps into culture medium. After allowing clumps to settle, supernatant lymphocytes were washed three times and diluted in medium to 2.5×10^6 viable (Trypan blue excluding) cells/ml. Aliquots (0.2 ml) were distributed into wells of microtiter plates. The medium used was supplemented RPMI 1640 (Microbiological Associates). Penicillin and streptomycin were added to cultures of lymphocytes from cephalosporin-treated mice but were not used in those experiments in which cephalosporins were directly added to the cultures. The mitogens, which were added at the initiation of culture, included phytohemagglutinin (PHA)-P 8.5 µg/ml (Difco); concanavalin A (Con A) 3 µg/ml (Sigma); pokeweed mitogen $^1/_{10}$ dilution (Grand Island Biological Co.); and lipopolysaccharide (LPS) (*E. coli* 0127:B8) 25 µg/ml (Sigma). Cultures were incubated at 37 °C in 5 °CO_2. At 48 h, 0.4 Ci (methyl[^{3}H])thymidine (2 Ci/mmol; New England Nuclear Corp.) was added to each culture. Cells were collected at 66 h onto fiberglass filters with a semiautomated harvester (Otto Miller), dried, and counted in a liquid scintillation counter.

Statistical Analysis. Data were analyzed by Student's *t*-test or the Duncan Multiple Range test [16]. All data values represent means of data from three separate experiments ± SD. There were at least four replicates per treatment group in each experiment and all lymphocyte cultures were run in triplicate.

Results

Effect of Adding Cephalosporins Directly to Cell Cultures. The responses of C3H/HeJ splenic lymphocytes to PHA in cultures containing cephalosporins are indi-

Table 1. Effect of cephalosporins in culture on responses of C3H/HeJ splenic lymphocytes to PHA

Antibiotic	100[a]	50	25	12.5
Cephalothin	0.7[b]	29.1	65.2	76.5
Cefazolin	65.0	109.4	140.4	115.7
Cefamandole	9.9	51.2	92.6	94.5
Cephalexin	0.2	3.9	23.5	50.8
Cephradine	1.1	10.1	35.7	66.5
Cephapirin	80.3	137.8	138.3	132.7
Cefoxitin	7.4	93.9	113.8	110.9

[a] Antibiotic concentration in culture (µg/ml).
[b] Results expressed as percentages of response in cultures without antibiotic ($18.1 \pm 3.0 \times 10^3$ cpm/culture).

Table 2. Effect of cephalosporins in culture on mitogenic responses of C3HeB/FeJ splenic lymphocytes

Antibiotic	PHA	Con A	PWM	LPS
Diluent	41.8 ± 5.0[b]	22.7 ± 2.0	35.4 ± 2.7	47.2 ± 1.3
Cephalothin[a]	49.7	4.2	55.9	85.9
Cefazolin	119.2	16.7	89.9	97.7
Cefamandole	84.7	17.2	69.8	90.7
Cephalexin	46.5	10.3	9.4	57.6
Cephradine	7.4	6.5	36.2	65.7
Cephapirin	68.9	13.3	48.2	76.2
Cefoxitin	93.7	123.3	67.1	82.8
Rifampin	126.5	37.8	38.1	65.1

[a] Drug concentration in culture = 25 µg/ml.
[b] Counts/min per culture × 10^{-3} ± SD.
Results expressed as percentages of responses in cultures without antibiotic.

cated in Table 1. The mean response of control cultures containing no cephalosporins, expressed as cpm/culture × 10^{-3} ± SD, is indicated in the footnote to Table 1. All other values represent percentages of responses in the control cultures. Decreased responses ($P < 0.01$) were seen in all cultures containing cephalexin or cephradine. Cephalothin also suppressed ($P < 0.05$) responses at all drug concentrations but not to the same extent as cephradine and cephalexin. Responses were also suppressed in cultures containing 50 µg/ml cefamandole ($P < 0.01$) or 100 µg/ml cefoxitin ($P < 0.01$). Cultures containing cefazolin (25 µg/ml) or cephapirin (12.5, 25, and 50 µg/ml), however, showed increased responses ($P < 0.01$) to PHA.

The effects of adding 25 µg/ml cephalosporins directly to cultured C3HeB/FeJ lymphocytes on responses to four different mitogens are shown in Table 2. Responses to PHA were again suppressed ($P < 0.01$) by cephalexin, cephradine, and cephalothin. Rifampin, used as a positive control, was always suppressive at 50 or 100 µg/ml (data not presented), but elevated responses were sometimes seen at lower concentrations of drug. Lymphocyte responses to Con A were suppressed to varying degrees by the tested cephalosporins, the most suppressive again being cephalexin, cephradine, cephalothin, and cephapirin. Cefoxitin, a cephamycin, was suppressive only at nontherapeutic levels (100 µg/ml). Rifampin suppressed responses to Con A, even at 12.5 µg/ml. Cephalexin, cephradine, cephalothin, cephapirin, and rifampin consistently suppressed lymphocyte responses to Pokeweed Mitogen (PWM) ($P < 0.01$) at 25 µg/ml. Suppression of responses to LPS was generally less impressive, but was observed in cultures containing 25 µg/ml cephalexin, cephradine, or rifampin ($P < 0.05$).

Effect of Injecting C3HeB/FeJ Mice with Cephalosporins on Lymphocyte Responses. Table 3 represents the serum levels achieved in C3H mice following i.v. injection with 14 mg/kg body wt. of the cephalosporins. Fifteen minutes after a single injection, serum levels ranged from 24 to 32 µg/ml. By 4 h, the antibiotics were undetectable.

Table 3. Serum levels achieved following injection[a] of mice with cephalosporins

Antibiotic[c]	15 min[b]	30 min	60 min	240 min
Cephalothin	28[c]	10	9.5	<1
Cefazolin	32	18	7.2	<1
Cefamandole	31	15	7.1	<1
Cephalexin	25	17	3.2	<1
Cephradine	24	18	6.5	<1
Cephapirin	26	12	6.0	<1
Cefoxitin	31	15	8.2	<1
Earles BSS (control)	<1	<1	<1	<1

[a] 14 mg/kg body wt. injected.
[b] Mice bled from heart at indicated times. Sera were pooled from both C3H/HeJ and C3Heb/FeJ mice (four mice/group).
[c] Antimicrobial level in micrograms per milliliter determined from zone diameter on Kirby-Bauer plates.

Table 4. Effect of injecting C3HeB/FeJ mice with cephalosporins on lymphocyte responses to mitogens

Antibiotic	PHA	Con A	PWM	LPS
Diluent	43.7±0.6[b]	90.7±1.6	19.7±1.2	24.7±1.2
Cephalothin[a]	54.2[c]	133.4	28.9	126.7
Cefazolin	68.6	118.0	100.0	94.3
Cefamandole	102.2	115.1	145.7	133.6
Cephalexin	48.0	52.6	25.4	100.0
Cephradine	51.9	22.0	75.6	136.4
Cephapirin	71.6	41.1	103.0	100.0
Cefoxitin	85.4	90.1	103.0	126.7
Rifampin	141.9	125.7	55.8	126.7

[a] 14 mg/kg body wt. administered every 6 h for 5 days.
[b] Counts/min per culture × 10^{-3} ± SD.
[c] Results expressed as percentages of responses by diluent controls.

Lymphocytes from mice pretreated with cephradine or cephalexin (Table 4) consistently showed decreased response to PHA, Con A, and PWM ($P<0.01$). Cells from mice pretreated with cephalothin had reduced responses to PHA and PWM ($P<0.01$). Pretreatment with cephapirin resulted in a suppressed response to Con A ($P<0.01$), and rifampin only suppressed the lymphocyte response to PWM ($P<0.01$). In no other treatment group were suppressed responses seen, but it was of interest to note elevated responses in mice pretreated with cefamandole (Con A, PWM, LPS), cephalothin (Con A, PWM), and rifampin (PHA, Con A, LPS).

Table 5 summarizes the effects of in vitro and in vivo cephalosporins on murine lymphocyte responses to mitogens. Only those drugs that consistently suppressed lymphocyte responses when added directly to cultures, i.e., cephalexin, cephradine, cephalothin, and cephapirin, had any suppressive effect on lymphocyte responses when administered to the mice.

Table 5. Summary of the effect of cephalosporins on mitogenic responses of C3Heb/FeJ lymphocytes

Antibiotic	PHA	Con A	PWM	LPS
Cephalothin	+	±	+	−
Cefazolin	−	±	−	−
Cefamandole	−	±	−	−
Cephalexin	+	+	+	±
Cephradine	+	+	+	±
Cephapirin	−	+	±	−
Cefoxitin	−	−	−	−
Rifampin	−	±	+	±

+, Lymphocyte responses suppressed following preinjection of mice with cephalosporins or when drugs are added to culture (25 μg/ml).
±, Lymphocyte responses suppressed only when cephalosporins are added to culture (25 μg/ml).
−, Lymphocyte responses not suppressed.

Table 6. Effect of cephalosporins on plaque-forming cells

Treatment group	Direct plaques (4 day)	Indirect plaques (7 day)
Cephalothin	2115 (306)[a]	1968 (28)
Cefazolin	2232 (410)	1563 (37)*
Cefamandole	2092 (515)	1742 (166)
Cephalexin	2200 (278)	1380 (143)*
Cephradine	1942 (138)	1468 (181)*
Cephapirin	1947 (185)	1688 (245)
Cefoxitin	2202 (231)	1485 (66)*
Rifampin	1520 (253)	1213 (309)*
Earles (control)	2165 (492)	1790 (171)

[a] Number of plaques/10^6 cells (SD).
* Significantly different ($p<0.05$) from control group.

Effect of Injections of Cephalosporins on Plaque-Forming Cell Responses. As the data in Table 6 indicate, no differences were seen between treatment groups in the number of direct PFCs 4 days after immunization, but comparison of 7-day indirect PFC responses revealed significant reduction ($P<0.05$) in those mice pretreated with cephalexin, cephradine, cefoxitin, cefazolin, or rifampin. Mice pretreated with cephalothin, cefamandole, or cephapirin did not differ from controls.

Effect of Pretreating with Cephalosporins on Delayed Hypersensitivity Response. Figure 2 shows the differences in footpad thickness in sensitized mice 24, 48, and 72 h after challenge with SRBCs. The prechallenge values (0 h) were measured immediately before injection of antigen. Footpad reactions reached a maximum at 24 h. Suppression ($P<0.05$) was seen in the response of most of the drug-treated animals at this time, with the greatest suppression seen in mice pretreated with cefamandole and moderate suppression in animals injected with cefazolin,

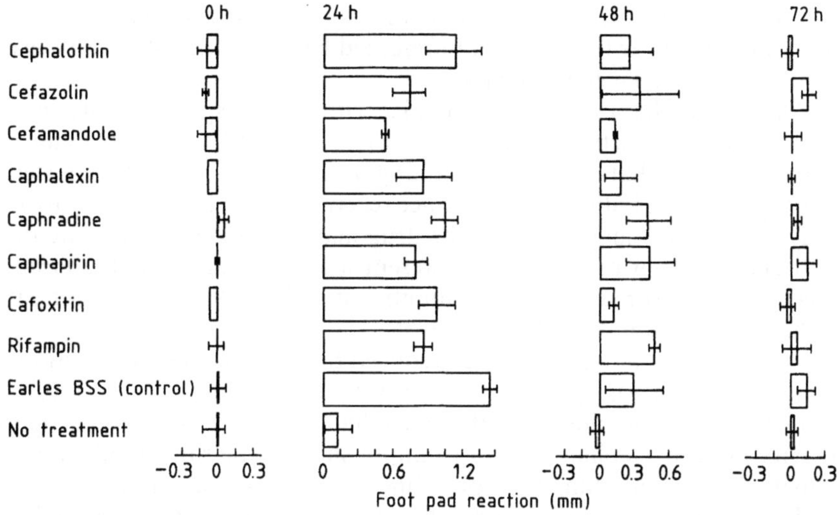

Fig. 2. Effect of pretreatment of Swiss Webster mice with cephalosporins on delayed footpad reaction. Values are expressed as the mean difference in footpad thickness (mm) between footpad, challenged with antigen and contralateral saline controls ± SD

cephapirin, cephalexin, or rifampin. At 48 h post challenge, there were no significant differences between treatment groups.

Discussion

The results of this study and reports of others [3] clearly demonstrate that cephalosporins can suppress in vitro responses of murine splenic lymphocytes. Although every drug tested suppressed the response to at least one mitogen, the overall pattern resembled that seen earlier with human lymphocytes [4]. Cephradine, cephalexin, and cephalothin were again found to be the most active and at the same dose levels in culture (≧25 μg/ml).

Reduced mitogenic responses of lymphocytes obtained from mice after injection with cephalosporins were most frequently seen in cultures from animals receiving cephalexin, cephradine, cephalothin, or cephapirin. The finding that these same drugs, which are suppressive when added directly to cultures, can produce similar effects when injected into animals gives support to the possibility that these findings may have clinical significance.

The mechanism for the augmented lymphocyte responses seen in mice pretreated with some of the cephalosporins is unclear. Cefazolin, which produced increased responses to Con A, has previously been reported to increase responses to PHA when added to cultures of human lymphocytes, a finding also seen when 25 μg/ml was added to cultured mouse lymphocytes. Responses to PWM or LPS were augmented in cells from mice pretreated with cefamandole, cephradine, or cefoxitin. This might be interpreted, at least for the first two agents, as a deregulation of B-cell responses to these mitogens resulting from the inhibitory action of cephalosporins on Con A responsive T-suppressor cells (cf. Table 2). It certainly would appear from the data presented here that cephalosporins exert their greatest effect on T-cell responses.

The finding that pretreatment of mice with cephalosporins results in a modest but significant reduction in indirect, but not direct, PFCs may be interpreted as further evidence that the drugs are acting on T cells. Gillissen [5] reported a similar suppression of indirect PFCs in mice receiving cephalothin on day 6 (30 mg/kg body wt. × 2) and suggested that the drug may be directly influencing the PFCs. Of the cephalosporins tested in the present study, cephalexin and cephradine produced the greatest reduction in the number of indirect PFCs. Mice pretreated with cephalothin did not differ from controls.

All of the cephalosporins tested reduced the delayed footpad reaction to some degree. It was surprising to note, however, that the greatest effect was seen in mice treated with cefamandole since this agent had shown almost no other suppressive activity in mice. Cephalexin and rifampin showed the same moderate degree of activity, but cephalothin and cephradine were only minimally suppressive.

Rifampin was selected as a positive control because of its reported ability to inhibit mitogenic responses. PFC formation, and DTH reactions [1]. Suppression of lymphocyte responses to mitogens were not always seen when 25 μg/ml rifampin was added to the cultures, but higher concentrations (50 μg/ml) always strongly inhibited the responses. The effects of pretreating mice with rifampin on PFC production and the DTH reaction in our study are in agreement with the results of others.

The results of this study are difficult to reconcile with the undeniable clinical effectiveness of the cephalosporins. There is little evidence for secondary infections associated with their use. Nevertheless, there are recent reports that cephalosporine are up to 20 times more effective than the penicillins in inhibiting both granulopoiesis in vitro [12] and generation of virus-specific cytotoxic T cells [6]. Since these effects were produced with clinically achievable levels of drug, further investigation of these agents is clearly indicated.

Summary

It has been shown that cephalosporins suppress [^{3}H]thymidine incorporation by human lymphocytes following stimulation with mitogens in vitro. We wished to determine whether the cephalosporins would also suppress (1) mitogen responses of murine splenic lymphocytes, (2) plaque-forming cells (PFCs) (direct and indirect), and (3) delayed-type hypersensitivity (DTH) responses to sheep red blood cells (SRBCs) after mice had been preinjected with the cephalosporins (14 mg/kg body wt. i.v. every 6 h for 5 days). Suppression of responses to PHA or Con A was observed in lymphocytes from mice pretreated with cephalexin, cephradine, or cephalothin. No suppression was seen in mice pretreated with cefamandole. Suppression of indirect PFCs was seen in mice pretreated with cefazolin, cefoxitin, cephradine, cephalexin, or rifampin, but not in animals pretreated with cephalothin, cefamandole, or cephapirin. No suppression of direct PFCs was observed. All of the cephalosporins tested suppressed the DTH footpad response to

SRBCs. The suppression of in vitro and in vivo responses of mice preinjected with cephalosporin doses comparable to those used therapeutically suggests that these results may have clinical significance.

References

1. Bassi L, Berardino LD, Arioli V, Silvestrio LG, Ligniere ELC (1973) Conditions for immunosuppression by rifampin. J Infect Dis 128:736–744
2. Bennett JV, Brodie JL, Benner EJ, Kirby WMM (1966) Simplified, accurate method for antibiotic assay of clinical specimens. Appl Microbiol 14:170–177
3. Borowski J, Jakoniuk P, Talarczyk J (1985) The influence of some cephalosporins on immunological response. Drugs Exp Clin Res 11(2):83–88
4. Chaperon EA, Sanders WE Jr (1978) Suppression of lymphocyte responses to cephalosporins. Infect Immun 19:378–384
5. Gillissen GJ (1982) Influence of cephalosporins on humoral immune response. In: Eickenberg HV, Hahn H, Opferkuch W (eds) The influence of antibiotics on host-parasite relationship. Springer, Berlin Heidelberg New York, pp 5–11
6. Huegin AW, Cerny A, Zinkernagal RM, Neftel KA (1986) Suppressive effects of beta-lactam antibiotics on in vitro generation of cytotoxic T cells. Int J Immunopharmacol 8(7):723–729
7. Jerne NK, Henry C, Nordin AA, Fuji H, Koros AMC, Lefkovits I (1974) Plaque forming cells: methodology and theory. Transplant Rev 18:130–191
8. Larson SE, DaMert GJ, Collins-Lech C, Sohnie PG (1980) Direct stimulation of lymphokine production by cephalothin. J Infect Dis 142:252–272
9. Liew FY (1977) Regulation of delayed-type hypersensitivity. I. T suppressor cells for delayed-type hypersensitivity to sheep erythrocytes in mice. Eur J Immunol 7:714–718
10. Manzella JP, Clark JK (1983) Effect of moxalactam and cefuroxime on mitogen stimulated mononuclear leukocytes. Antimicrob Agents Chemother 23:360–363
11. McCarthy RE, Arnold LY, Babcock GF (1977) Dextran sulfate: an adjuvant for cell mediated immune responses. Immunology 32:963–974
12. Neftel KA, Hauser SP, Muller MR (1985) Inhibition of granulopoiesis in vivo and in vitro by beta-lactam antibiotics. J Infect Dis 152:90–98
13. Roszkowski W, Ko HL, Roszkowski K, Jeljaszewicz J, Pulverer G (1985) Antibiotics and immunomodulation: effects of cefotaxime, amikacin, mezlocillin, pipericillin and clindamycin. Med Microbiol Immunol (Berl) 173(5):279–289
14. Sanders CC, Sanders WE Jr (1986) The cephalosporins and cephamycins. In: Peterson PK, Verhoef J (eds) Antimicrobial Agents Annual 1. Elsevier, Amsterdam, pp 66–90
15. Sanders CC, Sanders WE Jr (1987) The cephalosporins and cephamycins. In: Petersen PK, Verhoef J (eds) Antimicrobial Agents Annual 2. Elsevier, Amsterdam, pp 70–95
16. Snedecor GW, Cochran WG (1967) Statistical methods. 6th edn. Iowa State University, Ames, pp 258–298
17. Strong DM, Ahmed AA, Thuxman GB, Sell KW (1973) In vitro stimulation of murine spleen cells using a microculture system and a multiple automated sample harvester. J Immunol Methods 2:279–291

Effect of Trimethoprim/Sulfamethoxazole on Human Neutrophil Function and Survival of Mice Infected with Candida *

T. N. PATSELAS [1], G. W. SULLIVAN, and G. L. MANDELL

Introduction

Studies indicate that trimethoprim/sulfamethoxazole (TMP/SMX) may have beneficial actions on host defense against infection beyond its direct antimicrobial role. TMP/SMX has been reported to correct abnormalities of neutrophil motility in selected patients [3]. Futhermore, prophylactic treatment of patients with chronic granulomatous disease of childhood prolongs disease-free periods [7, 13] and TMP/SMX has been effective in reducing the number of infectious episodes in neutropenic patients [4–6]. These latter two observations may be due solely to the antimicrobial activity of TMP/SMX.

The purpose of this study was to investigate in vitro and in vivo effects of TMP/SMX using human neutrophils and a mouse model of *Candida* infection.

Materials and Methods

Trimethoprim/Sulfamethoxazole

Trimethoprim and sulfamethoxazole (supplied by Hoffmann-La Roche, Nutley, NJ, United States) were combined in proportions used in commercial preparations for the in vivo studies. This ratio of TMP to SMX was 1:5. The ratio used in the in vitro studies was 1:17, approximating that found in human serum. Trimethoprim was dissolved in 0.1 *N* lactic acid (2400 μg/ml) and sulfamethoxazole in 0.1 *N* sodium hydroxide (20000 μg/ml); both were diluted in normal saline or appropriate cell-suspending medium.

Polymorphonuclear Neutrophil Chemotaxis and Motility

Heparinized venous blood was drawn from healthy volunteers. Erythrocytes were allowed to sediment by gravity at room temperature for 1 h. The leukocyte-rich plasma was removed, polymorphonucelar neutrophils (PMN) washed, and the

* This study was supported in part by a grant from Hoffmann-La Roche, Nutley, NJ.
[1] *Present address:* Eastern Virginia Medical School Norfolk, VA, USA
Division of Infectious Diseases, Department of Internal Medicine, University of Virginia School of Medicine, Charlottesville, VA 22908, USA

The Influence of Antibiotics on the Host-Parasite Relationship III
Edited by G. Gillissen, W. Opferkuch, G. Peters, and G. Pulverer

concentration of PMNs adjusted to 5×10^7 PMNs/ml in Hank's balanced salt solution (HBSS, Microbiological Assoc., Bethesda, MD, United States).

Neutrophil chemotaxis was studied by the method of Nelson et al. [11]. PMNs were preincubated for 30 min with or without TMP/SMX at 37 °C in a shaking H_2O bath. After centrifugation for 5 min at 150 g, the cell pellet was resuspended in 0.1 ml supernatant to give a final concentration of 5×10^7 PMNs/ml.

The PMNs were placed in the center well of the triplet and nonchemotactic media in the inner well. The following chemoattractants were used in the outer wells: *n*-formyl methionyl leucyl phenylalanine (100 n*M*, FMLP) (Sigma Chemical, St. Louis, MO, United States), zymosan-activated serum (ZAS), and opsonized *Candida albicans*. ZAS was made fresh daily by tumbling zymosan, 1 mg/ml, (Sigma Chemical) for 30 min at 37 °C with fresh autologous serum containing 250 m*M* ε-aminocaproic acid (Sigma Chemical). The zymosan particles were removed by centrifugation at 3000 g for 5 min. Opsonized *C. albicans* (Strain B311, American Type Culture Collection, Rockville, MD #32354) was prepared by tumbling washed *C. albicans* (from a 24-h trypic soy broth culture) with 0.5 ml fresh autologous serum for 45 min at 37 °C [5×10^9 colony-forming units(CFUs)/ml].

Incubation of the agarose plates was carried out for 2 h at 37 °C in a humidified atmosphere containing 5% CO_2 in air. The plates were fixed with methanol, stained with Giemsa stain (Harleco, Gibbstown, NJ, United States), and the PMN migration zones measured. Directed migration was the distance in millimeters that neutrophils moved from the center well toward the chemoattractant in the outer well, and random migration was the distance moved toward a nonchemoattractive medium in the inner well.

Phagocytosis and Killing of Candida by Polymorphonuclear Neutrophils

A differential centrifugation method was used to determine the effect of TMP/SMX on the ingestion and killing of *C. albicans* by neutrophils. PMNs isolated from whole blood by dextran sedimentation were pretreated for 30 min with or without TMP/SMX and then tumbled with 3 to 4×10^6 CFUs/ml *C. albicans* (B311) at 37 °C in HBSS containing 10% normal pooled human serum. Samples were removed at specified times for determination of total, supernatant, and sediment-associated viable yeast [2].

Phagocytosis and killing of *Candida* was also investigated using the Geimsa stain technique described by Lehrer [8]. PMNs isolated by dextran sedimentation were pretreated for 30 min with or without TMP/SMX. Neutrophil monolayers prepared on glass coverslips were covered with 0.5 ml *C. albicans* suspension at 1×10^6 CFUs/ml and incubated for 0, 15, 30, 60, and 90 min at 37 °C. The glass coverslips were rinsed, fixed with methanol, and stained with Giemsa stain. Neutrophils were examined under 1000 X for intracellular yeast. Nonviable organisms were identified as "ghosts" by their absence of cytoplasmic basophilic stain and unaltered, viable yeast organisms were those that retained a deep-blue cytoplasmic stain. To express phagocytosis, results were reported as total *C. albicans*/100 PMNs. The percentage of intracellular *C. albicans* which were identified as "ghosts" was also recorded.

Superoxide Production

Polymorphonuclear neutrophils (0.5–1.5 × 10^6) in a total volume of 0.5 ml HBSS (Microbiological Associates, Bethesda, MD, United States) containing 120 μ*M* cytochrome c were agitated for 0 or 10 min at 37 °C in 5-ml plastic culture tubes (Falcon, Oxnard, CA, United States) in a shaking water bath. Superoxide dismutase (SOD, Sigma Chemical) (0.1 mg/ml) was added to the nonincubated 0-min samples. The reaction in the incubated samples was stopped by submerging the reaction tubes in an ice water bath for 10 min. The tubes were centrifuged at 3000 g × 5 min at 4 °C. The supernatants were decanted and their absorbance read at a wavelength of 550 nm with a Gilford model 2400 spectrophotometer (Gilford Instrument Laboratories, Oberlin, OH, United States). The nanomoles cytochrome c reduced was calculated per 1 × 10^6 PMNs using the formula:

(OD 37 °C–OD 4 °C)/(0.0185)/[PMN]

utilizing the extinction coefficient of 1.85 × 10^4

cm^2/mmol (reduced-oxidized) [10].

The possibility of TMP/SMX acting as an $O_{\bullet}^{-}$ scavenger was investigated. Superoxide was generated with xanthine (1.5 m*M*) and xanthine oxidase (50 mg/ml) for 5 min in a shaker bath at 37 °C in the presence of cytochrome c (120 mm). Catalase (500 U/ml) was added to prevent reoxidation of cytochrome c by H_2O_2. TMP/SMX at 120/2000 μg/ml was added and cytochrome c reduction was measured.

Minimal Inhibitory Concentration Determination

The MIC for TMP/SMX to *C. albicans* (B311) was determined using twofold serial dilutions of TMP/SMX in tryptic soy broth with an inoculum of 5 × 10^5 *C. albicans*/ml. The MIC was defined as the lowest concentration of drug that produced no turbidity after incubation for 24 and 48 h at 37 °C [12].

Mouse Survival

Fifty-seven 30-g ICR mice (Flow laboratories, Dublin, VA, United States) were pretreated with a single dose of TMP/SMX (2 and 10 mg/kg respectively) intravenously via the tail vein 30 min prior to i.v. infection with 3 × 10^5 to 9 × 10^6 CFUs *C. albicans* (strain B311). The mice were then treated with the same i.v. dose of TMP/SMX daily. An equal number of mice were sham treated with normal saline. The LD_{50} values with 95% confidence limits at 1, 2, 3, 4, 5, and 6 days postinfection were determined by the method of Litchfield and Wilcoxon [9].

Calculation and Expression of Results

Unless otherwise stated the results are expressed as the mean value ± standard error of the mean. Statistical evaluations were performed by the paired Student *t*-test.

Results

Polymorphonuclear Neutrophil Chemotaxis and Motility

Trimethoprim/sulfamethoxazole enhanced PMN random migration and directed migration to FMLP, opsonized *C. albicans,* and ZAS (Fig. 1). Random migration of PMNs was significantly increased by TMP/SMX at levels of 3/50 (μg TMP/μg SMX/ml respectively) and above ($P < 0.05$). TMP/SMX in concentrations of 30/500, 60/1000, and 120/2000 (μg TMP/μg SMX/ml respectively) significantly increased directed migration to two of the three chemoattractants ($P < 0.05$). TMP/SMX was not a chemotactic attractant for PMNs.

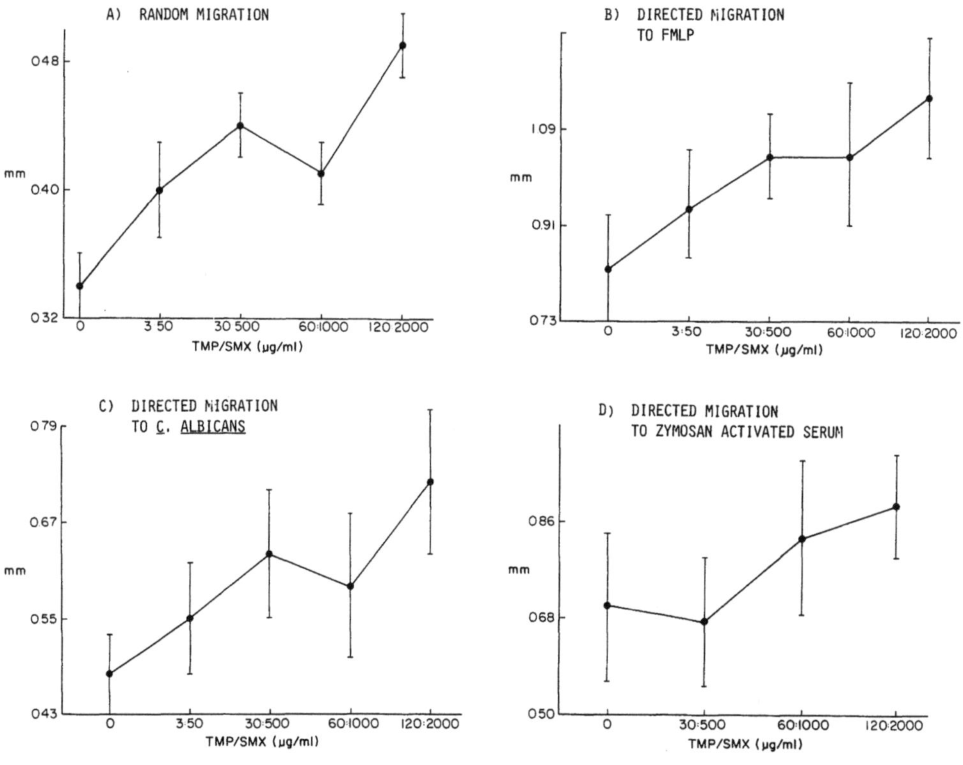

Fig. 1 A–D. Effect of TMP/SMX on PMN migration for 2 h under agarose. Random migration **A**; directed migration to FMLP (100 n*M*) **B**; *C. albicans* **C**; and zymosan-activated serum **D**. Mean ± SEM. Results are of four to five separate experiments

***Candida* Phagocytosis and Killing**

Differential Centrifugation Assay. There was no effect of TMP/SMX at 3 and 50 µg/ml respectively on ingestion or killing of *C. albicans*. High concentrations (120 and 2000 µg/ml respectively) did not alter ingestion but markedly decreased killing of ingested *C. albicans*. At 60 min 67% of all the cell-associated yeast (sediment) was alive in the TMP/SMX-treated suspension compared with only 18% of the cell-associated yeast viable in the untreated PMNs (Fig. 2).

Microscopic Assay. Results from experiments using glass-adherent PMNs supported the differential centrifugation assay results. Achievable serum levels of TMP/SMX (3 and 50 µg/ml respectively) did not significantly alter ingestion or

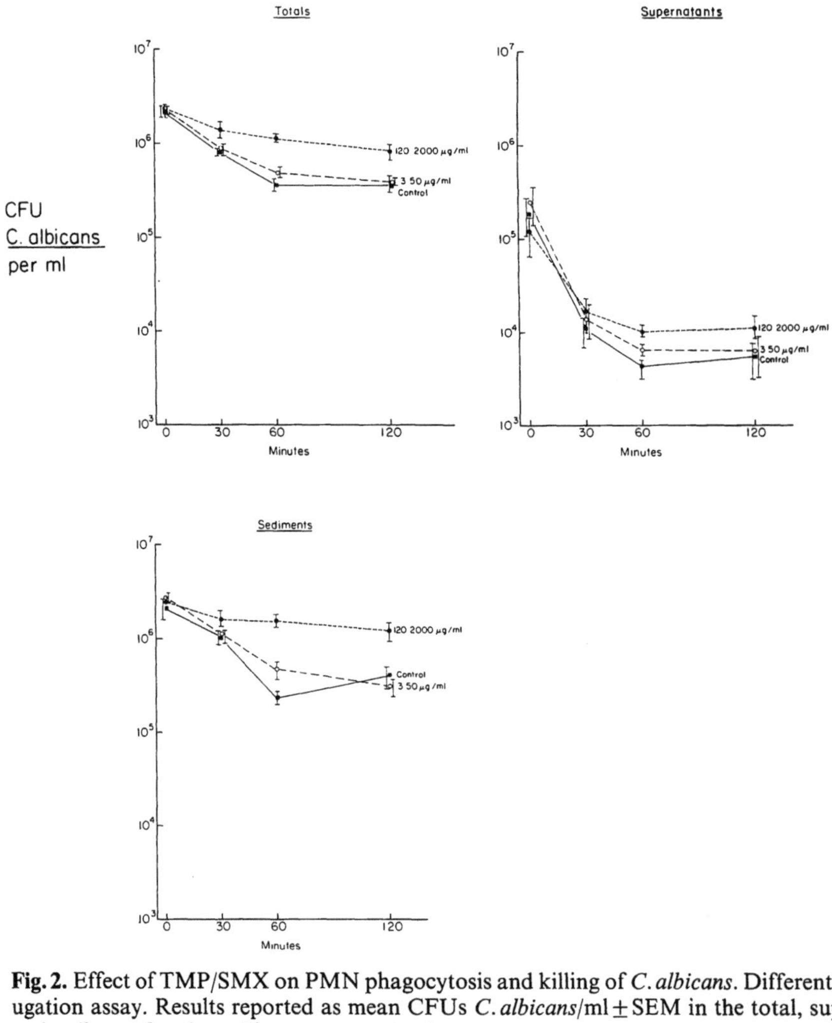

Fig. 2. Effect of TMP/SMX on PMN phagocytosis and killing of *C. albicans*. Differential centrifugation assay. Results reported as mean CFUs *C. albicans*/ml ± SEM in the total, supernatant, and sediment fractions. Five separate experiments

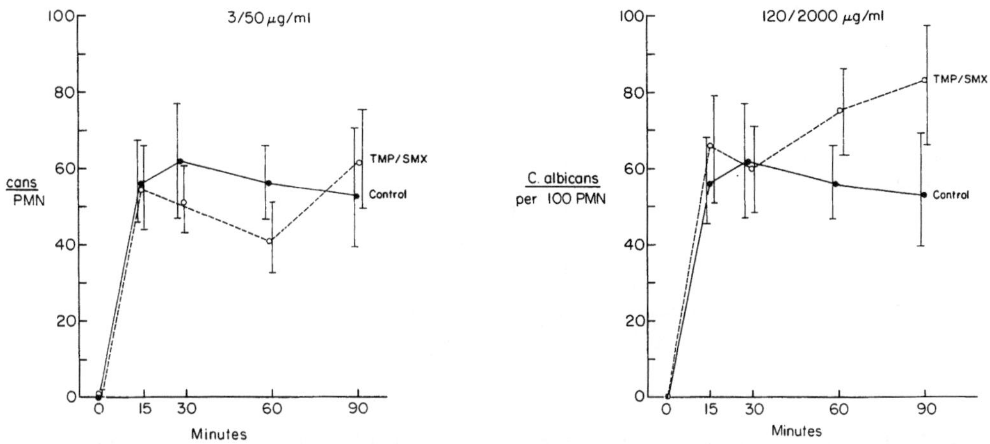

Fig. 3. Effect of two concentrations of TMP/SMX on PMN phagocytic index for *C. albicans*. Results are reported as *C. albicans*/100 PMN ± SEM (three to four separate experiments)

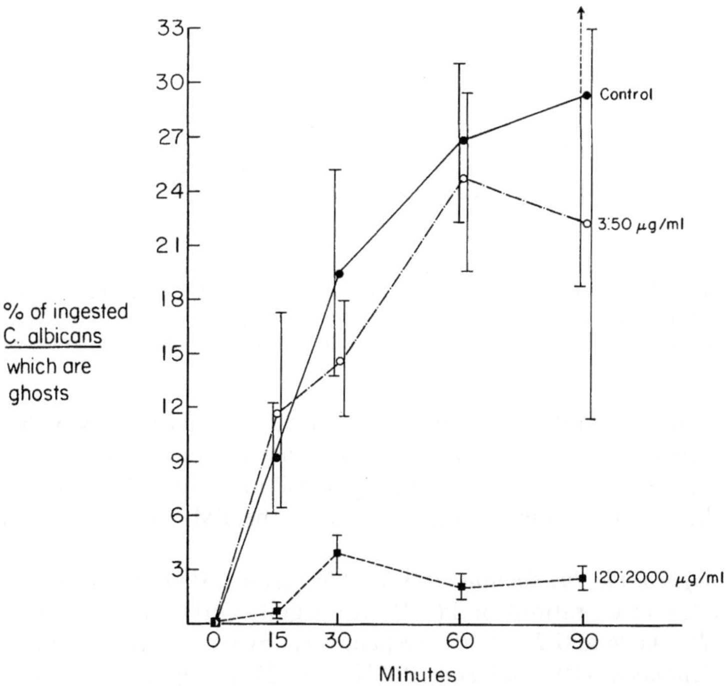

Fig. 4. Effect of TMP/SMX on killing of *C. albicans*. The results are reported as percentage of ingested *C. albicans* which are nonstaining (nonviable) "ghosts" ± SEM (three to four separate experiments)

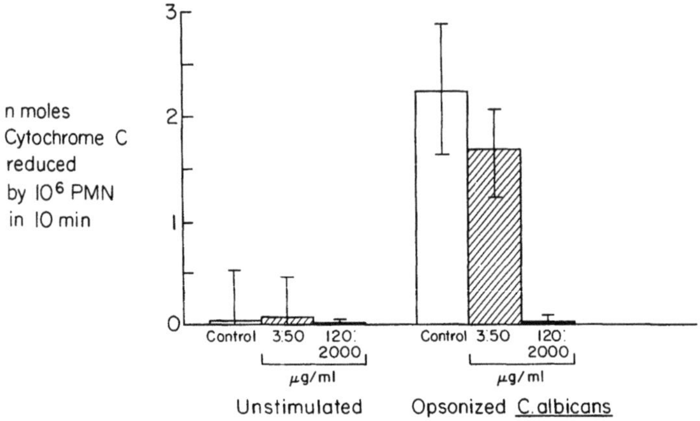

Fig. 5. Effect of TMP/SMX on PMN superoxide production by unstimulated PMNs and by PMNs incubated with *C. albicans*. The results are reported as nmol cytochrome c reduced by 10^6 PMNs in 10 min ± SEM (six separate experiments)

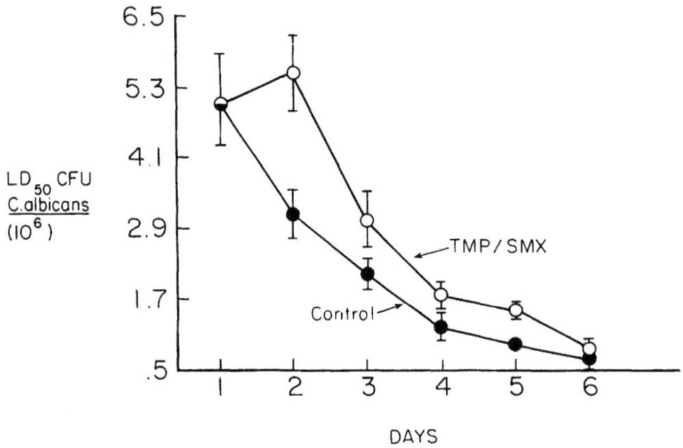

Fig. 6. Effect of TMP/SMX on mouse survival after i.v. infection with *C. albicans*. The results are reported as LD_{50} (CFUs *C. albicans*). TMP/SMX (2 mg/10 mg/kg, *open circles*) and untreated (*solid circles*). *Vertical bars* denote 95% confidence limits. Four separate experiments

killing of *C. albicans*. Higher concentrations of TMP/SMX did not affect phagocytosis (Fig. 3), but significantly decreased intracellular killing. At 60 min 27% of ingested organisms were dead "ghosts" in untreated PMNs, whereas only 2% of the ingested *Candida* were "ghosts" in the TMP/SMX-treated cells (Fig. 4).

Superoxide Production. Achievable serum (3/50 μg/ml) and high (120/2000 μg/ml) concentrations of TMP/SMX significantly inhibited superoxide production ($P = 0.026$ and $P = 0.001$, respectively) by neutrophils stimulated by ingestion of *C. albicans* (10 *C. albicans*/PMN) (Fig. 5). In separate experiments the same concentration of TMP/SMX did not scavenge O_2^- produced by the xanthine/xanthine oxidase reaction and pure opsonized *C. albicans* did not reduce cytochrome c.

Antimicrobial Activity. No inhibition of *C. albicans* growth was demonstrated at 64/1280 μg/ml TMP/SMX.

Animal Survival. Treatment of mice with TMP/SMX (2 and 10 mg/kg, respectively) improved mouse survival on subsequent challenge with *C. albicans* (Fig. 6). TMP/SMX significantly increased the LD_{50} of *C. albicans* for mice at 2, 3, 4, and 5 days after infection ($P<0.05$).

Discussion

High concentrations of TMP/SMX did increase both random and directed migration of PMNs in vitro to several chemoattractants including *C. albicans*. Levels of TMP/SMX similar to those achieved in serum with usual doses increased (but not significantly) directed migration and significantly increased random migration.

In vitro high TMP/SMX doses did not affect phagocytosis, but did significantly depress postphagocytic superoxide production as measured by cytochrome c reduction and microbicidal activity. Others have shown that sulfonamides reduce the ability of human PMNs to iodinate and kill *C. albicans* [8]. Anderson [1] and Siegel and Remington [14] demonstrated a decrease in postphagocytic protein iodination, H_2O_2 release, and chemiluminescence stimulated by yeast following in vitro TMP/SMX exposure. TMP/SMX did not suppress the oxidative burst in vivo [1].

The prophylactic effect of TMP/SMX in neutropenic patients may be due entirely to the antimicrobial activity of the combination. When a TMP/SMX-resistant organism is evaluated the data are inconclusive. Neutropenic patients on oral prophylactic TMP/SMX demonstrated higher rates of *Candida* colonization of the alimentary tract [4] and an equal number of disseminated candidiasis episodes [5] compared with control patients who did not receive prophylactic medications. In contrast, Kauffman et al. [6] report a reduction in *Candida* infections in TMP/SMX-treated neutropenic patients. Since the total number of *Candida* infections in all three of these studies was low it is difficult to draw definite conclusions.

Even though there was no discernable direct antimicrobial activity of TMP/SMX on *C. albicans*, TMP/SMX significantly increased the LD_{50} of mice acutely infected i.v. with *C. albicans*. A possible explanation is stimulation of mouse PMN function. Another possible mechanisms that could explain increased mouse survival following TMP/SMX treatment is prevention of secondary infections by TMP/SMX-sensitive organisms. Although TMP/SMX has only modest ability to alter PMN function at achievable serum levels, this may be of some importance in defense against infection.

Summary

Trimethoprim/sulfamethoxazole (TMP/SMX) has been reported to correct abnormalities of neutrophil chemotaxis in selected patients.

We examined the effect of TMP/SMX on chemotaxis and chemokinesis of normal human polymorphonuclear neutrophils (PMNs) under agarose. Therapeutic levels of TMP/SMX (3/50 μg/ml) had an in vitro stimulatory effect on random ($P = 0.049$) and a small but nonsignificant effect on directed migration to *f*-methionyl leucyl phenylalanine (FMLP) and *Candida albicans* ($P = 0.052$ and 0.073 respectively). Higher levels of TMP/SMX (30/500 μg/ml) significantly increased both random (0.34 ± 0.02 to 0.44 ± 0.02 mm, $P = 0.006$) and directed (0.48 ± 0.05 to 0.63 ± 0.08 mm, $P = 0.029$) migration to opsonized *C. albicans*. It similarly increased directed migration to FMLP- and zymosan-activated serum (both $P \leqq 0.02$).

Administration of 3/50 μg/ml and 120/2000 μg/ml TMP/SMX in vitro depressed the postphagocytic oxidative burst (24% and 100%, $P = 0.026$ and $P = 0.001$, respectively). Administration of 120/2000 μg/ml TMP/SMX but not 3/50 μg/ml diminished PMN candicidal activity ($P = 0.001$). Phagocytosis was not affected by TMP/SMX up to 120/2000 μg/ml.

Although TMP/SMX demonstrated no activity against *C. albicans* in vitro [minimal inhibitory concentration (MIC) >64/1280 μg/ml], daily i.v. doses of TMP/SMX (2/10 mg/kg) improved mouse survival after i.v. infection with *C. albicans*. TMP/SMX significantly increased the LD_{50} at days 2, 3, 4, 5, and 6 following infection ($P < 0.05$).

Since the *Candida* was not susceptible to the antimicrobial effect of TMP/SMX, we hypothesize that the increased survival of the infected mice may be related to enhanced neutrophil mobility.

References

1. Anderson R, Grabow G, Oosthaizen R, Theron A, Van Rensburg AJ (1980) Effects of sulfamethoxazole and trimethoprim on human neutrophil and lymphocyte functions in vitro: in vivo effects of co-trimoxazole. Antimicrob Agents Chemother 17:322–326
2. Bergman MJ, Guerrant RL, Murad F, Richardson SH, Weaver D, Mandell GL (1978) Interaction of polymorphonuclear neutrophils with *Escherichia coli*. J Clin Invest 61:227–234
3. De La Cruz A, Oleske J, La Braico J, Cooper R, Fishman D, Minnefor A, Lin R, Garcia R (1980) Correction of polymorphonuclear leukocyte chemotaxis defects with trimethoprim-sulfamethoxazole. Curr Chemother Infect Dis 12:185–186
4. Gualtieri RJ, Donowitz GR, Kaiser DL, Hess CE, Sande MA (1983) Double-blind randomized study of prophylactic trimethoprim/sulfamethoxazole in granulocytopenic patients with hematologic malignancies. Am J Med 74:934–940
5. Gurwith MJ, Brunton JL, Lank BA, Harding GKM, Ronald AR (1979) A prospective controlled investigation of prophylactic trimethoprim/sulamethoxazole in hospitalized granulocytopenic patients. Am J Med 6:248–256
6. Kauffman CA, Liepman MA, Bergman AG, Mioduszewski J (1983) Trimethoprim/sulfamethoxazole prophylaxis in neutropenic patients: reduction of infections and effect on bacterial and fungal flora. Am J Med 74:599–607
7. Kobayashi Y, Ammarro D, Ueda K, Kagosaki Y, Usui T (1978) Treatment of seven cases of chronic granulomatous disease with sulfamethoxazole-trimethoprim (SMX-TMP) Eur J Pediatr 127:247–254
8. Lehrer RI (1971) Inhibition by sulfonamides of the candidacidal activity of human neutrophils. J Clin Invest 50:2498–2505
9. Litchfield JT Jr, Wilcoxin F (1984) A simplified method of evaluting dose-effect experiments. Pharmacol Exp Ther 96:99–113

10. Margoliash E, Frohwirt N (1959) Spectrum of horse-heart cytochrome c. Biochem J 71:570–572
11. Nelson RD, Quie PG, Simmons RL (1975) Chemotaxis under agarose: a new and simple method for measuring chemotaxis and spontaneous migration of human polymorphonuclear leukocytes and monocytes. J Immunol 115:1650–1656
12. Peacock JE, Moorman DR, Wenzel RP, Mandell GL (1981) Methicillin-resistant *Staphylococcus aureus:* microbiologic characteristics, antimicrobial susceptibilities, and assessment of virulence of an epidemic strain. J Infect Dis 144:575–582
13. Regelmann W, Hays N, Quie PG (1983) Chronic granulomatous disease: historical perspective and clinical experience at the University of Minnesota Hospitals. In: Gallin JI, Fauci AS (eds) Advances in host defense mechanisms. Raven New York, pp 3–23
14. Siegel JP, Remington JS (1982) Effect of antimicrobial agents on chemiluminescence of human polymorphonuclear leukocytes in response to phagocytosis. J Antimicrob Chemother 10:505–515

Effects of Selected Antibiotics on Experimental Candidiasis in Cyclophosphamide-Treated Mice: An In Vivo Model to Evaluate the Antibiotic Effect on Granulocytopoiesis

M. C. Escande, C. Poyart-Salmeron, and P. H. Lagrange

Introduction

The level and duration of granulocytopenia in cancer patients treated with cytostatics drugs are the most important prognostic factors [3]. High dosages of beta-lactam antibiotics have been shown to have myelosuppressive effects [9], delaying or inhibiting the recovery of the polymorphonuclear phagocyte system. The underlying mechanisms of such adverse reactions are still a matter of debate, some authors being in favor of a peripheral immunopathological response with the production of specific antibiodies against the polymorphonuclear leukocytes (PMNs) [8], others favoring a direct toxicity to the bone marrow with a marked diminution of the well-differentiated myeloid cells associated with normal levels of immature myeloid precursor cells [9]. Since only in vitro models have been developed to examine the dose-dependent inhibition of granulopoiesis induced by beta-lactam antibiotics, it was decided to evaluate such potential adverse reactions in an in vivo model using neutropenic mice being treated with various antibiotics.

Cyclophosphamide (CY) was chosen as the agent of immunodepression because, with proper doses and appropriate timing, it induces a profound neutropenia, peaking between day 3 and 4, that is followed secondarily with a return to normal or above normal level within 1 week [10]. Since superinfections are usually associated with the delay of the bone marrow recovery after cytostatic treatment [3], a superinfection with *Candida albicans,* which is naturally resistant to the usual dose of beta-lactam, was performed in neutropenic mice being treated for varying periods with different beta-lactam antibiotics. In this infectious murine model, it was shown recently in our laboratory that the natural resistance against a high inoculum of *C. albicans* inoculated intravenously was exclusively mediated by the PMN system, related to the in vivo ability of the host to counteract the systemic spread of the intravenously injected yeast [5]. The depressive and enhancing effects of CY on resistance to *C. albicans* infection were associated with those cell populations recovering or rebounding in concurrence with the increase in resistance. Concurrent analysis of PMN counts in the peripheral blood and resistance after systemic infection were evaluated in groups of normal or CY-treated mice being treated daily with different antibiotics prior to the challenge. Three antibiotics were selected. Recently Gillissen [4] showed the opposite effect

Laboratoire Central de Microbiologie, Hôtel Dieu, 1, place du Parvis Notre Dame, 75181 Paris Cedex 04, France

The Influence of Antibiotics on the Host-Parasite Relationship III
Edited by G. Gillissen, W. Opferkuch, G. Peters, and G. Pulverer

of two cephalosporins (cefotaxime and cefoxitin) on the natural resistance of mice against *C. albicans* infection: mice treated with the former showed an increased resistance, mice treated with the latter a decreased resistance. We thus compare these two antibiotics and another: a new semisynthetic ureidopenicillin, piperacillin (PIP), which has been shown to have in vitro myelotoxic effects [3, 7], and which is regularly used as prophylactic treatment in febrile neutropenic patients in our hospital.

Material and Methods

Animals

Specific-pathogen-free, outbred, female Swiss OF1 mice were purchased from IFFA-CREDO (Domaine des Oncins, St Germain sur l'Arbresle, France). The mice were used at 6–8 weeks of age and were housed in our animal facilities and fed with sterile pellets and water.

Candida albicans

The *C. albicans* strain 3153 A, a reference strain, was grown in Sabouraud glucose broth at 37 °C until a stationary phase of growth was reached (about 24 h). Under these conditions, the culture gave a yield of approximately 2.5×10^8 cells/ml and the organism grew as essentially pure yeast phase population. Cells were then frozen and stored at -70 °C. Cells to be injected were cultured twice after thawing for 21 h at 37 °C in 10 ml Sabouraud glucose broth. Yeast cells from the second culture were washed three times in phosphate-buffered saline (PBS), and then adjusted to a concentration of 2×10^6 cells/ml with sterile nonpyrogenic saline, after counting in a hemacytometer. Each suspension was diluted further and spread onto Sabouraud agar plates to determine the viable counts. These counts were always $\pm 10\%$ of the hemacytometer counts.

For challenge, each mouse received around 1×10^6 *C. albicans* cells intravenously (i.v.) diluted in 0.5 ml sterile nonpyrogencic saline [5].

Drugs

Cyclophosphamide (CY) (CY, Asta, Laboratoire Lucien, Paris) was dissolved in 0.85% NaCl sterile solution immediately before use, membrane filtered (0.22 µm, Millipore Corps, United States), and injected intraperitoneally in a volume of 0.5 ml containing a dose of 1.5 mg/10 g body wt., at varying intervals, before the *C. albicans* challenge.

Antibiotics. The following antibiotics were included in our study: cefotaxime (CTX) (Laboratoires Roussel, Paris), cefoxitin (CXT) (Laboratoires Merk Sharp and Dohme, Paris), and piperacillin (PIP) (Laboratoires Lederlé, Paris). Separate groups of mice (10–20 animals/group) received the antibiotics once a day, injected subcutaneously in a volume of 0.5 ml 0.9% saline in the nape of the neck in varying concentrations, for 3, 7, or 15 consecutive days. Control mice received equal volume of saline.

Polymorphonuclear Leukocyte Index

Mice were bled from the retroorbital sinus. Cell counts were performed by diluting anticoagulated blood $^{1}/_{20}$ in Türk solution and counting the cells in a corpuscule-counting chamber. Differential cell counts were performed on blood smears after May-Grünwald-Giemsa staining by counting 200 leukocytes/slide. The results are expressed in terms of the PMN index, or as a percentage. The index was calculated by dividing the absolute number of PMNs found in treated mice by the mean number of PMNs in control mice. When the results are expressed as a percentage, the PMN index was multiplied by 100.

Mortality Rate

For estimation of mortality rate, the number of survivors was determined every day for 2 weeks. Using the 10^6 *C. albicans* challenge, very few survivors existed after this period: these surviving mice were assumed to be dead on day 15 for mean survival time (MST) estimations.

Statistical Analysis

Results are expressed as arithmetic means, and standard errors of the mean were calculated. Statistical significance was determined by Student's *t*-test for nonpaired data.

Results

Evaluation of CY-Treated Mice

Peripheral Blood Leukocytes. Total peripheral blood leukocytes were severely depressed after administration of one single injection of CY, but the effects of CY on different cell types were not equal (Table 1). The absolute number of PMNs was significantly lower in CY-treated mice 2 days after the injection of CY until the 5th day. The number of PMNs in CY-treated mice increased to normal levels by day 6–7 and above normal levels by day 8 or 9, returning to normal values with some fluctuations by day 15 (Table 2).

Mortality Rate after C. albicans Infection. Cyclophosphamide-treated mice were challenged with 2×10^6 *C. albicans* inoculated intravenously, either 3 or 7 days

Table 1. Absolute numbers (per cubic millimeter of blood) of total leukocytes, lymphocytes, and PMNs in cyclophosphamide (150 mg/kg)-treated and control mice, measured at varying intervals after CY treatment

Days after treatment	Control			Cyclophosphamide		
	Total	Lymphocytes	PMNs	Total	Lymphocytes	PMNs
0	5273±1578	4327±1413	756±162	3567± 994	2873± 961	675± 24
2	4433±1203	3777±1003	656±209	2133± 285	1852± 290	281± 6
3	5033±1071	4219±1054	815±166	1907± 684	1673± 597	242±141
4	4713± 142	4037± 137	675± 83	1890± 680	1568±1036	126± 98
5	3700± 152	2962± 27	741±160	1900± 208	1509± 115	180± 72
7	4433±1335	3798±1081	689±255	3100± 635	2453± 409	418±119
8	4133± 601	3312± 549	803± 64	5366±1397	3608± 804	1114±376

Table 2. Effect of time of CY administration[a] on PMN counts and on survival of OF_1 mice challenged IV with *C. albicans*[b]

Days from CY treatment	Absolute numbers of PMNs/mm³ (PMN index)[c]	Mean survival time (days)
J0	678±200 (1.00)	3.80±0.57 (0/10)[d]
J1	483±149 (0.71)	1.40±0.14[e] (0/10)
J4	77± 9[e] (0.11)	1.10±0.15[e] (0/10)
J6	112± 32[e] (0.16)	1.50±0.17[e] (0/10)
J8	1090±151[e] (1.60)	6.20±0.76[e] (1/10)
J11	810±176 (1.20)	5.80±0.54 (1/10)
J13	705±103 (1.03)	4.30±0.36 (0/10)
J15	421± 47 (0.62)	2.90±0.85 (1/10)

[a] All mice were inoculated with one single IP inoculation of 0.5 ml cyclophosphamide (150 mg/kg) on day 0.
[b] At varying intervals after Cy treatment, groups of ten mice were challenged by one IV injection of 0.9×10^6 live *C. albicans.*
[c] Absolute numbers of PMNs/mm³ were calculated from data on five mice/group, ± SEM.
[d] No. of days 15 survivors/No. of tested mice.
[e] $P<0.05$.

after CY inoculation. As shown in Fig. 1, all mice treated with CY 3 days prior to the challenge died within 24 h. In contrast, the mortality rate of the group of mice being treated with CY 7 days prior to the challenge did not differ significantly from those of the normal non-CY-treated group (2.4±0.6 and 2.8±0.6 days respectively). In another experiment, when separate groups of mice were challenged with $0{,}9 \times 10^6$ *C. albicans* at various intervals after CY inoculation, similar results were obtained, showing a good correlation between the kinetics of the absolute numbers of peripheral blood PMNs and the mean survival time (Table 2).

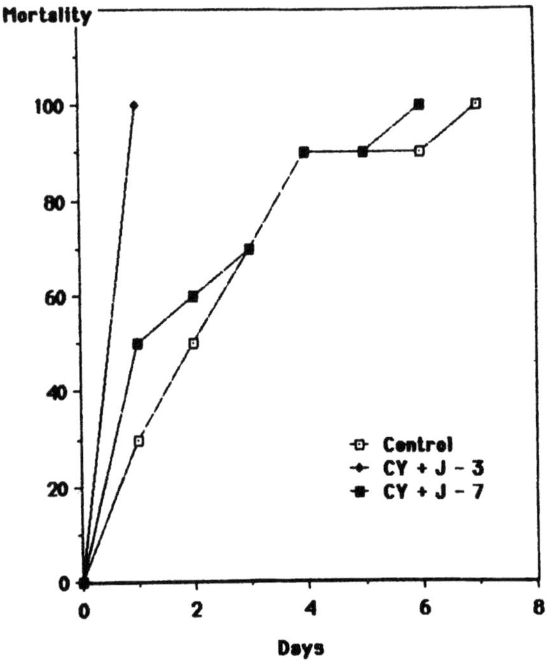

Fig. 1. Cumulative mortality rate after an intravenous injection of 2×10^6 live *C. albicans* in normal (control) and in mice being treated with a single intraperitoneal injection of cyclophosphamide (150 mg/kg) given 7 days (−7 CY) or 3 days (−3 CY) before the challenge. Groups of ten mice

Effects of Antibiotic Treatment of the C. albicans Infection in Normal and CY-Treated Mice

Antibiotic Treatment in Normal Mice. Three antibiotics were chosen, two cephalosporins (cefotaxime and cefoxitin) already described by Gillissen [4] as having the most contrasting effect on primary infection with *C. albicans,* and a new ureidopenicillin (piperacillin) used regularly in our hospital hematology unit for prophylactic antibiotherapy, in neutropenic febrile patients. Separate groups of normal mice were treated with daily s.c. injections of these three different antibiotics. As shown in Fig. 2, great individual variation occurs in the percentage of the PMN counts, but no significant variations were observed compared with the control groups during the first 5 days. This was followed with a slight decrease on day 7 and 8 in cefotaxime- and cefoxitin-treated mice. When similar groups of AB-treated mice were challenged with *C. albicans* on day 3 or 7 after AB treatments, no significant variation of the mortality rate was observed among the different groups. Only a slight increase of resistance was noted in mice treated for 3 days before challenge with cefotaxime and cefoxitin (Fig. 3 a), such effects disappearing when mice were treated for 7 days prior to the challenge (Fig. 3 b). The results of the calculated mean survival times in such groups of mice are shown in Table 3.

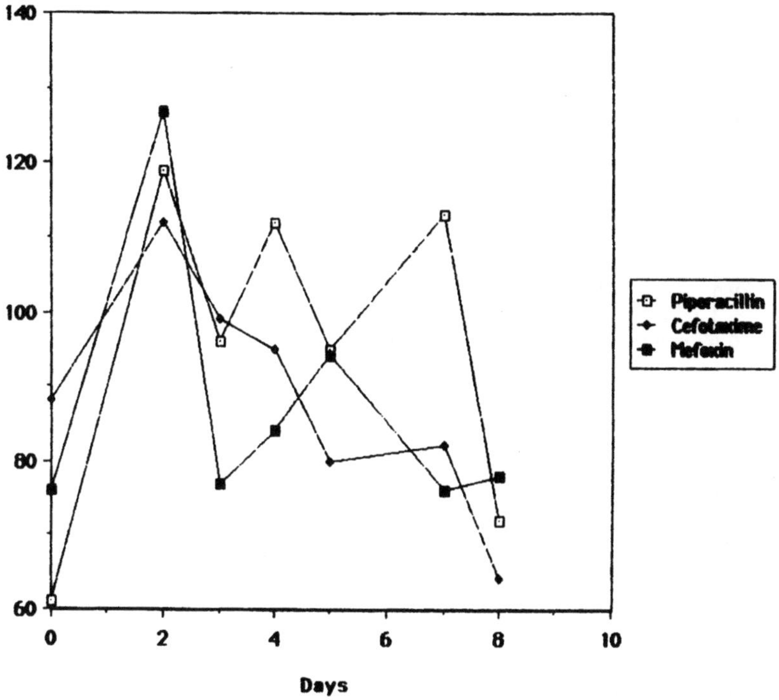

Fig. 2. Kinetics of the percentage of peripheral blood PMNs in separate groups of five mice each treated by one daily s.c. injection of piperacillin (250 mg/kg), cefotaxime (60 mg/kg), cefoxitin (mefoxin, 60 mg/kg), and saline (control)

Table 3. Effects of different antibiotics on the MST of *Candida albicans* infected[a], normal, or CY-treated mice

Treatment[b]	No. of days before challenge	MST (days) antibiotics used[c]			
		Piperacillin	Cefoxitin	Cefotaxime	Control
Control	3	2.5±0.4[d] (v=1.61)	3.9±0.5 (v=2.99)	3.4±0.5 (v=3.16)	2.8±0.6 (v=3.51)
	7	1.9±0.3 (v=1.43)	2.7±0.6 (v=4.01)	2.0±0.3 (v=1.11)	2.8±0.6 (v=3.51
Cyclophosphamide	3	1.0±0.0 (v=0)	1.0±0.0 (v=0)	1.0±0.0 (v=0)	1.0±0.0 (v=0)
	7	3.6±0.7 (v=5.38)	2.7±0.6 (v=4.23)	2.8±0.7 (v=5.07)	2.4±0.5 (v=3.16)

[a] All groups of mice were challenged by one injection of 2×10^6 live *C. albicans*.
[b] Mice were inoculated with one single injection of 0.5 ml saline with or without cyclophosphamide (150 mg/kg).
[c] Separate groups of mice were inoculated daily with one injection of piperacillin (250 mg/kg), cefoxitin (60 mg/kg), cefotaxime (60 mg/kg), or saline (control) for 3 or 7 days respectively before the challenge.
[d] Mean of ten mice per group ± SE of the mean (variance).

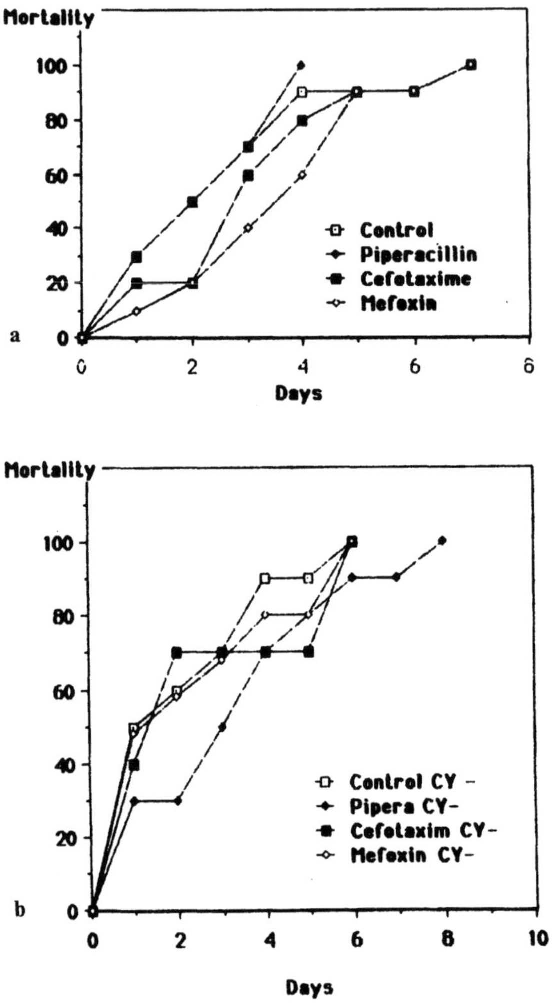

Fig. 3 a, b. Cumulative mortality rate in groups of mice inoculated with an intravenous injection of 2×10^6 live *C. albicans,* and being s.c. treated with injections of piperacillin, cefoxitin (Metoxin), cefotaxime, or saline (Control). **a** Separate groups of ten mice received four s.c. injections, at daily intervals, of PIP (250 mg/kg), cefoxitin (60 mg/kg), and cefotaxime (60 mg/kg) beginning 3 days prior to the challenge. **b** Separate groups of ten mice received eight s.c. injections, at daily intervals, of the same dosage of PIP, cefotaxime, and cefoxitin beginning 7 days prior to the challenge

Antibiotic Treatments in CY-Treated Mice. The same regimen of AB treatments was applied in mice which were pretreated on day 0 with one single inoculation of 150 mg/kg cyclophosphamide. The kinetics of the PMNs in AB-treated CY mice are shown in Fig. 4. It can be observed that the CY treatment induced a similar degree of profound granulopenia in all groups of mice, from day 3 to day 5.

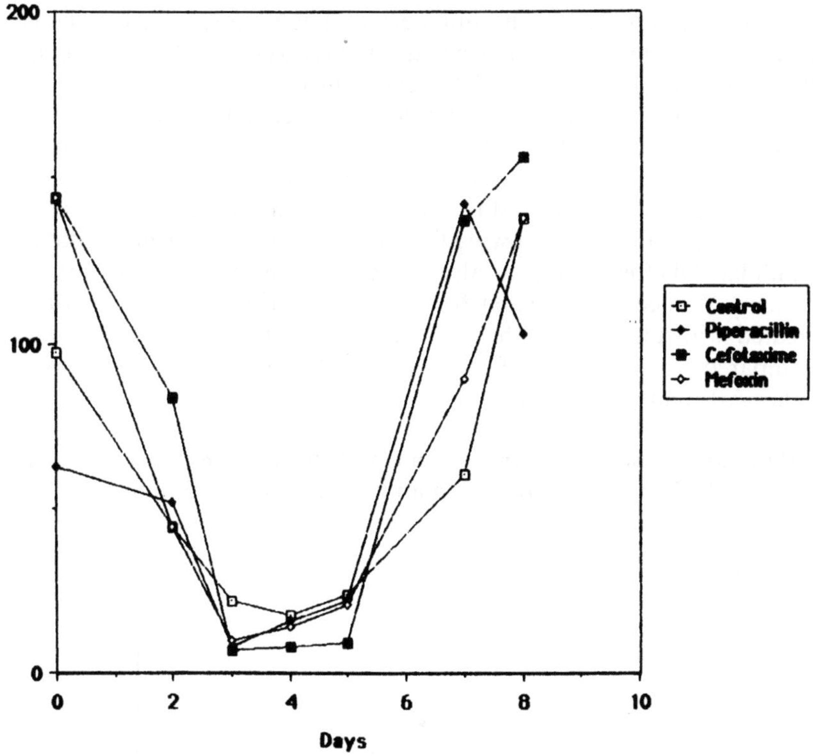

Fig. 4. Kinetics of the percentage of peripheral blood PMNs in separate groups of five mice each treated by one daily s.c. injection of piperacillin (250 mg/kg), cefotaxime (60 mg/kg), cefoxitin (Mefoxin, 60 mg/kg), or saline (control) from day 0 to day 8

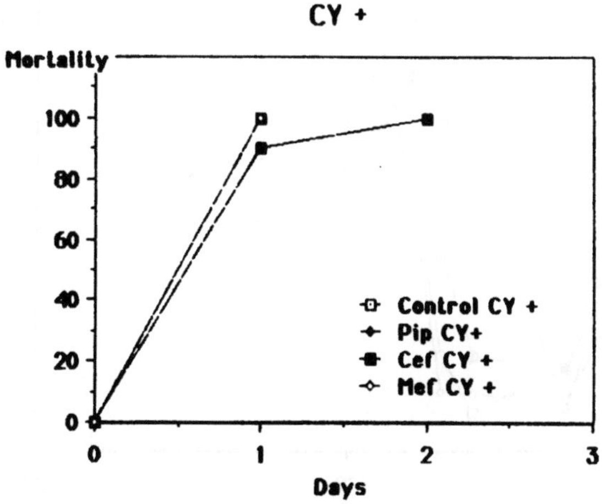

Fig. 5. Cumulative mortality rate after an intravenous injection of 2×10^6 live *C. albicans*, in separate groups (ten mice each) of normal or antibiotic-treated mice, both being pretreated with cyclophosphamide for 3 days before the challenge. The dose regimen of antibiotics and symbols used are the same as those described in Fig. 4

However, on day 7, the numbers of PMNs (expressed as percentages) in piperacillin and in cefotaxim treated CY mice were significantly higher ($P<0.05$) than in cefoxitin and control CY treated mice.

When similar groups of AB-treated CY mice were challenged i.v. with 2×10^6 *C. albicans* on day 3 or on day 7 after AB treatments, strikingly different results were observed. First as expected, in all AB-treated and control mice challenged 3 days after CY, the mortality rates were similar (Fig. 5), the great majority of mice dying within 24 h, showing that such in vivo AB treatments did not have any candidacidal effect alone, as already tested by in vitro tests (results not shown). When CY mice were treated for 7 days with these antibiotics, only the group treated with piperacillin showed a prolonged mean survival time (Table 3) as compared with the control. No significant difference was observed within the other AB-treated groups of mice.

Effects of Piperacillin Treatment in CY-Treated Mice. Since a quicker PMN rebound which was associated with an increased survival time was observed in the

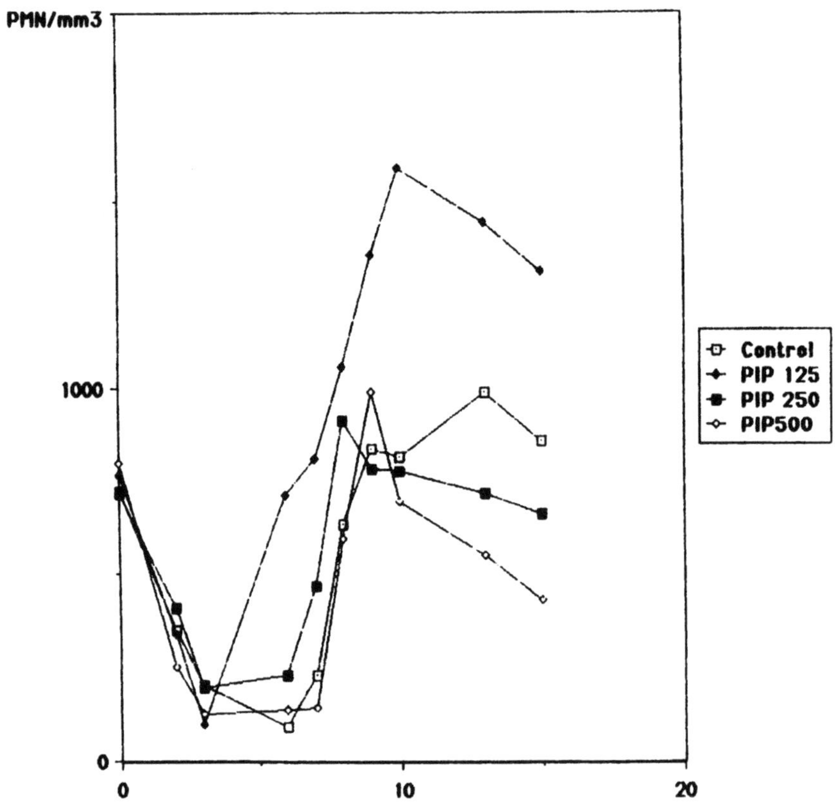

Fig. 6. Kinetics of the absolute numbers (per cubic millimeter) of peripheral blood PMNs harvested from separate groups of six CY-treated mice each, treated by one daily s.c. injection of piperacillin 125 mg/kg (250 mg/kg, 500 mg/kg), cefotaxime (60 mg/kg), cefoxitin (60 mg/kg), or saline (control) from day 0 to day 15

Table 4. Effect of time of administration of three different doses of piperacillin on the MST of OF1 mice challenged with *C. albicans*[a] after 8 or 15 days of AB treatment in CY-pretreated mice[b]

Groups of mice	MST (days) antibiotic treatment	
	8 days	15 days
Control 1 (CY−)	5.50±0.81 (1/10)[c]	5.50±0.83 (1/10)
Control 2 (CY+)	5.50±1.04 (2/10)	5.20±0.79 (1/10)
PIP 125 mg/kg	8.50±1.18 (4/10)	6.30±0.73 (1/10)
PIP 250 mg/kg	9.70±1.15[d] (5/10)	7.30±1.12 (3/10)
PIP 500 mg/kg	7.40±1.16 (3/10)	8.30±1.19[d] (4/10)

[a] All groups of mice were challenged by one injection of 0.9×10^6 live *C. albicans*, 8 or 15 days after CY-treatment.
[b] All groups of mice were inoculated with one injection of cyclophosphamide (150 mg/kg) on day 0, except the group control 1, which received an equal volume of saline.
[c] No. of survivors/No. tested mice on day 15.
[d] $P<0.05$.

group of CY mice treated with piperacillin, the next question was to determine whether a dose effect on the PMN counts and resistance might be detected after such AB treatment. As shown in Fig. 6, the numbers of PMNs in piperacillin-treated mice differed significantly from those of the non-AB-treated CY mice. Onset and level of the PMN rebound were significant quicker and higher in mice treated with the lowest dose of piperacillin (125 mg/kg) compared with the control group. However, as the administered doses increased, the onset of the PMN recovery was delayed, and from day 10 to day 15 a dose-dependent and inhibitory effect was observed in mice treated with doses equal to or higher than 250 mg/kg. Repeated experiments produced similar results.

The next experiments were then to test the *C. albicans* resistance in groups of CY mice receiving varying doses of piperacillin either for 8 days or for 15 days. In groups of mice treated with CY for 8 days and challenged with 0.9×10^6 *C. albicans,* the highest MST was observed in mice which received the median dose of piperacillin (250 mg/kg), mice which received 125 mg/kg or 500 mg/kg piperacillin showing less marked MST, but still higher than those found in control mice. In the three groups of mice treated with Piperacillin for 15 days before the challenge, a higher MST was observed compared with those observed in control mice, and a dose relationship was noticed (Table 4).

Discussion

In the present paper, we report on a series of studies aimed at assessing possible links betweens in vivo resistance of AB-treated immunodepressed mice to *C. albicans* challenge and the kinetics of the peripheral blood PMN counts. The antibiotics tested are those currently used in febrile neutropenic patients. As expected and in line with previous results [5], susceptibility to *C. albicans* appeared to be increased shortly (3–6 days) after CY exposure, and the antibiotic treatments during the granulocytopenia period did not modify the results. Indeed CY, given as a single dose of 100–200 mg/kg, affects most lymphoid cells, primarily B-lymphocytes [6], but also helper and suppressor cells [11] and rapidly dividing cells such as PMNs precursors [5]. It was not surprising, therefore, to find that the increase in susceptibility to *C. albicans* infection was associated with an immediate depression of peripheral blood leukocytes. A similar decrease was observed in mice treated for 3 days with the different antibiotics. However, the depression was somehow more marked in cefotaxime-treated mice (Fig. 4). Such an effect of CTX was also observed in normal non-CY-treated mice (Fig. 2), its maximum occurring after 8 days of treatment (a 36% of reduction was observed as compared with control mice). Such a partial reduction in PMN counts was associated only with a sligh increase in susceptibility (Table 3). Seven days after CY administration the in vivo resistance to *C. albicans* appeared unaffected (Fig. 1), at a time when PMNs were rebounding to normal or above normal levels (Table 1).

From day 8 through 11 after CY treatment, enhanced resistance was observed (Table 2), which was paralleled by a maximal increase in PMN counts. When CY-treated mice were daily inoculated with antibiotics, the PMNs rebounding appeared earlier in piperacillin and in cefotaxime-treated mice (Fig. 4). A direct relationship between the dose and the time of PMN recovery was observed in piperacillin-treated mice. The lower dose of piperacillin administered (125 mg/kg) for 7 days evoked a more rapid and higher rebound of peripheral blood PMN counts. When mice were treated by a two- or fourfold higher dose, the rebound was delayed accordingly. Morever, when such treatments were prolonged, the rebound was followed by a secondary decrease of PMN counts. It is quite possible that higher doses, such as 1000 mg/kg, might totally erase the rebound phenomenon and block the bone marrow recovery. This dose was shown to be the dose which inhibits 100% of in vitro colony formation of bone marrow culture [9]. However, when resistance of *C. albicans* was evaluated in such AB-treated mice, 8 or 15 days after CY pretreatment, no antibiotic dose relationships were observed; the increase resistance did not parallel the PMN levels found in different groups of mice. There are two possible nonexclusive explanations for such discrepancies. The first might be associated with a lower phagocytic and candidacidal activity of the rebounding PMNs in mice treated with 125 mg/kg piperacillin. Experiments are under way to clarify the issue. The second explanation might be the occurrence of a non-PMN-dependent increase of resistance as described recently by Bistoni et al. [2].

The peak of candidacidal activity occurred 12 days after CY-treatment. The candidacidal effector cells are cytotoxic cells to *C. albicans*. They lack the NK cell markers, and they are heterogeneous, largely nonadherent, and poorly phagocytic, as opposed to what happens with the candidacidal effectors present in the spleen of normal mice, which showed the functional patterns typical of mature macrophages [1]. Cells with different degrees of differentiation and/or phagocytic activity belonging to a monocyte macrophage lineage are probably responsible for the in vitro candidacidal activity, which correlates with the in vivo increase in resistance to *C. albicans* challenge. Such an increase in candidacidal activity seems to predominate over the yeast clearance capacity mediated by PMNs.

However, according to our observed results, it might be postulated that piperacillin treatment might then be able to induce an increase in proliferation and differentiation of such effector cytotoxic cells. Further experiments are needed to clarify this issue.

Summary

The effect of cefoxitin (CXT), cefotaxime (CTX), and piperacillin (PIP) on the natural resistance to *Candida albicans* infection has been evaluated in vivo, in normal and in neutropenic mice, in correlation with the polymorphonuclear (PMN) cell count in the peripheral blood. In neutropenic mice treated with PIP or CTX the PMN rebound occurred earlier and reached a higher level than in CXT-treated or control mice. A dose-dependent increase in resistance to *C. albicans* infection was observed in PIP-treated mice. It did not parallel the PMN levels found in the different experimental groups. Several hypotheses are discussed to explain the apparent dissociation of an increase in natural resistance with no concomitant increased number of the blood PMN.

References

1. Bacccarini M, Bistoni F, Pucetti P, Garaci E (1983) Natural cell mediated cytotoxicity against *Candida albicans* induced by cyclophosphamide: nature of the in vitro cytotoxic effector. Infect Immun 42:1–9
2. Bistoni F, Baccarini M, Blasi E, Marconi P, Puccetti P, Garaci E (1983) Correlation between in vivo and in vitro studies of modulation of resistance to experimental *Candida albicans* infection by cyclophosphamide in mice. Infect Immun 40:46–55
3. Bodey GP (1986) Infection in cancer patients. A continuing association. Am J Med 81 [Suppl IA]:11–26
4. Gillissen C (1985) Possible mechanisms of immunological side effects of antibiotics. Zentralbl Bakteriol [Suppl 13]:91–103
5. Hurtrel B, Lagrange PH, Michel JC (1980) Systemic candidiasis in mice: II. Main role of polymorphonuclear leukocytes in resistance to infection. Ann Inst Pasteur Immunol 131C:105–108
6. Lagrange PH, Mackaness GB, Miller TE (1974) Potentiation of T cell mediated immunity by selective suppression of antibody formation with cyclophosphamide. J Exp Med 139:1529–1539
7. Marie JP, Thevenin R, Zittoun R (1986) Inhibition de la granulopoiese in vitro par les β lactamines. Presse Med 15:2358–2361
8. Murphy MF, Chapman JF, Metcalf P, Waters AH (1985) Antibiotic induced neutropenia. Lancet II:1306–1307
9. Neftel KA, Hanser SP, Muller MR (1985) Inhibition of granulopoiesis in vivo and in vitro by β lactam antibiotics. J Infect Dis 152:90–98
10. Sher NA, Chaparas SD, Greenberg LE, Bernard S (1975) Effect of BCG, *Corynebacterium parvum* and methanol extraction residue in the reduction of mortality from *Staphylococcus aureus* and *Candida albicans* infections in immunosuppressed mice. Infect Immun 12:1325–1330
11. Turk JL, Poulter LW (1972) Selective depletion of lymphoid tissue by cyclophosphamide. Clin Exp Immunol 10:285–296

Immunomodulating Effect of Fosfomycin

G. Gillissen, M. Breuer-Werle, B. Melzer, and H. Ostendorp

Introduction

Antibiotics may influence immunological reactions. This has been shown with ex vivo and in vitro experiments using different parameters and experimental models [1, 4–6, 13]. The results, however, are not always in line with the immunological side effect of antibiotics in vivo as shown with experimental infections using primary resistant microorganisms [7].

In this context, it was of interest to know whether fosfomycin (FM), which has no structural resemblance to other antibiotics [10] and a particular mode of action of bactericidal activity [12, 15], is capable of modifying immune response parameters and if so whether there is a correlation between the results obtained with different experimental models. The influence of FM has, therefore, been examined in the course of experimental infections with *Candida*, on antibody formation in vivo and in vitro, on phagocytosis in vivo, and on mitogen-induced proliferation of lymphocytes whereby FM was either injected into cell donors or added in vitro together with mitogen to the test system.

Materials and Methods

For all assays "fosfocin pro infusione 3.0" (Boehringer, Mannheim, FRG) in dry form was used, containing 98.02% disodium salt of FM. Doses and concentrations were specified as FM representing on a weight basis 75.76% of the disodium salt. The contents of the infusion bottles, weighing 4.05 g, were dissolved in 100 ml distilled water, taking into account an excess of fosfomycin of 4.1%, and then further diluted with saline.

Experimental Infection

Inbred male Balb/cABOM mice weighing 20 ± 1 g (Bomholtgård, Ry, Denmark) were used for all assays. For infection, washed cells of the primary FM-resistant *Candida albicans* ATCC 10231 of the log growth phase in Sabouraud broth were injected intravenously in doses of 6×10^6 cells/0.25 ml pyrogen-free saline, corre-

Department of Medical Microbiology, Medical Faculty, Pauwelsstraße, 5100 Aachen, Federal Republic of Germany

The Influence of Antibiotics on the Host-Parasite Relationship III
Edited by G. Gillissen, W. Opferkuch, G. Peters, and G. Pulverer

sponding approximately to an ID_{75}. Treatment was performed by one intravenous injection of different doses of FM in 0.5 ml saline 1 h before infection with 25 animals/group.

Humoral Immunity

The influence of FM on antibody response in vivo and in vitro was evaluated by the number of IgM- and IgG-producing spleen cells, i.e., the direct and indirect plaque-forming cells (DPFC and IPFC) using the Jerne method [8, 9] modified by Cunningham [2, 3]. Mice were immunized with 2×10^8 washed sheep red blood cells (SRBCs), injected intraperitoneally in 0.5 ml saline, and the number of DPFC and IPFC was determined 3 and 7 days later respectively.

Fostomycin was given only once intravenously in doses of 0.6 or 1.0 mg in 0.25 ml saline (i.e., 30 mg and 50 mg/kg) either 1 h before sensitization or 1 day before evaluation, i.e., in the case of DPFC 2 days and in the case of IPFC 6 days after immunization.

A possible influence of FM on the expression of antibody response in vitro was examined by the addition of FM in concentrations of 7.5 μg and 120 μg/ml of the test system. For DPFC response, spleen cells were taken 3 days and for IPFC evaluation 7 days after sensitization of cell donors.

Phagocytosis In Vivo

The disappearance of microbial cells injected intraperitoneally within a short time was described as phagocytosis in vivo [11, 14], practically being a clearance reaction. Four hours after injection of 1×10^9 washed cells of *Candida albicans* ATCC 10231 taken from the log growth phase in Sabouraud broth and suspended in 0.5 ml of a 0.1% solution of casein-hydrolysate in distilled water, the peritoneal cavity was washed out with 3.0 ml saline containing 12.5 IU sodium heparinate (Liquemin, Roche, Switzerland) per milliliter. The clearance factor was calculated by dividing the ratio of recovered and injected cells – both determined as colony-forming units (CFUs) – in controls by that of recovered and injected CFUs in assays. Values over 1.0 indicated an enhanced disappearance of CFUs, i.e., a stimulation, and values below 1.0 an inhibition.

Fosfomycin was given intravenously once in doses of 0.6 mg or 1.0 mg/0.25 ml either 1 h or 1 day before infection.

Proliferation of Spleen Lymphocytes

Aseptically obtained spleens were minced by scissors and grinded down over a stainless steel sieve with Hank's 199 medium containing 10% fetal calf serum (Seromed, Biochrom KG, Berlin, FRG). After lysis of erythrocytes by hypotonic shock and washing lymphocytes, suspensions were given on cotton wool, filtered after an incubation for 30 min at 37 °C, washed twice with Hank's 199 medium with 10% fetal calf serum (Seromed), and resuspended in cell culture medium consisting of RPMI with 20% fetal calf serum, 100 m*M* L-glutamin and BME-Earl (Seromed).

For all assays, 2×10^6 lymphocytes/200 µl per well of microtiter plates were used (five assays in parallel) and stimulated by incubation for 3 days at 37 °C in an atmosphere of 5% CO_2 with different concentrations of purified phytohemagglutinin (PHA-P; Difco, Detroit, Michigan, USA). After the addition of [^{3}H]thymidine (0.5 µCi per well) and a further incubation over 16 h the activity uptake was measured.

The FM effect in vivo was investigated by treating the cell donors with different doses between 7.5 and 50 mg/kg given intravenously in 0.5 ml saline 1 day before the assay.

The influence of FM in vitro was evaluated by combining different concentrations of FM between 3.75 and 50 µg/ml dissolved in cell culture medium, and of PHA-P. The stimulation index was calculated by the ratio of assay and control.

Results

In experimental infections with an ID_{80} of the primary resistant *Candida,* FM induced a dose-dependent increase of survival rate with single doses between 7.5 and 30 mg/kg given 1 h before infection (Fig. 1). Higher doses of 50 mg/kg had no effect but were not inhibiting either.

Humoral immunity was evaluated by the PFC response. If FM was given once 1 h before immunization, the smaller dose of 0.6 mg/animal, i.e., 30 mg/kg, significantly increased the number of DPFC as well as IPFC (Fig. 2). In contrast, the dose of 1.0 mg/animal or 50 mg/kg induced a significant reduction of DPFC and IPFC relative to controls. If the animals were not treated with FM before immunization but only 1 day before testing, the smaller dose of 30 mg FM/kg again stimulated the DPFC as well as the IPFC response significantly. The higher dose of 50 mg, however, did not reduce the number of DPFC as observed in the case

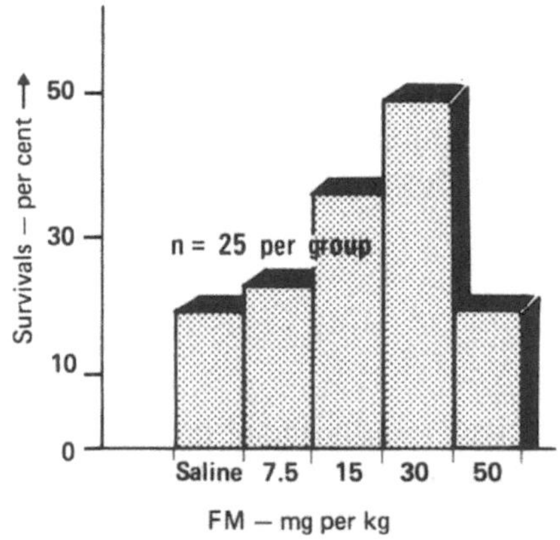

Fig. 1. Fosfomycin effect on survival rate in experimental infection with *Candida albicans.* FM was given once 1 h before infection. Twenty-five animals per group

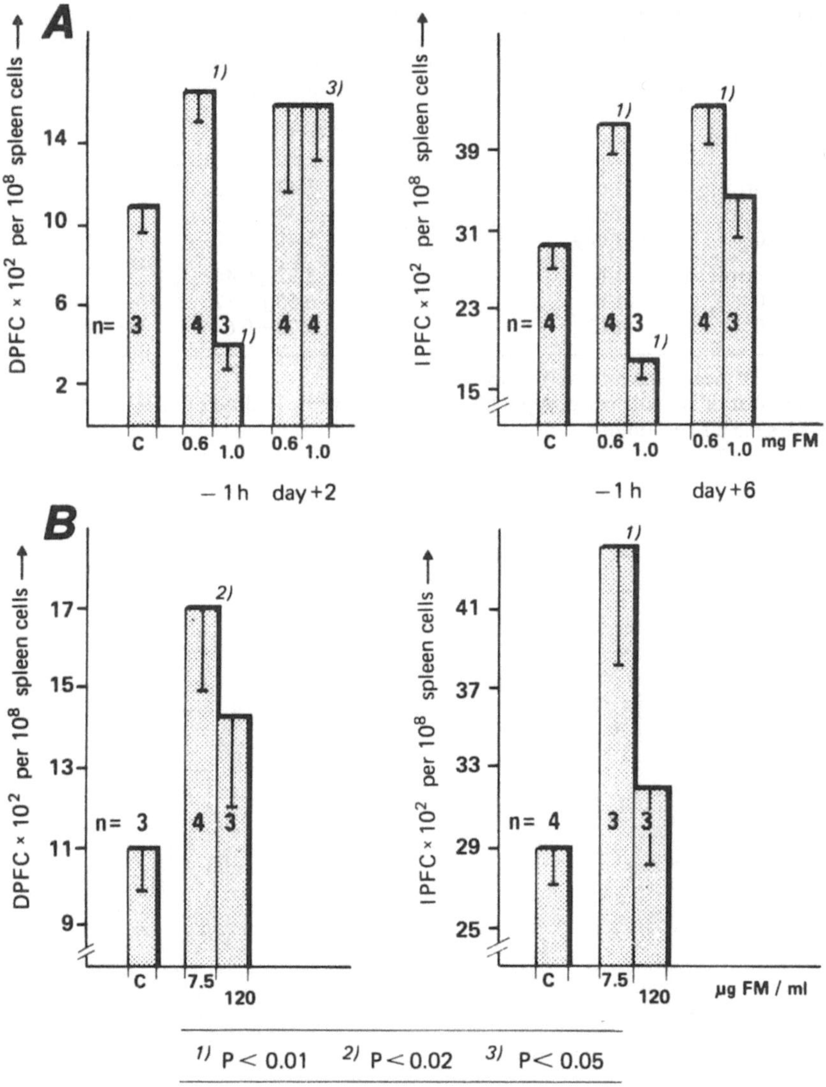

Fig. 2 A, B. Influence of FM on PFC response: **A** in vivo, **B** in vitro. *n*, number of animals/group. −1 h and day +2 = time of treatment relative to sensitization

of pretreatment but increased it. With the same experimental design and at 50 mg/kg, the number of IPFC was only slightly but not significantly higher than the control values.

In vitro, FM also enhanced the expression of DPFC and IPFC in concentrations of 7.5 µg/ml. Higher concentrations of 120 µg/ml only had a slight stimulating effect (Fig. 2).

Phagocytosis in vivo (clearance reaction) was influenced neither by 30 mg FM/kg nor by 50 mg/kg if given the day before infection with *Candida*. If, however,

Table 1. Phagocytosis in vivo (clearance test) – evaluation 4 h after intraperitoneal infection

Treatment		n	CFUs × 10^{-6}/ animal recovered	P	Index
Dose FM (mg/kg)	Time[a]				
A. Control	−1 day	6	5.43 ± 0.65	–	–
30.0	−1 day	6	5.38 ± 0.27	NS	1.01
50.0	−1 day	6	5.41 ± 0.72	NS	1.00
B. Control	−1 h	6	8.32 ± 0.44	–	–
30.0	−1 h	6	6.65 ± 1.12	<0.01	1.25
50.0	−1 h	6	9.20 ± 0.68	<0.05	0.90

[a] Time of treatment relative to time of infection.
n, number of animals per group; NS, not significant; A, B, dose of infection 1.07 and 1.13 × 10^9 CFUs/0.5 ml per animal.

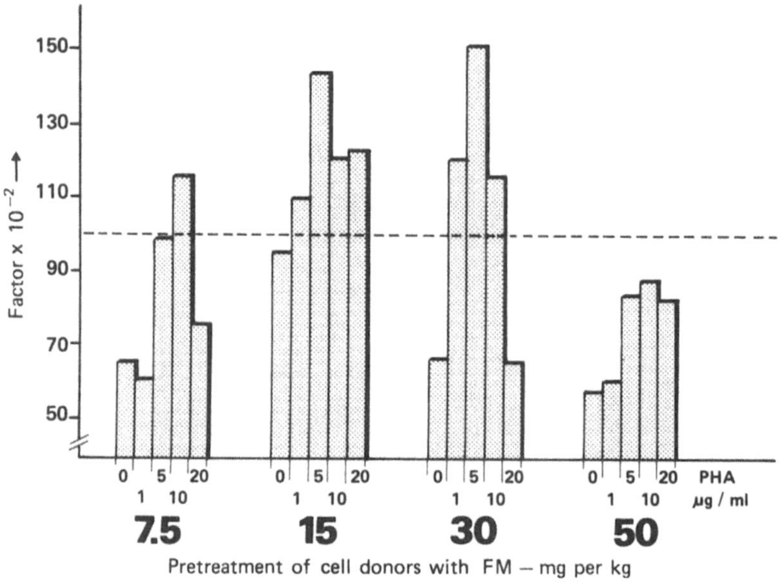

Fig. 3. Significance of FM treatment on PHA-induced proliferation of spleen lymphocytes

FM was given only 1 h before, then the smaller dose of 30 mg/kg was significantly stimulating and the higher one of 50 mg/kg was inhibiting (Table 1).

The PHA-P-induced proliferation of spleen lymphocytes was modulated by FM treatment of cell donors but also in vitro if added to the medium in transformation assays.

Pretreatment of cell donors with up to 30 mg/kg FM resulted in a dose-dependent increase of lymphocyte reactivity, whereas the higher dose of 50 mg/kg was inhibitory (Fig. 3). These results are principally in line with those obtained with other experimental models.

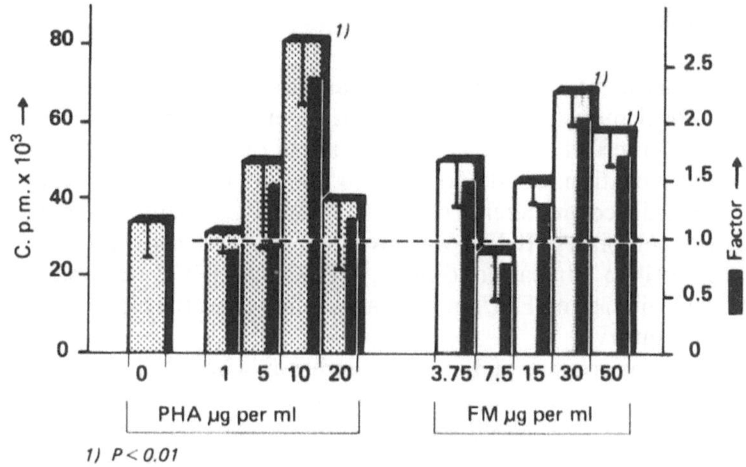

Fig. 4. In vitro influence of FM on transformation rate of spleen lymphocytes

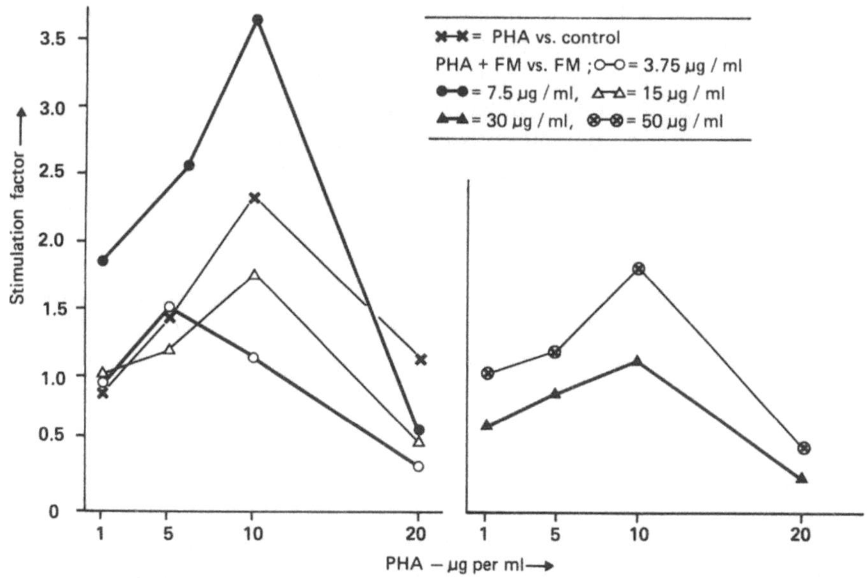

Fig. 5. Phytohemagglutinin-induced proliferation rate of spleen lymphocytes in the presence of FM

In vitro, FM alone, i.e., in the absence of PHA-P, stimulates proliferation, but significantly only with the higher concentrations of 30 and 50 µg/ml (Fig. 4). The combination of different concentrations of PHA-P and FM in vitro allows the calculation of the effect of PHA in the presence of FM (PHA-P + FM versus FM alone). Figure 5 shows that the mitogenic effect is dependent on the concentration of PHA-P and of FM as well. Only the values of the optimal concentration of PHA-P alone are considerably increased by 7.5 µg FM/ml. Every other PHA-P/FM ratio is less effective.

Discussion

The experiments showed that FM has a distinct immunomodulating effect which could be demonstrated with different experimental models. The direction and extent of this effect are, however, dependent on doses and application time relative to immunization. Single doses of 30 mg FM/kg injected shortly before immunization induced an increase of DPFC and IPFC, whereas the higher dose of 50 mg/kg was inhibitory. If FM was given days after sensitization, which corresponds fairly well to clinical conditions, DPFC and IPFC responses were equally enhanced with 30 mg FM/kg. In this case, however, the higher dose of 50 mg/kg was not inhibitory.

The importance of the administration schedule for FM was demonstrated with the in vivo phagocytosis model. Similarly to the PFC assay, the smaller dose of 30 mg FM/kg induced a stimulation and the higher one of 50 mg/kg an inhibition. This, however, could only be seen if FM was given shortly before immunization. No significant effect was observed if FM was given the day before.

These results correspond with the FM effect on mitogen-induced transformation of lymphocytes. Here again the smaller dose of 30 mg/kg enhanced and the higher one of 50 mg/kg inhibited the PHA-P reactivity of the cells.

These observations suggested that it would be possible to obtain comparable results in experimental infection with *Candida*. This was, indeed, the case insofar as single doses of FM up to 30 mg/kg given shortly before infection increased the dose-dependent survival rate. The higher dose of 50 mg/kg, however, had no effect if compared with controls, but was not inhibiting either. This means that FM stimulates defense mechanisms in infection and even the higher dose of 50 mg/kg is not inhibiting in spite of such an effect in other experimental models.

Another question is the influence of FM on immune parameters in the case of an immunodeficient state. Preliminary experiments showed that FM treatment with adequate doses may reduce the immunodepressing effect of corticoids or of cyclophosphamide.

Summary

Fosfomycin (FM) enhanced host resistance in experimental infections with primary resistant *Candida albicans* gradually up to 30 mg/kg. Higher doses had no effect. Direct and indirect plaque-forming cell (DPFC and IPFC) responses were also stimulated if FM was given in a dose of 30 mg/kg shortly before immunization, but the higher dose of 50 mg/kg was inhibiting. After single administrations of FM some days after sensitization, both doses increased the number of DPFC and IPFC. In vitro, FM enhanced the expression of DPFC and IPFC with a concentration of 7.5 μg/ml. The stimulation observed with 120 μg/ml was not significant. Phagocytosis in vivo was stimulated by FM in doses of 30 mg/kg but not by 50 mg/kg, the latter, however, only given shortly before infection. Mitogen-induced lymphocyte proliferation increased by pretreatment of cell donors with FM up to 30 mg/kg. Higher doses were inhibitory. Also in vitro, FM modulated the proliferation rate depending of the FM/mitogen ratio.

References

1. Adam D, Hahn H, Opferkuch W (1985) The influence of antibiotics on the host-parasite relationship II. Springer, Berlin Heidelberg New York
2. Cunningham AJ (1965) A method of increased sensitivity for detecting single antibody-forming cells. Nature 207:1106–1107
3. Cunningham AJ, Szenberg A (1968) Further improvements in the plaque technique for detecting single antibody-forming cells. Immunology 14:599–600
4. Eickenberg HH, Hahn H, Opferkuch W (1982) The influence of antibiotics on the host-parasite relationship. Springer, Berlin Heidelberg New York
5. Gillissen G (1980) Antibiotika und Immunantwort – Begleiteffekt der Chemotherapie. Immun Infekt 8:79–88
6. Gillissen G (1982) Non-specific influence of antibiotics on the course of infectious processes. Infection 10:128–130
7. Gillissen G (1985) Possible mechanisms of immunological side-effects of antibiotics. Zbl Bakt Hyg [A] Suppl 13:91–103
8. Jerne NK, Nordin AA (1963) Plaque formation in agar by single antibody-producing cells. Science 140:405
9. Jerne NK, Henry C, Nordin AA, Fuji AM, Koros C, Lefkovits I (1974) Plaque forming cells: methodology and theory. Transplant Rev 18:130–191
10. List WF (1983) Probleme der Antibiotikatherapie auf einer operativen Intensivstation. In: Spitzy KH, Adam D (eds) Fosfomycin – ein neuartiges Antibiotikum. Pmi – pharmacological and medical information, Frankfurt/M, pp 109–111
11. Mediaris DN, Kenny JF (1986) Observations concerning the pathogenesis of *E. coli* infections in mice. J Immunol 101:534–540
12. Peters G, Schumacher-Perdreau F, Pulverer G (1980) Vergleich der Staphylokokken- und Mikrokokken-Wirksamkeit von Fosfomycin- Oxacillin und Penicillin G. Dtsch Med Wochenschr 105:1541–1543
13. Pulverer G, Jeljaszewicz J (1985) Chemotherapy and immunity. Zbl Bakt Hyg [A] Suppl 13:1–245
14. Pusztai-Markos ZS (1977) Failure of correlation between in vitro and in vivo effect of T and B cell mitogen in the mouse. Z Immunitätsforsch 153:60–73
15. Vömel W (1982) Bakteriologische und pharmakologische Grundlagen der klinischen Anwendung von Fosfomycin. In: Linzenmeier G (ed) Aktuelle Aspekte zur bakteriologischen Resistenzbestimmung und der Resistenzsituation. Braunschweig, pp 57–72

Effects of Antibiotics on Resistance to Colonization with Enteric Pathogens in Mice

D. J. HENTGES [1], W. W. MARSH [2], S. H. DOUGHERTY [3], W. R. THAL [1], and M. K. ADAMS [1]

There is considerable evidence that the administration of large quantities of antibiotics to experimental animals greatly increases their susceptibility to colonization with exogenous organisms. When the antibiotics are given perorally, the intestinal flora is frequently disrupted and the animals are easily colonized with enteric pathogens. This was demonstrated some time ago by Freter [3, 4], who gave Swiss mice and guinea pigs high concentrations of antibiotics, rendering the animals susceptible to infection with antibiotic-resistant strains of *Shigella flexneri* and *Vibrio cholerae*. At about the same time, Bohnhoff et al. [1] reported that peroral administration of streptomycin to mice greatly increased their susceptibility to *Salmonella enteritidis* infection. The antibiotic lowered the ID_{50} of *Salmonella enteritidis* from 1 million viable bacteria to fewer than 10 bacteria [2]. Data from in vitro studies indicated that disruption of the flora resulted in a decrease in volatile fatty concentrations and an increase in the pH of intestinal contents, providing conditions that favored multiplication of *Salmonella enteritidis*.

The protection against colonization of the intestinal tract afforded by the intact flora was termed "colonization resistance" by van de Waaij et al. [9]. These investigators studied colonization resistance in mice before, during, and after peroral administration of streptomycin and neomycin in quantities that eliminated the aerobic components of the intestinal flora. The animals were challenged intragastrically with *Escherichia coli, Klebsiella pneumoniae,* or *Pseudomonas aeruginosa* during each of the three experimental periods. Before antibiotic administration, colonization resistance was high and the animals gradually eliminated the challenge organisms from their intestinal tracts. During administration, there was a precipitous decrease in resistance to colonization and the antibiotic-resistant challenge organisms were retained in the intestinal tract for the duration of the experiments. After cessation of antibiotic administration, colonization resistance was gradually restored concomitant with the repopulation of the intestinal tract with anaerobic components of the intestinal flora that had survived exposure to streptomycin and neomycin. Gnotobiotic mice colonized with these anaerobes displayed a high level of resistance against the challenge strain of *E. coli,* suggesting a critical role for anaerobes in the maintenance of colonization resistance. On the basis of these and similar observations, van de Waaij [8] developed the concept of selective decontamination of the intestinal tract, namely, the

[1] Department of Microbiology and [2] Department of Pediatrics, Texas Tech University, Health Sciences Center, Lubbock, TX 79430, USA
[3] Department of Surgery, Texas Tech University, Health Sciences Center, El Paso, TX 79905, USA

The Influence of Antibiotics on the Host-Parasite Relationship III
Edited by G. Gillissen, W. Opferkuch, G. Peters, and G. Pulverer

elimination of the potentially pathogenic aerobic bacteria and the retention of protective anaerobic bacteria. Antibiotics particularly effective in this regard were polymyxin B, trimethoprim-sulfamethoxazole, and nalidixic acid in combination with amphotericin B or nystatin.

We assessed the effects of administering, individually to mice, high concentrations of ampicillin, clindamycin, kanamycin, metronidazole, and streptomycin on colonization resistance against peroral challenge with *P. aeruginosa* [5]. Despite differences in spectra of activity, all of the antibiotic decreased the resistance of the animals to intestinal colonization with *P. aeruginosa*. Streptomycin, which was most effective in reducing colonization resistance, was investigated further.

Streptomycin-treated mice and untreated control mice were challenged with *P. aeruginosa*, representing an opportunistic organism, *Salmonella typhimurium*, representing an enteric pathogen [7], or *Streptococcus faecalis* representing a common intestinal flora organism which frequently overgrows during antibiotic therapy. All of these organisms were resistant to high concentrations of streptomycin. The treated mice were given 5 mg/ml streptomycin sulfate (Sigma Chemical, St. Louis, USA) in their drinking water for a period of 2 weeks. One week after initiation of antibiotic treatment, treated and untreated animals were challenged perorally with 10^8 viable *P. aeruginosa*, 10^3 viable *Salmonella typhimurium*, or 10^6 viable *Streptococcus faecalis*. Seven days after challenge the animals were killed and counts of the challenge organisms in homogenates of various organs were determined.

The cecum and small intestine of all streptomycin-treated mice were colonized with *P. aeruginosa* and the oganism translocated to the mesentery, liver, or spleen of the majority of these animals [6]. None of the untreated mice were colonized. Although the *Salmonella typhimurium* challenge dose was much smaller than the *P. aeruginosa* dose, the cecum, small intestine, and extraintestinal organs of all streptomycin-treated mice were colonized with the organism. *Salmonella typhimurium* failed to colonize untreated mice. Similarly, *Streptococcus faecalis* colonized the cecum and small intestine of all streptomycin-treated mice and the extraintestinal organs of the majority of the animals. The organs of 10% of untreated mice harbored *Streptococcus faecalis*, however. Streptomycin administration therefore greatly decreased the resistance of mice to intestinal colonization with *P. aeruginosa*, *Salmonella typhimurium*, and *Streptococcus faecalis* and facilitated translocation of the organisms to extraintestinal sites.

In all of these studies, the principal interest was the protective role of the indigenous intestinal flora against colonization by exogenous organisms. Very large quantities of antibiotics were given in order to greatly perturb the intestinal flora and determine how this ecological upset influenced colonization resistance. However, almost nothing is known about the effects of antibiotics administered at therapeutic levels on colonization resistance against enteric pathogens. When an individual is taking antibiotics, is the natural protection provided by the intestinal flora diminished, thus facilitating colonization by antibiotic-resistant pathogens?

Using Swiss white mice, we are currently examining the influence of several oral antibiotics, administered at therapeutic levels, on colonization resistance against enterotoxigenic *E. coli*, *Salmonella typhimurium*, and *Shigella flexneri*.

The antibiotics selected for the study are commonly given to infants and small children in developing countries to treat a variety of infections. Streptomycin, which was administered at high concentration, was included as a control. The quantities of the antibiotics used in the animal experiments (Table 1) were identical, on a body weight basis, to the quantities recommended for administration to infants and small children. Experiments on the influence of the antibiotics on the implantation dose$_{50}$ (ID_{50}) of the pathogens for the mice were performed first. The antibiotics were introduced directly into the stomach, using a thin plastic feeding tube connected to a syringe, three times a day for a period of 3 days. One day later, the animals were challenged perorally with pathogens in doses ranging from one organism to 10^{10} organisms. Ten mice were challenged with each dose. Three days after challenge, fecal specimens, obtained from the mice, were homogenized in phosphate-buffered saline, serially diluted, and plated on MacConkey's agar containing 1 mg/ml streptomycin sulfate, which was selective for the streptomycin-resistant pathogens. The presence or absence of the pathogens in the feces was then recorded and the ID_{50} for each pathogen calculated.

The results, illustrated in Table 2, demonstrate that untreated mice were very resistant to colonization with *Shigella flexneri* but were relatively susceptible to

Table 1. Quantities of antibiotics administered intragastrically to mice

	μg/g body wt./day
Amoxicillin	40
Chloramphenicol	50
Erythromycin	40
Penicillin V	50
Sulfamethoxazole[a]	50
Trimethoprim[a]	10
Streptomycin (control)	500

[a] These antibiotics were administered concomitantly.

Table 2. Influence of antibiotic administration on the ID_{50} values of intestinal pathogens for mice

Treatment	*Salmonella typhimurium*	*Shigella flexneri*	*Escherichia coli*
Untreated	5.4×10^3	1.9×10^8	2.7×10^7
Amoxicillin	1.2×10^5	8.9×10^8	2.4×10^7
Chloramphenicol	2.4×10^4	2.2×10^9	1.2×10^5
Erythromycin	2.7×10^4	1.0×10^9	1.4×10^4
Penicillin V	8.0×10^3	1.7×10^8	2.8×10^4
TMS[a]	1.4×10^5	$>3.7 \times 10^9$	3.0×10^7
Streptomycin (control)	<1	<1	<1

[a] Trimethoprim-sulfamethoxazole.

Table 3. Influence of antibiotic administration on colonization resistance against intestinal pathogens in mice

Treatment	*Salmonella typhimurium*	*Shigella flexneri*	*Escherichia coli*
Amoxicillin	↑↑[b]	↑	NC
Chloramphenicol	↑	↑	↓↓
Erythromycin	↑	↑	↓↓↓
Penicillin V	NC[c]	NC	↓↓↓
TMS[a]	↑↑	↑↑	NC
Streptomycin (control)	↓↓↓↓	↓↓↓↓	↓↓↓↓

[a] Trimethoprim-sulfamethoxazole.
[b] The arrows indicate the effects of the antibiotic on colonization resistance; ↑ indicates an increase and ↓ a decrease in resistance. The greater the number of arrows the more pronounced the effect.
[c] NC indicates no change in colonization resistance.

colonization with *Salmonella typhimurium*. Enterotoxigenic *E. coli* occupied an intermediary position in this regard. Predictably, streptomycin, administered in high concentration, rendered the animals exceedingly susceptible to colonization with the three pathogens. When the antibiotics were administered at therapeutic levels, colonization resistance was diminished in some cases, was unaffected in other cases, or else it was enhanced (Table 3).

Enhancement of resistance was apparent when the mice were given erythromycin, amoxicillin, chloramphenical, or trimethoprim-sulfamethoxazole and were challenged with either *Salmonella typhimurium* or *Shigella flexneri*. Penicillin V did not influence colonization resistance against these two pathogens. Administration of erythromycin, chloramphenicol, or penicillin V decreased colonization resistance against enterotoxigenic *E. coli*, on the other hand. Amoxicillin and trimethoprim-sulfamethoxazole had no effect on colonization resistance against this pathogen.

The enhancement of resistance after antibiotic administration was unexpected. Presumably, perturbation of the ecology of the gastrointestinal tract by antibiotics sometimes results in an environment that is more hostile to pathogens than before treatment. In every case where an antibiotic produced an effect, resistance to colonization with *Salmonella typhimurium* and *Shigella flexneri* was enhanced. However, the situation with *E. coli* was the reverse. When an effect was observed, the antibiotic decreased resistance to colonization with this pathogen.

The responses of *Salmonella typhimurium* and *Shigella flexneri* to the ecological changes in the intestine induced by antibiotics were essentially the same. *E. coli* responded in a totally different fashion. Therefore, identical factors appear to regulate colonization of the intestine by *Salmonella typhimurium* and *Shigella flexneri*. These factors differ from those that regulate the colonization of the intestine by *E. coli*. This provides strong evidence that a universal mechanism governing colonization resistance against pathogens in the intestinal tract does not exist.

Summary

There is evidence that peroral administration of high concentrations of antibiotics disrupts the intestinal flora and greatly increases the susceptibility of experimental animals to colonization with exogenous organisms, including enteric pathogens. When Swiss white mice were given large quantities of streptomycin, they became susceptible to intestinal colonization with *Pseudomonas aeruginosa, Salmonella typhimurium,* and *Streptococcus faecalis.* These organisms translocated extraintestinally and were isolated from the mesentery, liver and spleen. Varied results were obtained when antibiotics were administered at therapeutic levels and mice were challenged with enterotoxigenic *E. coli, Salmonella typhimurium,* or *Shigella flexneri.* Enhancement of resistance occurred when erythromycin, amoxicillin, chloramphenicol, or trimethoprim-sulfamethoxazole were given and the animals were challenged with *Salmonella typhimurium* or *Shigella flexneri.* Penicillin V did not influence colonization resistance against these two pathogens. Administration of erythromycin, chloramphenicol, or penicillin V decreased colonization resistance against enterotoxigenic *E. coli.* Amoxicillin and trimethoprim-sulfamethoxazole had no effect on colonization resistance against this pathogen. The similar response of *Salmonella typhimurium* and *Shigella flexneri* to changes induced by antibiotics and the different response of enterotoxigenic *E. coli* suggests that a universal mechanism governing colonization resistance in the intestinal tract does not exist.

Acknowledgment. This research was supported in part by a grant from the Thrasher Research Fund, Salt Lake City, Utah, USA.

References

1. Bohnhoff M, Drake BL, Miller CP (1954) Effect of streptomycin on susceptibility of intestinal tract to experimental *Salmonella* infection. Proc Soc Exp Biol Med 86:132–137
2. Bohnhoff M, Miller CP (1962) Enhanced susceptibility to *Salmonella* infection in streptomycin-treated mice. J Infect Dis 111:117–127
3. Freter R (1955) The fatal enteric cholera infection in guinea pig, achieved by inhibition of normal enteric flora. J Infect Dis 97:57–65
4. Freter R (1956) Experimental enteric *Shigella* and *Vibrio* infections in mice and guinea pigs. J Exp Med 104:411–418
5. Hentges DJ, Stein AJ, Casey SW, Que JU (1985) Protective role of intestinal flora against infection with *Pseudomonas aeruginosa* in mice: influence of antibiotics on colonization resistance. Infect Immun 47:118–122
6. Hentges DJ, Que JU, Casey SW (1985) The influence of streptomycin on the ecology of the intestine and resistance to infection. In: Adam D, Hahn H, Opferkuch W (eds) The influence of antibiotics on the host-parasite relationship II. Springer, Berlin Heidelberg New York, pp 267–276
7. Que JU, Hentges DJ (1985) Effect of streptomycin administration on colonization resistance to *Salmonella typhimurium* in mice. Infect Immun 48:169–174
8. van der Waaij D (1982) Colonization resistance of the digestive tract: clinical consequences and implications. J Antimicrob Chemother 10:263–270
9. van der Waaij D, Berghuis de Vries JM, Lekkerkerk van der Wees JEC (1971) Colonization resistance of the digestive tract in conventional and antibiotic-treated mice. J Hyg 69:405–411

Influence of Antibiotics on Biochemical Intestinal Microflora-Associated Characteristics in Man and Animals

T. MIDTVEDT

Normally, humans harbor an intestinal microflora that numbers 10^{13}–10^{14} bacteria, a population equaling or exceeding the total number of cells comprising the human body. This population forms dynamic ecosystem(s), governed by a wide variety of host- and microflora-derived physiochemical conditions, including pH, redox potential, nutrient availability, peristalsis, and transit time; and the flora influence a large series of physiological and biochemical functions in the host. From a host defense point of view, it is generally assumed that a normal intestinal flora represents a very valuable defense mechanism.

Every time a human or another mammalian organism receives an antimicrobial agent, a series of exceedingly complex alterations and interactions are established. Since the introduction of the first antibiotic more than 40 years ago, there have been many reports dealing with disturbances in the normal distribution and balance of the intestinal flora administration of such agents. However, in contrast, rather few reports have appeared dealing with problems more directly related to antibiotic-induced functional alterations in the microbial flora, causing host/flora interactions.

In such research, one approach of increasing importance is to study mammals with no bacterial flora, i. e., germ-free animals and newborns, thereby establishing values with regard to anatomical structures, and physiological and biochemical functions in the host per se. When such baselines are first established, the normal influence(s) of the flora as well as alterations in these influences are more easily worked out. With a slight travesty of the well-known terminology introduced by Claude Bernhard, the mammalian organism itself can be characterized as the *milieu interieur,* the normal flora as the *milieu exterieur,* and the mammalian organism and its microbial ecosystems as the *milieu total.* When studying such ecosystems, two new terms – MAC and GAC – have been shown to be of considerable value [1]. A MAC (microflora-associated characteristic) can be defined as the recording of any anatomical structure, or physiological or biochemical function in a macroorganism, which has been influenced by the microflora. When microbes actually influencing the parameter under study are absent – as in germ-free animals, newborns, and/or in relation to ingestion of antibiotics – the recording of a MAC can be defined as a GAC (germ-free animal characteristic). Table 1 lists some of the intestinal structures and functions which are known to be influenced by the intestinal flora. Additionally is quoted some data concerning the most active part (species when known) of the flora.

Department of Medical Microbial Ecology, Karolinska Institutet, Box 60400, 10401 Stockholm, Sweden

The Influence of Antibiotics on the Host-Parasite Relationship III
Edited by G. Gillissen, W. Opferkuch, G. Peters, and G. Pulverer

Table 1. Some intestinal structures and functions influenced by the microflora

Parameter	MAC	GAC	Microbes involved
Intestinal wall	Thick lamina propria Irregular villi High cell turnover	Thin lamina propria Regular villi Low cell turnover	Unknown Unknown Unknown
Cecum size	Normal	Enlarged	Unknown
Intestinal smooth muscle activity	Vivid spontaneous contractions	Markedly reduced contractions	Unknown
Sensitivity toward biogenic amines	Normal	Markedly reduced	Unknown
Amounts of biogenic amines	MAC=GAC	GAC=MAC	
Bile acid metabolism	Deconjugation Dehydrogenation Dehydroxylation	No deconjugation No dehydrogenation No dehydroxylation	Several species Several species Few species, mostly anaerobic, non-spore-forming, gram+rods
Bilirubin metabolism	Deconjugation Urobilinogen formation	Little deconjugation No urobilinogen formation	Several species *Clodstridium ramosum*
Cholesterol	Mainly coprostanol	Only cholesterol	An *Eubacterium* species
Dipeptidases (such as beta-aspartylglycine)	Absent	High amounts	Unknown
Intestinal gases	H_2, CH_4, CO_2	No H_2 or CH_4 Reduced CO_2	Unknown
Mucus	Absent in feces	High amount	Several species, such as *Peptostreptococcus micros, Bacteroides ruminococcus,* and *Bifidobacterium*
SCFAs	High amounts Several acids	Small amounts Few acids	Probably several species
Tryptic activity in feces	Little or no activity	High activity	Unknown

Thus, accepting the fact that many *interieur* structures and functions are acted upon by the normal flora, the possibility exists that ingestion of antibiotics into conventional mammals may switch one or more of these parameters "back" to the levels, found in germ-free individuals. Recently, we have investigated the effect of ten orally given antimicrobial agents upon some MACs in human volunteers. The following drugs were given for 6 days to groups of six to seven volunteers: ampicillin 500 mg q.i.d.; bacitracin 25000 IU q.i.d; clindamycin 150 mg q.i.d; cotrimoxazole 160/800 mg b.i.d; doxycycline 200 mg on the 1st day, thereafter 100 mg daily; erythromycin 250 mg q.i.d; metronidazole 400 mg t.i.d; nalidixic acid 500 mg q.i.d; ofloxacin 200 mg b.i.d.; and vancomycin 240 mg q.i.d. Fecal samples were taken twice before, on day 3 and 6 during, and weekly to monthly after administration of the drugs. All samples were frozen within 10 min after delivery, and they were investigated in a blind fashion. The study was performed according to the revised Helsinki Declaration; no serious side effects were observed.

Of the many MACs to be studied, we decided to concentrate on the following: conversion of cholesterol to coprostanol, dehydroxylation of cholic acid to deoxycholic acid, and transformation of conjugated bilirubin to urobilinogen in order to elucidate some of the major aspects of hepatic/intestinal interactions and enterohepatic circulation; inactivation of tryptic activity in order to study a pancreatic/intestinal cofunction; breakdown of mucin in order to study an intestinal function of major importance for the preservation of the integrity of the intestinal mucosa; and absence of beta-aspartylglycine and presence of short-chain fatty acids (SCFAs) in order to elucidate the microbial interaction with compounds mainly deriving from the diet.

The results from this investigation are currently being published. Table 2 summarized some of the data obtained [5–10], together with the results of some other investigations of the effect of antimicrobial drugs upon MACs in man and rat. In general, the influences have been found to be more long-lasting in rat than in man. The reason for this difference is unknown. However, it might be reasonable to assume that a human, eating a varied diet and daily coming into contact with several people, is exposed to far more microbial species than a laboratory rat, daily eating the same sterilized diet and being exposed to a very limited number of humans or other animals. Therefore, the chance of a rat randomly picking up an eradicated species is probably far smaller than for a healthy man. The situation in rats resembles that in patients kept under isolation conditions.

Of the parameters studied, significant alterations were found in all except two, i.e., presence of beta-aspartylglycine [17] and alterations in fecal tryptic activity [18]. Of the ten antibiotics included in the study, bacitracin, clindamycin, and vancomycin caused significant alterations in more than half of the MACs. Ampicillin, doxycycline, erythromycin, and metronidazole caused significant alterations in less than half the MACs, whereas cotrimoxazole, nalidixic acid, and ofloxacin caused MAC alterations in some individuals only. In most cases, the MAC disturbances were normalized within 6 weeks. However, in four individuals, production of coprostanol was still zero, even after 6 weeks (unpublished results).

Taken together, our results indicate that drugs with an anaerobic, gram-positive "profile" (such as bacitracin, clindamycin, and vancomycin) interact more seriously with the physiologically active part of the gastrointestinal flora than drugs acting mainly upon aerobic, gram-negative organisms (such as cotrimoxazole, nalidixic acid, and ofloxacin).

The possible influence(s) of these intestinal microbial interactions upon functions to be performed in other places of the body have only recently been recognized. Many of the substances produced in the intestine by the microbes present are parts of enterohepatic feedback systems, and intestinal alterations in production may influence (regulatory) functions in other places of the body, thereby also interfering with the organism's capability to defend itself against "the microbial world." In fact, the possible influence of any microbial interference with the *milieu interieur* should be analyzed according to the scheme outlined in Table 3. As an example, data concerning possible influences of SCFAs (which are nearly ex-

Table 2. Influence of antibiotics upon microflora-associated characteristics (MACs)

Species [reference]	Characteristic	Agent	Effect
Man [2]	Coprostanol	AMP, CLI, OXI, NEO/BAC	GAC pattern
		PEN V, DOX	No effect
Man [3]	H_2 production	MET, PEN V	Reduction
		DOX	No effect
	CH_4 production	MET	Reduction
		DOX, PEN V	No effect
Man [4]	SCFAs	CO-TRI	Reduced
Man [5]	Coprostanol	CLI, MET	Major effect
	Bilirubin	CLI, MET	Major effect
	Urobilinogen, SCFAs	AMP, CLI	Major effect
	Mucin	CLI	Major effect
	Trypsin, beta-asp-glycine	AMP, CLI, MET	No effect
Man [6]	Mucin	BAC, CLI, VAN	GAC pattern
		AMP, DOX, ERY, MET, NAL	Minor effect
		CO-TRI, OFL	No effect
Man [7]	SCFAs	AMP, CLI	Major effect
		MET	No effect
Man [8]	SCFAs	BAC, VAN	Major effect
		ERY	Minor effect
		CO-TRI, DOX, NAL, OFL	No effect
Man [9]	Bilirubin	AMP, BAC, CLI, ERY, VAN	Major effect
		CO-TRI, DOX, MET, NAL, OFL	No effect
Man [10]	tα-Dehydroxylation	CLI	Major effect
		AMP, MET	No effect
Rat [11]	Bile acids:	ERY, NEO/BAC	GAC pattern
	deconjugation/	NEO, PEN G	GAC pattern
	dehydroxylation	MET	Minor effect
Rat [12, 13]	Coprostanol/	AMP, COL, ERY	GAC pattern
	urobilinogen/	NEO/BAC, NEO	GAC pattern
	mucin/trypsin	PEN G	GAC pattern
		MET	Minor effect
Rat [14]	Trypsin	AMP, CLI	GAC pattern
		DOX, PEN G	GAC pattern
Rat [15]	Coprostanol/ urobilinogen/mucin/ trypsin	CLI	GAC pattern
Rat [16]	Mucin/coprostanol/	CLI	Major effect
	trypsin/SCAFs	CLI	Major effect
	Beta-aspartylglycine	CLI	No effect

AMP, ampicillin; CLI, clindamycin; COL, colistin; CO-TRI, cotrimoxazole; DOX, doxycycline; ERY, erythromycin; MET, metronidazole; NEO/BAC, neomycin/bacitracin; NEO, neomycin; PEN G, benzylpenicillin; PEN V, phenoxymethylpenicillin; OXI, oxytetracycline.

Table 3. Example of consequence analysis of one MAC

Statement:			SCFAs are normally produced in high amounts by the intestinal flora; they are partly absorbed and partly excreted in feces
Mechanism behind possible consequenes		Biochemical:	SCFAs are involved in several metabolic pathways
		Immunological:	Uncertain
Place:		Locally:	In the intestinal lumen At the mucosa surface Within the mucosa cells
		Distant:	In the liver, pancreas, brain, etc.
Form:	Direct:	Locally:	Main anions in intestinal content Growth promotion of some microbes Growth suppression of others Growth regulation of mucosa cells
		Distant:	Energy supply to the general metabolism
	Indirect:	Locally:	"Promoted" microbes produce suppressive bacteriocins Direct suppression provides niches for other microbes to grow
		Distant:	Metabolic alterations act on production of insulin, etc.
Consequences:		Physiological:	Locally the SCFAs are parts of direct/indirect regulatory mechanisms for water and electrolyte absorption; the net effect is antidiarrheic. Involved in regulation of mucosa cell turnover, they take part in regulation of carbohydrate metabolism, etc.
		Pathophysiological:	Involved in hepatic coma. Probably involved in colonic cancer, ulcerative and pseudomembraneous colitis, etc.

clusively produced by the intestinal flora) are listed in Table 3. However, it has to be underlined that several other parameters, such as bile acids, cholesterol, bilirubin, and mucin, might be of equal physiological and pathophysiological importance.

In this paper I have focused on the philosophy behind our ongoing work on the influence of antibiotics on biochemical intestinal microflora-associated characteristics. The results can be found in the papers mentioned in the reference list. The need for further investigations is obvious. It must also be underlined that in the near future more drugs will enter the antimicrobial market than ever before. However, before the wave of new and very potent penems, penams, cephems, cephams, macrolides, etc. "floods down" the intestinal tract of our patients, it might be wise to start thinking about possible interactions with the physiological part of the flora and short- and long-term consequences of these interactions. The flora and its functions create an important part of the host's defense systems, not to be disturbed too much by the drugs given.

Summary

From a host defense point of view, a normal intestinal flora represents a valuable defense mechanism. Alterations in this flora resulting from administration of antibiotics can be studied by following alterations in intestinal structures and functions which are normally influenced by the microflora. In our ecological studies we have investigated the influence of several antibiotics upon a long list of such so-called microflora-associated characteristics (MACs) in man and rat. Several antibiotics may alter the findings so that they are similar to those obtained in germ-free animals (germ-free animal characteristics/GACs). Each antibiotic may create its own MAC/GAC profile, partly reflecting the characteristics of the microbial species, and partly its antibacterial spectrum and concentration in the intestinal tract. Such MAC/GAC alterations may interact to affect functions outside the gastrointestinal tract.

References

1. Midtvedt T, Björneklett A, Carlstedt-Duke B, Gustafsson BE, Höverstad T, Lingaas E, Norin KE, Saxerholt H, Steinbakk M (1985) The influence of antibiotics upon microflora-associated characteristics in man and mammals. In: Wostmann BS (ed) Germfree research: microflora control and its application to the biomedical sciences. Alan R Liss, New York, pp 241–244
2. Midtvedt T, Frederichsen P (1977) Influence of antibiotics on microbial intestinal transformation of cholesterol to coprostanol in man. Scand J Gastroenterol 12:669–672
3. Björneklett A, Midtvedt T (1981) Influence of three antimicrobial agents – penicillin, metronidazole, and doxycycline – on the intestinal microflora of healthy humans. Scand J Gastroenterol 16:473–480
4. Höverstad T, Björneklett A, Fausa O, Midtvedt T (1985) Short-chain fatty acids in the small-bowel bacterial overgrowth syndrome. Scand J Gastroenterol 20:492–499
5. Midtvedt T, Carlstedt-Duke B, Höverstad T, Lingaas E, Norin E, Saxerholt H, Steinbakk M (1986) Influence of peroral antibiotics upon the biotransformatory activity of the intestinal microflora in healthy subjects. Eur J Clin Invest 16:11–17
6. Carlstedt-Duke B, Höverstad T, Lingaas E, Norin KE, Saxerholt H, Steinbakk M, Midtvedt T (1986) Influence of antibiotics on intestinal mucin in healthy subjects. Eur J Clin Microbiol 5:634–638
7. Höverstad T, Carlstedt-Duke B, Lingaas E, Midtvedt T, Norin KE, Saxerholt H, Steinbakk M (1986) Influence of ampicillin, clindamycin and metronidazole on fecal excretion of short-chain fatty acids in healthy subjects. Scand J Gastroenterol 21:621–626
8. Höverstad T, Carlstedt-Duke B, Lingaas E, Norin E, Saxerholt H, Steinbakk M, Midtvedt T (1986) Influence of oral intake of seven different antibiotics on faecal short-chain fatty acid excretion in healthy subjects. Scand J Gastroenterol 21:997–1003
9. Saxerholt H, Carlstedt-Duke B, Höverstad T, Lingaas E, Norin KE, Steinbakk M, Midtvedt T (1986) Influence of antibiotics on the faecal excretion of bile pigments in healthy subjects. Scand J Gastroenterol 21:991–996
10. Andreasson K, Norin KE, Midtvedt T (1988) Influence of ampicillin, clindamycin or metronidazole upon the 7α-dehydroxylation of bile acids in the human intestine. Curr Microbiol 16:329–331
11. Gustafsson BE, Norin KE (1977) Development of germ-free animal characteristics in conventional rats by antibiotics. Acta Pathol Microbiol Scand Sect B 85:1–8
12. Gustafsson BE, Midtvedt T, Strandberg K (1977) Effects of microbial contamination on the cecum enlargement of germ-free rats. Scand J Gastroenterol 5:309–314
13. Gustafsson BE, Gustafsson J-Å, Carlstedt-Duke B (1977) Prolonged induction of germfree bile acid pattern in conventional rats by antibiotics. Acta Med Scand 201:155–160
14. Genell S, Gustafsson BE (1977) Impaired enteric degradation of pancreatic endopeptidases in antibiotic-treated rats. Scand J Gastroenterol 12:801–809
15. Carlstedt-Duke B, Gustafsson BE, Midtvedt T (1985) Clindamycin-induced alterations in intestinal microflora-associated characteristics in rats. Scand J Gastroenterol 20:92–98

16. Carlstedt-Duke B, Alm L, Höverstad T, Midtvedt A-C, Norin KE, Steinbakk M, Midtvedt T (1987) Influence of clindamycin, administered together with or without lactobacilli, upon intestinal ecology in rat. FEMS Microbiol Ecol 45:251–259
17. Norin E, Carlstedt-Duke B, Gustafsson A, Höverstad T, Lingaas E, Midtvedt A-C, Saxerholt H, Steinbakk M, Midtvedt T (1987) Absence of β-aspartylglycine in feces – a microflora-associated characteristic, MAC (abstr) IX International Symposium on Gnotobiology, Versailles, France, June 1987
18. Norin KE, Carlstedt-Duke B, Höverstad T, Lingaas E, Saxerholt H, Steinbakk M, Midtvedt T (1988) Faecal tryptic activity in humans: influence of antibiotics on microbial intestinal degradation. Microbial Ecology in Health and Diseases 1:65–68

Antibiotics and the Host-Parasite Relationship in Cystic Fibrosis

J. A. Raeburn, R. Sutherland, R. T. Cullen, and A. Greening

Introduction

Patients with cystic fibrosis (CF) have repeated pulmonary infections which lead to chronic bronchiectasis and other forms of lung damage. Although the causative gene has now been located on chromosome 7, and DNA sequences of that gene are being analysed, the reason for the recurrent respiratory infection is not known. Treatment with high doses of appropriate antibiotics, often for several weeks or even on a long-term basis, plays a most important part in management. However, despite newer antibiotics and, in particular, agents with much greater activity against *Pseudomonas aeruginosa,* many patients with antibiotic-sensitive bacteria in the sputum continue to suffer progressive lung damage.

Studies of the host-parasite relationship in CF of a decade ago sought to identify a specific gap in host defense which might explain recurrent respiratory infection. No consistent primary defect was found although some patients had secondary changes in phagocytic cells [7] or in immunoglobulins [5]. It was considered that these changes might explain the chronicity of infection after the initial triggering factor. Wilson et al. [9] showed that monocytes from CF patients, or from obligate carriers, differed from those of normal subjects in that they secreted substances in vitro which had numerous biological functions; in particular they were stimulants of neutrophil chemotaxis. The reason for poor responses to antibiotic therapy in CF, despite sensitivity of the organisms in vitro, is also not fully understood, but lack of antibiotic penetration through mucus (of either human or bacterial origin) is thought to play a part. It is clear that cystic fibrosis is a condition in which antibiotic interactions with the host defences could be of great importance and we have therefore carried out a series of studies to monitor these aspects.

Patients and Methods

Patients attending the adult CF clinic at the Western General Hospital were studied during follow-up of their respiratory condition. In general each patient is seen monthly and undergoes clinical, respiratory function and immunological moni-

University Department of Medicine, Western General Hospital, Edinburgh, EH4 2XU, United Kingdom

The Influence of Antibiotics on the Host-Parasite Relationship III
Edited by G. Gillissen, W. Opferkuch, G. Peters, and G. Pulverer

toring. Standard methods were used for measurement of total and differential leucocytes, immunoglobulins and forced respiratory volume (FEV1). Chemiluminescence studies were performed by the method described by Kowolik et al. [4].

Results

Figure 1 shows the serial leucocyte counts, throughout life, of an 11-year-old boy who died of cystic fibrosis. In the last 4 years of his life there was a steep rise in total leucocytes due entirely to an increase in granulocytes. This pattern is typical of the white cell changes in CF patients who die of respiratory infection. The time at which the rise in granulocytes begins is, however, extremely variable. Table 1 shows some of the main findings of the comparisons between CF subjects and controls. There were significant differences between patients and controls in re-

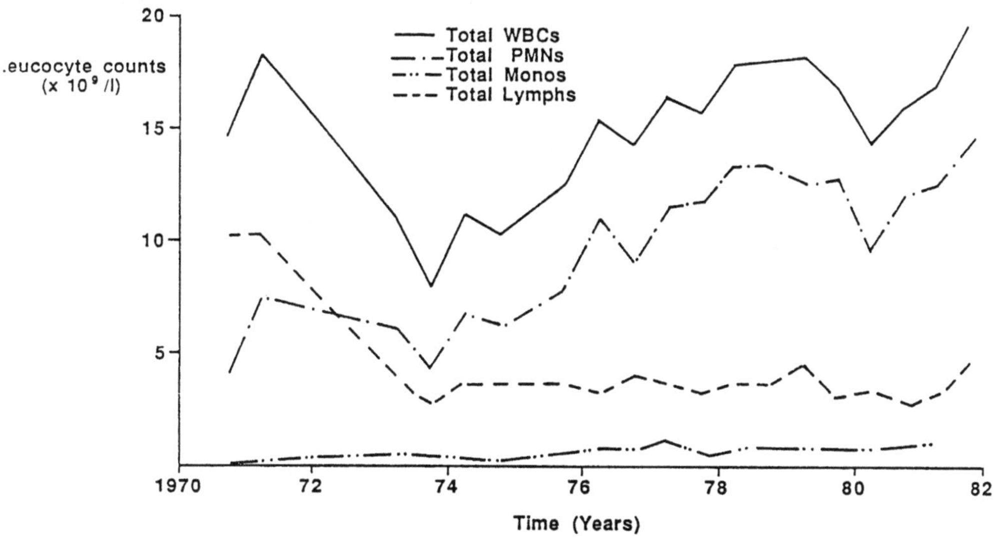

Fig. 1. Serial leucocyte counts in CF (in a boy who died at age 11 years)

Table 1. Comparisons between CF patients and controls

	Mean value of				
	Lyz	Lum-CL	LUC-CL	MPO	Neutrophils
CF	5.36	591	394	0.074	6.96
Control	3.81	402	368	0.100	3.63
P value	<0.01	< 0.05	NS	NS	NS

Lyz, serum lysozyme level (μg/ml); Lum-CL, chemiluminescence response to zymosan challenge using luminol enhancement (mV); LUC-CL, chemiluminescence response to zymosan challenge using lucigenin enhancement (mV); MPO, neutrophil myeloperoxidase activity (units/10^6 cells per minute); Neutrophils, absolute neutrophil count ($\times 10^9$/liter); NS, differences not significant.

Table 2. Serial measurements of leucocytes, forced expiratory volume, immunoglobulins and chemiluminescence in response to PMA or staphylococcal stimulation in a 16-year-old male with CF. During the period of study he received ciprofloxacin for a total period of 8 weeks, clindamycin for 4 weeks and prednisolone (15 mg/day) for 6 weeks. The main infecting organism was *Staphylococcus aureus*

Date	8/86	11/86	2/87	4/87	6/87
WBCs	9.5	15.6	7.2	10.2	13.0
PMNs (%)	61	76	45	41	70
FEV1	1.7	1.65	1.92	2.62	2.75
IgG	325	238	235	174	171
IgA	281	273	266	194	196
CL-PMA	162	1542	2185	–	3556
CL-SA		129	143		53

WBCs, total leucocyte count $\times 10^9$/liter; PMNs %), granulocytes as a percentage of the total leucocytes; FEV1, forced expiratory volume in litres per second; CL-PMA, chemiluminescence response to phorbol myristate in a luminol-enhanced system; CL-SA, chemiluminescent response to opsonized *Staphylococcus aureus* using lucigenin enhancement.

Table 3. Serial measurements of leucocytes, forced expiratory volume, immunoglobulins and chemiluminescence in response to PMA or staphylococcal stimulation in a 16-year-old male with CF. During the period of study he received ciprofloxacin almost continuously, four courses of ceftazidime plus tobramycin each for 3 weeks, clindamycin for 4 weeks and prednisolone (15 mg/day) for 18 weeks. The main infecting organism was *Pseudomonas aeruginosa*

Date	8/86	11/86	2/87	5/87	7/87
WBCs	12.1	7.4	12.2	13.1	26.1
PMNs (%)	78	52	73	63	88
FEV1	0.35	0.55	0.61	0.45	0.48
IgG	245	154	171	138	154
IgA	328	268	252	274	381
IgM	314	292	307	309	196
CL-PMA	1223	1624	1696	3061	3314
CL-SA	54	100	136	102	86

WBCs, total leucocyte count $\times 10^9$/liter; PMNs %), granulocytes as a percentage of the total leucocytes; FEV1, forced expiratory volume in litres per second; CL-PMA, chemiluminescence response to phorbol myristate luminol-enhanced system; CL-SA, chemiluminescent response to opsonized *Staphylococcus aureus* using lucigenin enhancement.

spect of serum lysozyme levels and in chemiluminescence responses to challenge with zymosan. Tables 2–4 show some serial alterations in values in three individuals with respiratory damage due to CF. The patient whose data is summarized in Table 2 had relatively good respiratory function results. He had large numbers of *Staphylococcus aureus* in the sputum (10^7/ml) with *Pseudomonas aeruginosa* at a lower level (10^5/ml). Antibiotic treatment against both these organisms from 8/86 to 2/87 produced a small fall in IgG and IgA and a slight improvement of respiratory function. When prednisolone therapy was given (from 2/87 to 4/87) there were much greater changes in these measurements which persisted after cessation

Table 4. Serial measurements of leucocytes, forced expiratory volume, immunoglobulins and chemiluminescence in response to PMA or staphylococcal stimulation in a 16-year-old female with CF. During the period of study she received ciprofloxacin almost continuously, five courses of tobramycin and ceftazidime for 3 weeks each, aztreonam, azlocillin and clindamycin for 4 weeks each and prednisolone (15 mg/day) for 6 months. The main infecting organism was *Pseudomonas aeruginosa*

Date	11/87	12/87	2/87	3/87	6/87
WBCs	6.7	8.9	13.5	10.9	10.8
PMNs (%)	70	67	81	72	74
FEV1	0.65	0.75	0.4	0.62	0.5
IgG	217	184	181	178	127
IgA	225	210	214	211	222
IgM	173	122	190	176	166
CL-PMA	–	2478	1759	2653	3921
CL-SA	–	102		194	84

WBCs, total leucocyte count $\times 10^9$/liter; PMNs %), granulocytes as a percentage of the total leucocytes; FEV1, forced expiratory volume in litres per second; CL-PMA, chemiluminescence response to phorbol myristate in a luminol-enhanced system; CL-SA, chemiluminescent response to opsonized *Staphylococcus aureus* using lucigenin enhancement.

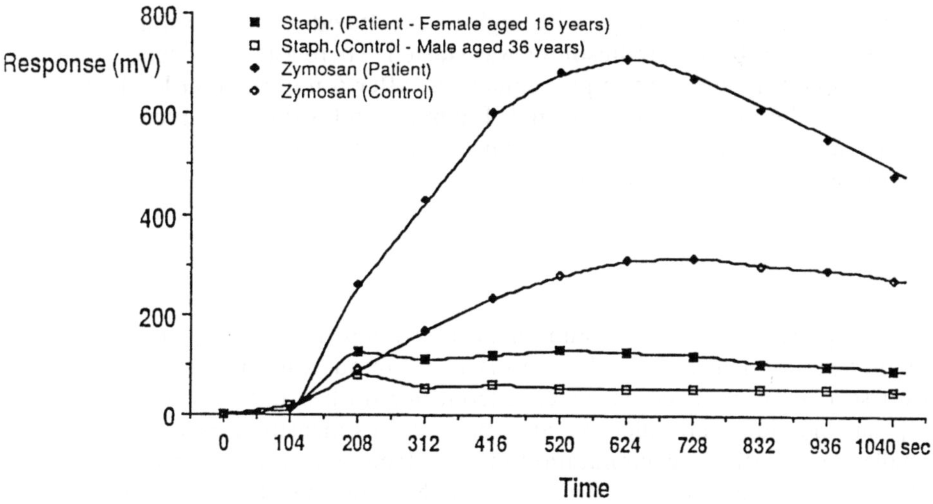

Fig. 2. Lucigenin-enhanced chemiluminescence in CF

of steroid therapy when antibiotics were given only for documented sputum infection. Table 3 summarizes data from a 16-year-old male with respiratory function which was always less than 20% of the predicted normal value for age and weight. His *P. aeruginosa* infection ($>10^7$/ml sputum) required frequent intensive antibiotic therapy. From 8/86 to 11/86 this produced a fall in total leucocytes and granulocytes, IgG, IgA and IgM and a modest rise of forced expiratory function. Then prednisolone therapy was started (in 11/86). There was very little change in most parameters but the WBCs, PMNs, and chemiluminescence responses in-

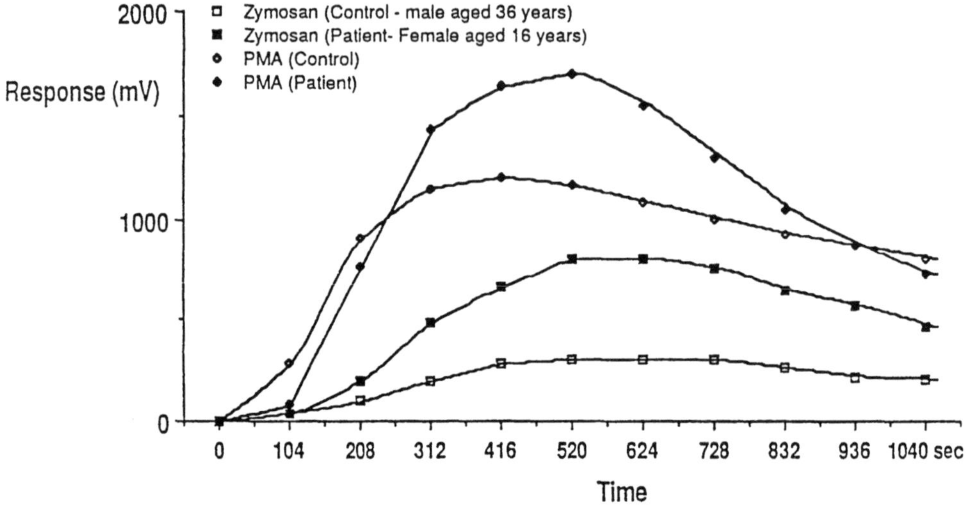

Fig. 3. Luminol-enhanced chemiluminescence in CF

creased. Table 4 shows similar results from a 16-year-old female with severe lung damage. After initial therapy with high-dose ceftazidime and tobramycin for 3 weeks (11/86 to 12/86) prednisolone was started. There was no evidence of significant respiratory function improvement but after 6 months IgG levels had decreased to the lower limit of normal. Figures 2 and 3 show the typical patterns of increased chemiluminescence response to in vitro challenge of a CF patient, in comparison to a healthy control.

Discussion

The CF patient with chronic pulmonary infection usually has elevated peripheral blood levels of neutrophils: often this is a continuous abnormality which persists over several years. There is evidence from our studies and those of Graft et al. [3] that individual granulocytes are "primed," as measured by the response to challenges in vitro in chemiluminescence systems. Recently increased monocyte chemiluminescence was also demonstrated [8]. Thus the CF subject has in his circulation excess numbers of phagocytic cells which individually will react excessively, thus producing greater amounts of reactive oxygen species. These could well exacerbate, or be the cause of, inflammation in the lungs. Since antibiotics may influence the host responses, their use in high doses over long periods could affect the course of cystic fibrosis by that mechanism as well as by merely inhibiting bacterial activities. An antibiotic effect which enhances chemiluminescence [2] could in this situation be deleterious.

Our studies of individual subjects show how variable some of the parameters which are measurable can be, during a series of repeated infections and intensive treatment of cystic fibrosis. These are complicated more if steroid or other immunosuppressive therapy is used, treatment which is now being investigated more systematically [1, 6]. Many more studies of the host defence system in CF are indicated. However, our preliminary data suggest that intensive antibiotic therapy plus steroids will be more effective if administered prior to major decrease of respiratory functions.

Summary

Most patients with CF suffer repeated chest infection and require treatment with antibiotics, in high doses, for long periods. There are no consistent host defence defects but in vitro tests from CF patients often show significantly different mean values and also a greater variance than do those of control subjects. These changes could result from the disease itself, from infection, or from therapy. In some patients we have observed that ceftazidime treatment increases chemiluminescent (CL) responses to zymosan and other stimuli [2]. Other antibiotics (e.g. tobramycin) can reduce CL responses.

There is now evidence that lung damage in CF may be related to an excessive neutrophil influx to inflamed alveoli. These phagocytes may then produce abnormally high levels of reactive oxygen species, with a potential to cause lung damage. Monitoring of host defence functions during therapy in CF is therefore important. We have made serial measurements of total WBCs, CL responses to specific stimuli and immunoglobulins in CF patients receiving appropriate antibiotic therapy and (occasionally) during steroid treatment. There are no consistent host-defence changes, but the mangitude of alteration in some individuals suggests a pathogenetic role in the causation of subsequent lung damage.

References

1. Auerbach HS, William M et al. (1985) Alternate day prednisolone reduces morbidity and improves lung function in cystic fibrosis. Lancet II:686–688
2. Cullen RT, McCrae WM, Govan JRW, Raeburn JA (1983) Ceftazidime in cystic fibrosis; clinical, microbiological and immunological studies. J Antimicrob Chemother 12 [Suppl A]:369–375
3. Graft DF, Mischler)E et al. (1982) Granulocyte chemiluminescence in adolescent patients with cystic fibrosis. Amer Rev Respir Dis 125:540–543
4. Kowolik M, Raeburn JA, Grant M (1982) In vivo effect of ampicillin and cefaclor on blood and gingival crevicular neutrophil myeloperoxidase activity. In: Eichenberg H, Opferkuch W (eds) The influence of antibiotics on the host-parasite relationship. Springer, Berlin Heidelberg New York, pp 56–66
5. McCrae WM, Raeburn JA (1974) Patterns of infection in cystic fibrosis. Scott Med J 19:187–193
6. Pantin CFA, Stead et al. (1986) Presdnisolone in the treatment of airflow obstruction in adults with cystic fibrosis. Thorax 41:34–38
7. Raeburn JA, McCrae WM (1976) Immune responses to bacteria in cystic fibrosis. Proceedings of the 7th international congress of cystic fibrosis. Paris, pp 541–544
8. Regelman WE, Lunde NM et al. (1986) Increased monocyte chemilumiscence in cystic fibrosis patients and their parents. Pediatr Res 20:619–622
9. Wilson GB, Fudenberg HH et al. (1981) Effects of ciliary dyskinesia substances on neutrophil movement in vitro. J Clin Invest 68:171–183

Absence of a Postantibiotic Effect in Experimental Left-Sided *Streptococcus faecalis* Endocarditis Treated with Penicillin Plus Gentamicin

M. T. Hessen, P. G. Pitsakis, and M. E. Levison

In ongoing experiments, the pharmacodynamic effects of antibiotics have been evaluated in the rat model of aortic valve *Streptococcus faecalis* endocarditis.

This model is appropriate to demonstrate pharmacodynamic effects as the aortic valve vegetation is a protected site in which the host defense mechanisms apparently are of little importance in eliminating bacteria.

In this model the right carotid artery of a rat is cannulated, and the catheter is advanced into the left ventricle. Twenty-four hours later 10^9 colony-forming units (CFUs) *S. faecalis* are injected into the tail vein. All rats infected with this inoculum develop endocarditis on the aortic valve. Eighteen hours later, rats are treated i.m. with one or more doses of antibiotic. Bacterial counts and antibiotic concentrations in vegetations of these rats are then determined at various times after injection of antibiotic in order to correlate the response of the bacterial population to the concentration of the antimicrobial agent in the vegetation. Clearance of organisms from the vegetation is related to the rate and extent of the bactericidal effect and the duration of a post antibiotic effect (PAE), the PAE being defined as the persistence of inhibitory activity following brief exposure of bacteria to an antibiotic.

A small bactericidal effect following a dose of antibiotic would require the cumulative effect of multiple doses to reduce significantly the bacterial population in the vegetation. The additional absence of a PAE would require relatively short dosing intervals to maintain tissue antibiotic concentrations above the minimal inhibitory concentrations (MIC) and thereby prevent bacterial regrowth in the latter portions of each dosing interval. In contrast, a rapid and large bactericidal effect following a single dose of antibiotic would reduce the bacterial population in the vegetation to relatively low numbers. This small residual bacterial population would require a relatively long interval to recover to its original numbers. The additional presence of a long PAE in vivo would extend the inhibitory effect on the small residual population and allow use of long antibiotic dosing intervals, during which tissue drug levels could fall below the MIC without loss of efficacy.

Enhancement of the rate and extent of bactericidal activity is one of the indications for use of the combination of penicillin plus gentamicin in the therapy of enterococcal endocarditis. In addition, a PAE has been demonstrated in vitro for

Division of Infectious Diseases, Department of Medicine, Medical College of Pennsylvania, 330 Henry Avenue, Philadelphia, PA 19129, USA

The Influence of Antibiotics on the Host-Parasite Relationship III
Edited by G. Gillissen, W. Opferkuch, G. Peters, and G. Pulverer

S. faecalis exposed to penicillin, gentamicin and the combination of penicillin plus gentamicin in the following experiments.

The initial bactericidal and PAEs were determined in vitro by the method of McDonald et al. [1] in broth suspensions of 10^7 CFUs *S. faecalis*/ml following a 2 h exposure to penicillin (20 μg/ml) and gentamicin (3, 6, 12, and 24 μg/ml), each alone, and the combination of penicillin (20 μl/ml) plus gentamicin (3 and 6 μg/ml). Repeated washing was used for drug removal. Five blood culture isolates of *S. faecalis* from patients with endocarditis were studied. The MIC of each strain was 3.1 μg/ml for penicillin and 6.3 μg/ml for gentamicin. The mean PAE for penicillin 20 μg/ml alone was 1.8 h. Increasing concentrations of gentamicin caused both an increased rate of bactericidal action and increased duration of PAE from 0.5 to 3.7 h. The combination of penicillin plus gentamicin showed both more rapid killing than that of penicillin or gentamicin alone and a prolongation of the PAE. The PAE for penicillin and gentamicin, 3 μg/ml, was 2.9 h; and for penicillin plus gentamicin 6 μl/ml, 3.3 h. If present in vivo the prolongation of the PAE with the combination of penicillin plus gentamicin should permit antibiotic levels to fall such that antibacterial activity could be absent for a considerable portion of the dosing interval without altering drug efficacy.

Indeed, the duration that antibiotic levels exceed the MIC plus the duration of the PAE in some cases could be longer than the conventional dosing interval for these drugs. In this case, antibacterial activity of antibiotics administered at the usual intervals might be affected by the PAE induced by a previous dose, as has been described for other antibiotic-organism combinations. To assess bactericidal activity during a PAE induced by a prior 2-h exposure to gentamicin 3 μg/ml (PAE 0.7 h), penicillin 20 μg/ml (PAE, 1.8 h), or penicillin 20 μg/ml plus gentamicin 3 μg/ml (PAE, 3.5 h), we exposed the persisting organisms (after removal of prior antibiotic by washing) to penicillin 20 μg/ml or penicillin 20 μg/ml plus gentamicin 3 μg/ml. Changes in enterococcal counts were similar for organisms previously exposed to gentamicin or no antibiotic (i.e., about 1.0 $\log_{10}$ CFUs/ml fall with subsequent exposure to penicillin 20 μg/ml, and about a 4.0 $\log_{10}$ CFUs/ml fall with subsequent exposure to penicillin 20 μg/ml plus gentamicin 3 μg/ml). However, bactericidal activity of both penicillin and penicillin plus gentamicin was diminished by prior exposure to either penicillin or penicillin plus gentamicin. Inhibition of bactericidal activity was greater following prior exposure to penicillin plus gentamicin than penicillin alone.

One possible explanation for resistance to the bactericidal activity of penicillin plus gentamicin during the PAE could be the absence of renewed synthesis of penicillin-binding protein molecules following antibiotic removal.

In order to determine whether these phenomena occur in vivo, we treated experimental enterococcal endocarditis in rats with a single injection of the combination of penicillin plus gentamicin in doses that resulted in vegetation antibiotic concentrations similar to those in the in vitro experiments.

Penicillin concentrations in vegetation were 2.7 μg/g or greater, that is above the MIC, for 3 h after aqueous penicillin, 50 mg/kg i.m. The gentamicin concentration was about 2 μg/g.

Figure 1 shows the pharmacodynamic effects following single doses of aqueous penicillin G plus gentamicin in rats with experimental enterococcal endocarditis.

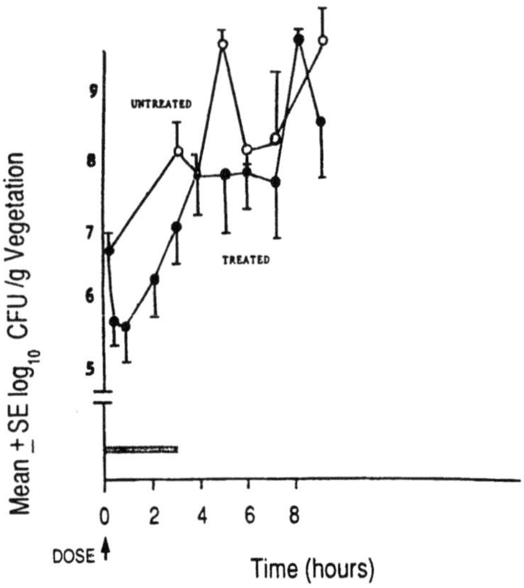

Fig. 1. Pharmacodynamic effects following a single IM dose of aqueous penicillin G plus gentamicin in rats with experimental *Streptococcus faecalis* aortic valve endocarditis. Mean ± S.E. vegetation bacterial counts are presented for treated and untreated rats. Vegetation concentrations of penicillin exceed the MIC of the organism for the time period indicated by the hatched horizontal bar

In contrast to the in vitro study in which there was a prolonged PAE of 3.5 h, vegetation enterococcal counts rose rapidly after an initial decline and exceeded pretreatment enterococcal counts at 3 h after treatment, despite vegetation penicillin levels above the MIC of the organism. Vegetation enterococcal counts in both treated and untreated rats continued to rise rapidly in parallel fashion. Thus, no PAE was demonstrated in the rat endocarditis model.

It is unlikely that the experimental model itself is a factor, for ciprofloxacin exhibited a PAE versus *Pseudomonas aeruginosa* in this model, whereas β-lactams, with or without gentamicin, did not, as will be described later. An alternative explanation may be that the metabolic state of the organisms in vivo is different from that in vitro so that rapid resynthesis of penicillin-binding proteins occurs in vivo, allowing immediate regrowth of tissue organisms following drug removal.

In summary, for whatever reason, an in vitro PAE for enterococci induced by the combination of penicillin plus gentamicin does not predict the presence of an in vivo PAE in experimental enterococcal endocarditis.

Summary

A persistent suppression of bacterial growth following brief exposure to an antibiotic (postantibiotic effect or PAE) has been described for a variety of antibiotics and microorganisms. If present in vivo, a PAE may allow antibiotic tissue levels at the site of infection to fall below the minimal inhibitory concentration (MIC) without loss of efficacy due to bacterial regrowth in the latter portion of the dosing intervals. In the present studies, a PAE was sought in vitro and in vivo for penicillin G plus gentamicin vs. *S. faecalis*. The studies demonstrated that increasing concentrations of gentamicin caused an increased rate of bactericidal action and an increasingly prolonged PAE in vitro. The combination of penicillin plus gentamicin, in addition to more rapid killing, exhibited a more prolonged PAE than did penicillin or gentamicin alone. The bactericidal activity of both penicillin and penicillin plus gentamicin in vitro was found to be diminished during the PAE induced by prior exposure to penicillin plus gentamicin. However, unlike these in vitro findings, no PAE could be demonstrated in vivo in rats with experimental, left-sided, enterococcal endocarditis treated with penicillin plus gentamicin. This would suggest that antibiotic vegetation levels should be maintained above the MIC throughout the dosing interval to prevent loss of efficacy due to bacterial regrowth.

Reference

1. McDonald PS, Craig WA, Kunin CM (1977) Persistent effect of antibiotics on *Staphylococcus aureus* after exposure for limited periods of time. J Infect Dis 135:217–223

Absence of a Postantibiotic Effect in Experimental Left-Sided *Pseudomonas Aeruginosa* Endocarditis Treated with Imipenem with or Without Gentamicin *

M. T. Hessen, P. G. Pitsakis, and M. E. Levison

In ongoing experiments, the pharmacodynamic effects of antibotics have been evaluated in the rat model of aortic valve *Pseudomonas aeruginosa* endocarditis.

In this model the right carotid artery of a rat is cannulated and the catheter advanced into the left ventricle. Twenty-four hours later 10^7 colony-forming units (CFUs) *P. aeruginosa* are injected into the tail vein. All rats infected with this inoculum develop endocarditis on the aortic valve. Eighteen hours later, rats are treated i.m. with one or more doses of antibiotic. At various times after injection of the antibiotic, rats are killed. Bacterial counts and antibiotic concentrations in the vegetations of these rats are then determined in order to correlate the response of the bacterial population to the concentration of the antimicrobial agent in the vegetation. Clearance of organisms from the vegetation is related to the rate and extent of the bactericidal effect and the duration of a post antibiotic effect (PAE), the PAE being defined as the persistence of inhibitory activity following brief exposure of bacteria to an antibiotic.

A PAE has been noted in vitro and in vivo with several antibiotic-bacteria combinations. However, beta-lactam antibiotics fail to produce a PAE against most gram-negative bacteria.

In prior experiments with the rat model of *P. aeruginosa* endocarditis, the pharmacodynamic effects of BMY, a ceftazidime-like beta-lactam, were compared with those of ciprofloxacin. The rapid bactericidal effect after one dose of ciprofloxacin resulted in a large reduction in the bacterial vegetation population in the 4-h interval during which vegetation ciprofloxacin levels exceeded the minimal inhibitory concentration (MIC).

The additional presence of a long in vivo PAE with ciprofloxacin for another 4 h resulted in superior efficacy of this agent when compared with BMY, for a second dose of ciprofloxacin, 8 h after the first dose, was sufficient to sterilize the vegetations. To be equally efficacious, the β-lactam antibiotic, which exhibited slow bactericidal activity and no PAE, had to be given in multiple doses at relatively short intervals.

Because an in vitro PAE has been described for imipenem, as well as aminoglycosides, versus *Pseudomonas aeruginosa,* we evaluated the pharmacodynamic effects of imipenem, with or without gentamicin, versus *P. aeruginosa* in vitro and in vivo in experimental aortic valve *P. aeruginosa* endocarditis in the rat.

* This study was supported in part by grants from Merck, Sharp and Dohme, West Point, PA, USA.

Division of Infectious Diseases, Department of Medicine, Medical College of Pennsylvania, 3300 Henry Avenue, Philadelphia, PA 19129, USA

The Influence of Antibiotics on the Host-Parasite Relationship III
Edited by G. Gillissen, W. Opferkuch, G. Peters, and G. Pulverer

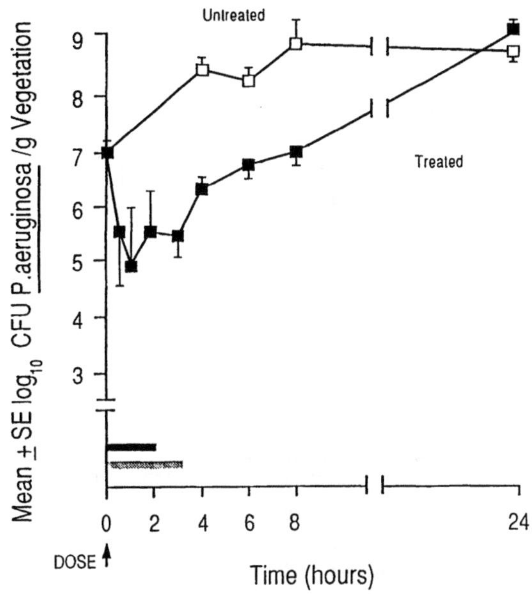

Fig. 1. Pharmacodynamic effects following a single IM dose of 120 mg/kg imipenem/cilastatin in rats with experimental *P. aeruginosa* aortic valve endocarditis. Mean counts of bacteria in vegetation ± SE are shown by *points with bars* for treated rats (*closed boxes*) and untreated rats (*open boxes*). *Bold horizontal bars* represent periods during which the level of imipenem in vegetations exceeds the MIC (solid) and MBC (hatched)

An isolate from the blood of a patient with *P. aeruginosa* endocarditis was used. The mean MIC and minimal bactericidal concentration (MBC) for imipenem was 1.9 and 14.9/μg per milliliter, respectively, and for gentamicin 3.1 and 6.3/μg per milliliter, respectively.

The initial bactericidal and PAEs were determined in vitro by the method of McDonald et al. [1] in broth suspensions of $10^{6.5}$ CFUs *P. aeruginosa*/ml following a 2-h incubation in either antibiotic-free (Mueller-Hinton broth MHB or MHB containing imipenem (30 μg/ml) or gentamicin (1 or 3 μg/ml). The size of the inoculum was similar to the bacterial counts in vegetations, and the concentrations of antibiotics were similar to those present in vegetations of rats 30–60 min after dosing. Gentamicin 3 μg/ml alone caused a 1.8 $\log_{10}$ CFU/ml fall in bacterial count and a 1.4-h PAE. Imipenem alone caused a 1.3 $\log_{10}$ CFU/g fall in bacterial count and about a 3-h PAE. The addition of gentamicin to imipenem enhanced both the bactericidal action and the PAE. For example, imipenem plus gentamicin 1 μg/ml caused a 2 $\log_{10}$ CFU/ml fall and a 5.4-h PAE; and imipenem plus gentamicin 3 μg/ml caused a 4 $\log_{10}$ CFU/ml fall and a 4.6-h PAE.

In rats with *P. aeruginosa* endocarditis, vegetation imipenem levels after one i.m. dose of imipenem/cilastatin, 120 mg/kg, were approximately 1.5 × MBC at peak and remained in excess of the MBC for 2 h. At 3 h vegetation levels were below the MBC, but above the MIC. At 4 or more h vegetation levels were estimated to be only slightly above or below the MIC in most rats.

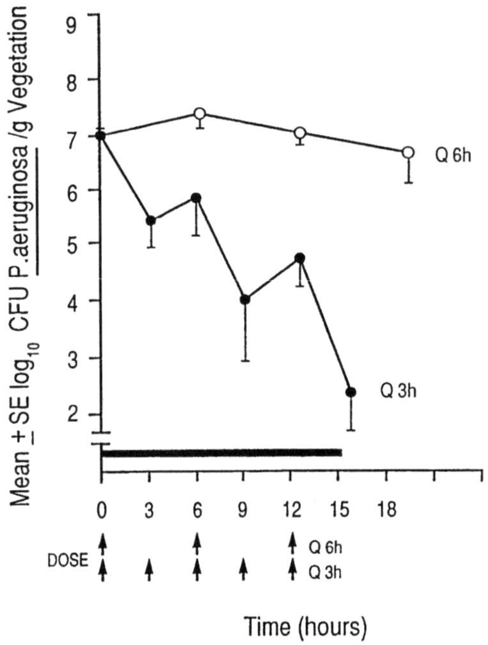

Fig. 2. Pharmacodynamic effects following an IM dose of 120 mg/kg imipenem/cilastatin either every 3 h (*closed circles*) or every 6 h (*open circles*) in rats with experimental *P. aeruginosa* aortic valve endocarditis. Mean counts of bacteria in vegetations ± SE are represented by *points with bars*. The *bold horizontal bar* represents the period during which the level of imipenem in vegetations exceeds the MIC in rats receiving the 3 h regimen

Figure 1 shows the pharmacodynamic effects following a single i.m. dose of 120 mg/kg imipenem/cilastatin in rats with experimental *P. aeruginosa* aortic valve endocarditis.

After the one dose of imipenem/cilastatin, bacterial counts fell 2 $\log_{10}$ CFUs/g vegetation during the 1st h, when vegetation imipenem levels were in excess of the MBC. During the next 2 h, when vegetation imipenem levels were still in excess of the MIC, vegetation counts remained stable. However, after 3 h, when vegetation imipenem levels were at or below the MIC in most rats, vegetation bacterial counts rose exponentially.

Thus, no in vivo PAE could be demonstrated for imipenem in this model.

Figure 2 shows the pharmacodynamic effects following an i.m. dose of 120 mg/kg imipenem/cilastatin either every 3 or every 6 h in rats with experimental *P. aeruginosa* aortic valve endocarditis.

In the group treated at 3-h intervals, vegetation concentrations remained in excess of the MIC during the entire dosing interval. In the group treated at 6-h intervals, trough vegetation levels were not measurable.

In the group treated at 3-h intervals, after five doses, mean vegetation bacterial counts dropped 4.6 $\log_{10}$ CFUs/g, from 7.2 $\log_{10}$ CFUs/g to 2.6 $\log_{10}$ CFUs/g. In the group treated at 6-h intervals, mean vegetation bacterial counts remained stable (range 6.7 to 8.4 $\log_{10}$ CFUs/g) throughout the 15-h treatment

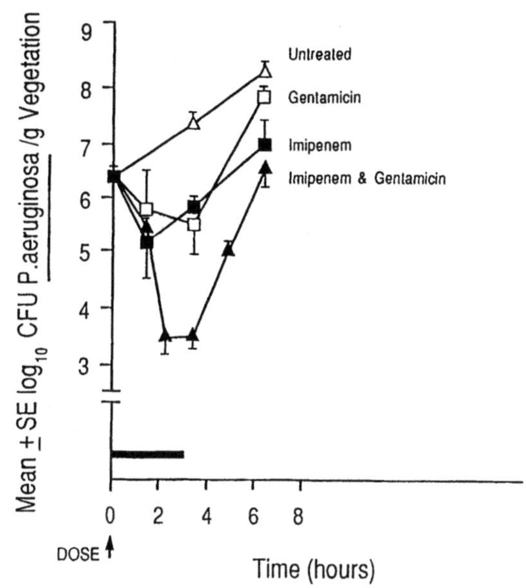

Fig. 3. Pharmacodynamic effects following a single IM dose of 120 mg/kg imipenem/cilastatin and 3 mg/kg gentamicin, each alone or in combination, in rats with experimental *P. aeruginosa* aortic valve endocarditis. Mean bacterial counts in vegetations ± SE are represented by *points with bars* for untreated rats *(open triangles)*, and for rats treated with imipenem/cilastatin *(closed boxes)*, gentamicin *(open boxes)*, and imipenem plus gentamicin *(closed triangles)*. The *bold horizontal bar* represents the period during which the level of imipenem in vegetations exceeds the MIC

period. Thus, though a bactericidal action occurred in the first 3 h of the 6-h dosing interval, the absence of a PAE allowed regrowth in the latter half of the dosing interval and resulted in loss of efficacy.

Figure 3 shows the pharmacodynamic effects following a single i.m. dose of 120 mg/kg imipenem/cilastatin plus 3 mg/kg gentamicin, each alone or in combination, in rats with experimental *P. aeruginosa* aortic valve endocarditis.

In the groups treated with imipenem plus gentamicin, vegetation concentrations of imipenem were similar to those in the prior experiments. The mean gentamicin vegetation level at 1 h was 1.7 µg/g and was similar to concentrations that both enhanced the bactericidal effect of imipenem and caused a 5-h PAE in vitro.

However, in the group treated with imipenem plus gentamicin, vegetation counts dropped from 6.4 to 3.6 $\log_{10}$ CFUs/g at 1 h, stabilized at 3.6 $\log_{10}$ CFUs/g for another hour, then rose exponentially during the next 3 h, at a time when imipenem levels were at or below the MIC.

Thus in *P. aeruginosa* aortic valve endocarditis treated with imipenem alone or in combination with gentamicin, no in vivo PAE was demonstrated, despite the presence of an in vitro PAE. This lack of concordance between in vitro and in vivo results could not be attributed to factors such as drug concentration, duration of drug exposure, the presence of serum, or the inoculum size. The inability to demonstrate an in vivo PAE with imipenem is also unlikely to reside in the model itself, as ciprofloxacin did induce a PAE in this endocarditis model.

Nevertheless, from these data, it is apparent that the absence of a significant in vivo PAE with imipenem versus *P. aeruginosa* may require frequent administration of this antibiotic to maintain tissue levels above the MIC for the pathogen when devising treatment schedules for experimental endocarditis and presumably clinical infection.

Summary

A persistent suppression of bacterial growth after limited exposure to an antibiotic in vivo (i.e., postantibiotic effect) would allows imipenem tissue levels to fall below the minimal inhibitory concentration (MIC) between doses without loss of efficacy. Because a postantibiotic effect has been described in vitro for imipenem, as well as for aminoglycosides, vs. *Pseudomonas aeruginosa,* we evaluated imipenem with and without gentamicin vs. *P. aeruginosa* in vitro and in vivo in experimental *P. aeruginosa* endocarditis in the rat. The in vitro, postantibiotic effect with imipenem alone lasted 3 h; with gentamicin, about 1.4 h; and with imipenem plus gentamicin, about 5-h. When rats with *P. aeruginosa* endocarditis were treated with imipenem alone or in combination with gentamicin, an initial rapid bactericidal effect in the vegetations was observed but was followed by a rapid rise in *P. aeruginosa* vegetation counts as soon as the imipenem levels in the vegetation fell below the MIC, i.e., no in vivo postantibiotic effect was demonstrated. Gentamicin levels in the vegetation were similar to concentrations that both enhanced the bactericidal effect of imipenem and caused a 5 h postantibiotic effect in vitro. Thus, an in vitro postantibiotic effect for imipenem or imipenem plus gentamicin vs. *P. aeruginosa* does not necessarily predict its presence in vivo in *P. aeruginosa* endocarditis in the rat.

Reference

1. McDonald PJ, Craig WA, Kunin CM (1977) Persistent effect of antibiotics on *Staphylococcus aureus* after exposure for limited periods of time. J Infect Dis 135:217–223

Influence of Mezlocillin Administration to Pregnant Mice on the Immune System of Their Offspring

W. Roszkowski [1], B. Wesokowska [1], H. L. Ko [2], K. Roszkowski [1], P. Ciborowski [3], J. Jeljaszewicz [3], and G. Pulverer [2]

Introduction

Effects of mezlocillin on the function of the immune system of mice have been demonstrated in previous studies [2, 3, 6, 7]. Experiments performed in vivo revealed that mezlocillin given systemically or orally to Balb/c mice caused a significant depression of the delayed-type hypersensitivity reaction as well as of IgM and IgG responses. This was accompanied by a decrease in the proliferative activity of lymphocytes. Similar treatment with mezlocillin given repeatedly after grafting of murine transplantable tumor (sarcoma L-1) caused a statistically significant prolongation of Balb/c mice survival and reduction of tumor size [2, 3].

Recently we have studied the effects of mezlocillin treatment on the digestive tract microflora of Balb/c mice [3]. We found that subcutaneous administration of this antibiotic led to a rapid elimination from the serum and to concentration of mezlocillin in the colon, followed by fast bacterial decontamination of the digestive tract microflora. All the pharmacological phenomena mentioned above were strictly correlated with bacterial decontamination of the colon of Balb/c mice. Therefore we concluded that the immunosuppressive and antitumor properties of mezlocillin observed are related to the eradication of endogenous bacterial microflora rather than to the direct effects of this antibiotic.

In the present paper basic immune parameters of progeny of mezlocillin-treated mice are studied. Besides the evaluation of weight and cell content of lymphatic organs we have used the lymphocyte-induced angiogenesis (LIA) test, which is recommended as a reliable and sensitive test for the local graft-versus-host reaction. This test represents the activity of T-lymphocytes. The ability to produce anti-(SRBC = sheep red blood cells)antibodies has been used for the evaluation of specific humoral responses.

Material and Methods

Experimental

The study was performed on 30-day-old offspring of inbred 3-month-old C3HW mice. Prospective mothers were treated with mezlocillin (experimental group) or

[1] Institute of Lung Diseases, Warsaw, Poland
[2] Hygiene Institute, University of Köln, 5000 Köln, Federal Republic of Germany
[3] National Institute of Hygiene, Warsaw, Poland

The Influence of Antibiotics on the Host-Parasite Relationship III
Edited by G. Gillissen, W. Opferkuch, G. Peters, and G. Pulverer

saline (controls) during the last 7–9 days of gestation. Mice of the experimental group received subcutaneously 300 mg mezlocillin/kg body weight or 150 mg/kg body weight orally. Thirty days after delivery some offspring were killed and the angiogenic potential of the lymph node and spleen lymphocytes estimated by the LIA test. In some mice the weight and cell content of lymph nodes, thymus, and spleen were studied as well as that of Thy-1,2-positive cells. Finally, some of these mice received SRBC injections to study the humoral immune response.

Lymphoid Cell Suspension

Axillary, inguinal, and brachial lymph nodes were pressed through a nylon blood filter in cold Parker medium (TC 199, Gibco Co.). Cells were washed twice and resuspended in a concentration of 10^7 cells/ml of the TC 199 medium (for the LIA test) or 5×10^6 cells/ml of TC 199 medium supplemented with 3% calf serum (for the cytotoxic test with anti Thy-1,2 antibodies). Spleen was pressed through the nylon blood filter and suspended in 2 ml TC 199 medium. Lymphocytes were isolated from this suspension by superimposing 2 ml upon 1 ml of the Ficoll-Uropoline mixture. After centrifugation over 7–10 min at 1400 g the cells obtained in the interface were washed twice and resuspended in TC 199 medium in a concentration of 10^7 cells/ml. The viability of cells isolated was assessed in all cases by trypan-blue dye exclusion. The percentage of viable cells was always greater than 90%.

Estimation of Angiogenic Potention of Splenic and Lymph Node Lymphocytes

Lymphocyte-induced angiogenesis assays were performed according to Sidky and Auerbach [9]. Preparation of cell suspensions and all infections were carried out under sterile conditions. Briefly: 10^6 cells in 0.1 ml TC 199 medium were injected into 6- to 8-week-old Balb/c mice. Animals before injections were immunosuppressed by total body X-ray exposure (700 cGy, Mueller RT 1100 apparatus; cathode current, 10 mA; accelerating voltage, 70 kV, 1.25 Al filter, 100 cGy/min in air). All injections were performed intracutaneously. Trypan blue was added to the tested inocula in order to facilitate the location of injection sites later on. As a control, 0.1 ml TC 199 medium alone was injected. Three days after injection, mice were killed by cervical dislocation and their skin was dissected from underlying muscles. The sites of angiogenic reaction of the inner skin surface were examined with the dissecting microscope at 32 × magnification. All newly formed blood vessels were identified and counted.

Two-Stage Cytotoxic Test

Thy-1,2-positive cells in cell suspensions of lymph nodes were identified by monoclonal antibodies (Maus Hybridoma Myeloma N5-1 + AkR/y spleen, clone TS Ig class: IgM from Miles Laboratory) following the technique of Sachs et al. [8].

Briefly: 2.5×10^5 lymphocytes were incubated with 50 µl monoclonal antibody (anti Thy-1,2) at a dilution of 1:40 for 30 min at 37 °C. The cells were pelleted and resuspended in equal volumes of guinea pig complement (Biomed) at a dilution of 1:5 and incubated for 30 min at 37 °C. After incubation, samples were centrifuged, the supernatant was discarded, and 0.1% trypan blue was added to the pellets. The percentage of blue-stained dead cells was scored by counting at least 200 cells from each sample.

Evaluation of Anti-SRBC Response

Mice were intraperitoneally injected with 10^8 sheep red blood cells (SRBCs). After 7 days they were bled from the retroorbital plexus. Sera were separated, heat inactivated, and scored for the level of hemagglutinating antibodies. Briefly: serial twofold dilutions of sera (100 µl) were mixed with equal volumes of 2% SRBCs. Samples were incubated at 37 °C for 30 min and centrifuged for 5 min at 110 g. Thereafter the erythrocytes were resuspended by vigorous shaking. Hemagglutination was scored under a microscope. Results were expressed as the reciprocal of the mean end point hemagglutination dilution.

Cellularity of Lymphatic Organs

Thymus, spleen, and two inguinal lymph nodes were isolated and weighed, then pressed through the nylon blood filter, and resuspended in 0.6 ml saline. The number of cells in the suspension was the same as that for the method used for the white blood cell count. The cellularity of organs was calculated by division of total cell count in organs studied by their weight in milligrams.

Statistical Analysis of Results

In all cases the statistical significance of values obtained was calculated with the help of Student's *t*-test.

Results

Examination of lymphatic organs in all groups of mice was performed on the 30th day of their life; the results are shown in Tables 1–3. The offspring of mezlocillin-treated mothers showed a significantly lower thymus, spleen, and lymph node weight. Significant increase of relative cellularity was observed in thymus and lymph nodes. However, in all cases the absolute lymphocyte count was decreased. These phenomena were observed in offspring of mothers treated by mezlocillin subcutaneously or orally. Table 4 shows the results of LIA induced by lymphocytes from the progeny of mezlocillin-treated mice and the reaction from control animals. Significantly lower LIA was observed after injecting the material (splenic

Table 1. Weight and cellularity of thymus

Offspring of mothers treated with	No. of mice	Relative thymus weight ± SD	Cell number/ mg × 10^6
Saline (control)	29	2.7 ± 0.21	0.60 ± 0.08
Mezlocillin s.c.[a]	23	1.1 ± 0.15*	1.05 ± 0.10*
Mezlocillin p.o.[b]	25	1.3 ± 0.17*	1.16 ± 0.13*

[a] 300 mg/kg body weight daily over 7–9 days.
[b] 150 mg/kg body weight daily over 7–9 days.
SD, standard deviation; * $P < 0.05$.

Table 2. Weight and cellularity of spleen

Offspring of mothers treated with	No. of mice	Relative organ weight ± SD	Cell number/ mg × 10^6
Saline (control)	24	3.0 ± 0.19	0.50 ± 0.04
Mezlocillin s.c.[a]	21	2.0 ± 0.10*	0.56 ± 0.09*
Mezlocillin p.o.[b]	19	1.8 ± 0.12*	0.65 ± 0.07*

[a] 300 mg/kg body weight daily over 7–9 days.
[b] 150 mg/kg body weight daily over 7–9 days.
SD, standard deviation; * $P < 0.05$.

Table 3. Weight and cellularity of inguinal lymph nodes

Offspring of mothers treated with	No. of mice	Relative organ weight ± SD	Cell number/ mg × 10^6
Saline (control)	24	2.29 ± 0.02	0.40 ± 0.03
Mezlocillin s.c.[a]	24	0.21 ± 0.03*	0.73 ± 0.09*
Mezlocillin p.o.[b]	20	0.19 ± 0.04*	0.76 ± 0.08*

[a] 300 mg/kg body weight daily over 7–9 days.
[b] 150 mg/kg body weight daily over 7–9 days.
SD, standard deviation; * $P < 0.05$.

Table 4. Angiogeneic activity of lymphocytes from mice born from mothers treated with mezlocillin during gestation as measured by the number of newly formed blood vessels ± SD

Mothers treated with	Cell source	
	Spleen	Lymph nodes
Saline (control) ($n = 10$)	17.3 ± 0.7 ($n = 17$)	22.3 ± 0.3 ($n = 19$)
Mezlocillin s.c.[a] ($n = 10$)	11.0 ± 0.6* ($n = 16$)	12.4 ± 0.8* ($n = 17$)
Mezlocillin p.o.[b] ($n = 10$)	10.4 ± 0.4* ($n = 18$)	11.3 ± 1.0* ($n = 17$)

[a] 300 mg/kg body weight daily over 7–9 days.
[b] 150 mg/kg body weight daily over 7–9 days.
SD, standard deviation; * $P < 0.05$.

Table 5. Percentage of Thy-1,2-positive lymphocytes present in lymph nodes of mezlocillin-treated mice progeny

Mothers treated with	% of Thy-1,2-positive lymphocytes ± SD
Saline (control) ($n=13$)	71 ± 1.8
Mezlocillin s. c.[a] ($n=14$)	47 ± 1.9 *
Mezlocillin p. o.[b] ($n=14$)	43 ± 4.1 *

[a] 300 mg/kg body weight daily over 7–9 days.
[b] 150 mg/kg body weight daily over 7–9 days.
SD, standard deviation; * $P<0.05$.

Table 6. Hemagglutination response of mice born by mothers treated with saline or mezlocillin during gestation (response against 10^8 SRBCs)

Mothers treated with	$\log_2$ titer ± SD
Saline (control) ($n=11$)	2.71 ± 0.27
Mezlocillin s. c.[a] ($n=12$)	1.09 ± 0.31 *
Mezlocillin p. o.[b] ($n=13$)	1.23 ± 0.35 *

[a] 300 mg/kg body weight daily over 7–9 days.
[b] 150 mg/kg body weight daily over 7–9 days.
SD, standard deviation; * $P<0.05$.

and lymph node lymphocytes) from mice born from mezlocillin-treated mothers. The results presented in Table 5 indicate that offspring from mice treated with mezlocillin have a decreased percentage of Thy-1,2-positive cells in their lymph nodes.

Table 6 presents the results of the humoral anti-SRBC response. A significantly lower concentration of hemagglutinating anti-SRBC antibodies was found in the sera of progeny of mezlocillin subcutaneously and orally treated mice.

Discussion

Our previous studies showed that some penicillins like mezlocillin and piperacillin possess potent and long-lasting immunosuppressive effects when given in vivo. However, the mechanisms of immunosuppression are still not clear. We found that the immunopharmacological effects of these antibiotics are strictly correlated with decontamination of digestive tract flora; this strongly indicates indirect mechanisms of mezlocillin-induced effects. This suggestion was confirmed by results obtained after oral treatment with mezlocillin, which is nonabsorbable from the digestive tract. We think that similar mechanisms are responsible for antitumor effects observed during and after mezlocillin treatment. In the present paper we found that general and oral treatment of pregnant mice with this antibiotic may significantly affect the function and development of the lymphatic system of their progeny.

Generally penicillins are believed not to affect the immunity of adult organisms [1]. We can only agree with such suggestions when direct interactions between antibiotics and immune cells are considered. Our present results show that the administration of mezlocillin – besides impairment of immunofunctions in adult animals – causes potent effects on their progeny. We observed not only a reduction in relative thymus, spleen, and lymph node weight, but also a significant depression of the cellular immune response measured by the LIA test. Similar findings were observed for humoral immunity, and once again indirect effects of mezlocillin are postulated. This is due to the fact that in all the experiments performed similar immunopharmacological effects were observed, despite the different route of mezlocillin administration (s.c. or oral). Nondetectable levels of mezlocillin in serum after oral administration [3–5] practically eliminate the possibility of a direct mezlocillin influence on the fetus and its immune system.

Summary

Oral as well as subcutaneous administration of mezlocillin to pregnant C3HW mice during the last 7–9 days of gestation induced immunosuppressive effects in their offspring. Thirty days after delivery the weight of their spleen, thymus, and lymph nodes was significantly decreased as well as the percentage of Ty-1,2-positive cells within their lymph nodes and their humoral immune response. Offspring from mezlocillin-treated mice produced significantly lower LIA test results in Balb/c mice.

References

1. Hauser WE, Remington Js (1982) Effect of antibiotics on the immune response. Am J Med 72:711–716
2. Roszkowski K, Ko HL, Roszkowski W, Jeljaszewicz J, Pulverer G (1985) Effect of some antimicrobial antibiotics on sarcoma L-1 tumor growth in mice. Zbl Bakt Hyg [A] Suppl 13:199–218
3. Roszkowski K, Ko HL, Van der Waaij D, Roszkowski W, Jeljaszewicz J, Pulverer G (1987) Antibiotic treatment, intestinal aerobic microflora and experimental sarcoma L-1 growth in Balb/c mice. Zbl Bakt [A] 265:378–384
4. Roszkowski K, Roszkowski W, Pulverer G, Jeljaszewicz J (1986) The influence of antimicrobial antibiotics on antitumor immunity. Ann Immunol Hung 26:369–388
5. Roszkowski K, Roszkowski W, Pulverer G, Jeljaszewicz J (1986) Antibiotic and antitumor immunity. In: Jeljaszewicz J, Pulverer G (eds) Antimicrobial agents and immunity. Academic Press, London New York, pp 67–87
6. Roszkowski W, Ko HL, Roszkowski K, Jeljaszewicz J, Pulverer G (1985) Antibiotics and immunomodulation effects of cefotaxime, amikacin, mezlocillin, piperacillin and clindamycin. Med Microbiol Immunol (Berl) 173:279–289
7. Roszkowski W, Ko HL, Roszkowski K, Jeljaszewicz J, Pulverer G (1985) Effects of selected antibiotics on the cellular and humoral immune response in mice. Zbl Bakt Hyg [A] Suppl 13:59–70
8. Sachs DH, Winn HJ, Russel PS (1971) The immune response to xenografts. Recognition of mouse H-P histocompatibility antigens by the rat. J Immunol 107:481–489
9. Sidky YA, Auerbach R (1975) Lymphocyte induced angiogenesis and quantitative and sensitive assay for the graft-vs-host reaction. J Exp Med 141:1084–1091

Changes in the Immune Parameters of Antibiotic-Bacterial Interactions Induced by Hypothalamic and Other Electrolytic Brain Lesions Produced Through Stereotaxically Implanted Depth Electrodes

J. SZENTIVANYI [1], A. SZENTIVANYI [2], P. SCHULTZE [3], G. FILIPP [3], and O. HEIM [3]

In the years of 1952 through 1958, in a series of papers, Szentivanyi et al. [12, 11, 27, 31, 10, 32, 33, 26, 9, 30, 20] first described the critical role played by hypothalamic structures in the regulation and expression of immunologic inflammation, immunity, and hypersensitivity reactions. More recently rapidly growing extensive evidence demonstrated that neural and hormonal signals generated outside the immune system do indeed significantly contribute to immune homeostasis. These findings led to the identification of immune neuroendocrine circuits that are based on a bidirectional flow of information between the immune, endocrine, and nervous systems [13, 3, 19, 16]. These data also confirmed the conclusions reached in the earlier-mentioned works of Szentivanyi et al. that a critical integrative level of this complex regulatory network is the hypothalamus [23, 7, 6, 35, 34, 1, 18, 17, 22].

In the studies described here, with the use of permanently implanted depth electrodes placed in specific hypothalamic and extrahypothalamic areas of the brain, various nuclear groupings were electrolytically eliminated in guinea pigs that were given graded numbers of *Escherichia coli* pretreated with subinhibitory concentrations of ampicillin. These lesioned animals were then administered the pretreated organisms and the immunogenicity of the bacteria tested by a variety of immune parameters.

Experimental Design

Particolored 173 male guinea pigs, averaging 400–600 g weight and kept on a common diet, were used throughout the experiments. The animals were anesthesized with an intraperitoneal injection of 30 mg/kg chlorohydrate and placed in a modified Horsely-Clarke stereotaxic apparatus specially designed for this species. The animal's head was immobilized by introducing conic screws into the external auditory canals and fixing the incisors on a gliding bridge. The head was then depressed by steel springs in order to maintain contact between the incisors and the gliding bridge. The back of the animal's muzzle was also held in place by screws. The skull was trephined with an electric dental drill with a spherical bit. The bilateral electrolytic focal lesions were produced through a unipolar needle

Departments of Pharmacology and Therapeutics [2] and Comprehensive Medicine [1], University of South Florida College of Medicine, Box 9, Tampa, FL 33612–4799, USA Faculty of Medicine [3], University of Saarland, Homburg, Federal Republic of Germany

The Influence of Antibiotics on the Host-Parasite Relationship III
Edited by G. Gillissen, W. Opferkuch, G. Peters, and G. Pulverer

electrode insulated to its tip by glass casing. A direct current of 1.5 mA for 15 s using a Grass S48 stimulator was used for lesioning. One focus was placed to the right and one to the left of the median line.

Measurements of the various hypothalamic and other brain regions were previously carried out on the head of a guinea pig fixed in formalin. After placing the animal's head into the correct position as stated above, and incising the skull, the crosswise suture at the junction of the sagittal and coronary sutures afforded a fully visible basic point. The tip of the electrode being accurately placed on the intersection of the two sutures, its position was exactly gauged in all three directions of space. Reading of the coordinates was carried out with the help of Nonius scales. Subsequently, the cranial lid being taken off, a median-sagittal cutting was excised from the brain. After this intervention the point of the electrode was directed to the brain area selected for destruction with the location of the electrode checked once again on the Nonius scales. According to these coordinates, the electrode located 4 mm behind the intersection of the two sutures, penetrated to a depth of 13 mm, 1 mm both to the right and left of the median, was positioned to destroy the central section of the tuber cinereum serving as a point of orientation. Two sets of transverse microscopic arrangements forwarded the electrode into all directions of space and guided it to the appropriate hypothalamic or other nuclear group. These movements were also controlled on the Nonius scales. In the case of the sham-operated controls the electrodes were implanted in the same areas but without producing electrolytic lesions (no electric current applied). Upon completion of the lesioning procedure the skin was closed and the animals placed in a conventional infant incubator.

Animals were killed by cervical dislocation 6 or 14 days after lesioning. At the time of death the brains were removed, fixed in 4% formaldehyde, and sectioned in the coronal plane. Sections stained with hematoxylin and eosin were examined for placement and extent of lesions. Lesion size and location were determined by microscopic inspection. All animals whose lesions did not fall within the designated nuclei were excluded from the study. Mortality was less than 10% and essentially confined to the first postoperative day. Beyond that, all groups appeared healthy in terms of body weight, temperature, and food and water intake.

In assessing the various parameters of immunogenicity of *E. coli,* essentially the procedures described in a companion chapter of this volume (Friedman et al., p 263) were used. Thus, for direct examination of the immunogenic potential of ampicillin, exposed *E. coli* were injected in normal guinea pigs, that is *E. coli* which were treated for 2 h in vitro with subinhibitory doses of ampicillin as compared with untreated *E. coli* incubated for the same length of time in medium alone without ampicillin. As previously described, blood was obtained from each animal by cardiac puncture at varying times thereafter, usually on the 6th or 14th days and anti-*E. coli* agglutinin titer determined in the serum by standard agglutination tests in microtiter plates. Also the ability of *E. coli* to induce normal spleen cells to produce anti-*E. coli* plaque-forming cells (PFCs) was determined by the standard plaque assay of viable *E. coli* in agar plates as described previously.

The ability of ampicillin-pretreated *E. coli* to stimulate normal spleen cell blastogenic responses was also studied as follows. Briefly, 10^6 or 10^8 washed *E. coli* either untreated or at various times after exposure to graded amounts of ampicillin, followed by washing and resuspension in saline, were assessed for this activity by the standard spleen cell blastogenic procedure. Heat-killed bacteria (80 °C for 30 min) were added to cultures of 10^6 spleen cells from rats in 0.5 ml medium in well Linbro plates. The plates were incubated for 56 h at 37 °C in a 5% CO_2-air atmosphere then pulsed with 0.25 µCi tritiated thymidine (specific activity 6.7% Ci/mmol) added in a volume of 10 µl. The cells were harvested 18 h later using an automatic cell harvester and the tritiated thymidine incorporation into DNA was assayed by liquid scintillation counting. The stimulation index (SI) was calculated as counts per minute (CPM) for stimulated cultures minus CPM for control cultures divided by CPM for control cultures × 100.

Lymphocytic cyclic nucleotides were assayed by the radioimmunoassay procedure of [24] as modified by acetylation of the antigen with acetic anhydride in aqueous solution to increase the sensitivity of the assay [15]. Isolation of blood lymphocytes was carried out with the procedure of [5]. To measure lymphocytic beta-adrenergic receptor densities, the procedures of [36] and [4] were used. The binding data so obtained were analyzed for equilibrium dissociation constants (K_d) and maximum binding (B_{max}) using a Fortran IV G SCAFIT data processing program written by Faden and Rodbard [14] (Hancock et al., 1979), obtained through Biomedical Computing Technology Information Center (Nashville, Tennessee) and run on an IBM 3033 mainframe computer. Also, the binding data were tested for statistical significance using SAS computer programs for analysis of variance (ANOVA) coupled with Duncan's New Multiple Range Test by SAS Institute Incorporated (Cary, North Carolina).

Delayed cutaneous hypersensitivity to picryl chloride and tuberculin as well as passive cutaneous anaphylaxis were produced and evaluated 1 week postoperatively as described by [20, 21].

Results

Table 1 provides a comprehensive summary of the effects of bilateral hypothalamic and other brain lesions on parameters of immunogenecity of *E. coli* pretreated with subinhibitory concentrations of ampicillin. The first vertical column lists these parameters, whereas the second column shows the corresponding findings obtained on sham-lesioned guinea pigs injected with heat-killed bacteria but without in vitro pretreatment with ampicillin, indicating no significant change from normal controls with or without sham lesions or the administration of heat-killed bacteria. The third vertical column indicates where there was a statistically significant change relative to values obtained in sham-lesioned animals injected with heat-killed bacteria with no in vitro pretreatment with ampicillin. It appears that the ampicillin pretreatment of these animals resulted in statistically significant increased humoral and cellular immune responses without, however, any change in the concentration of lymphocytic cyclic nucleotides or β-adrenergic receptors. The group of animals with electrolytic lesions in the anterior and ventromedial hypothalamus showed an identical pattern of responses. Both groups relative to the pattern of reactivity obtained in the sham-lesioned ampicillin-pre-

Table 1. Effect of bilateral hypothalamic and other brain lesions on parameters of immunogenicity of *E. coli* pretreated with subinhibitory concentrations of ampicillin

Parameters	Sham lesion untreated	Sham lesion ampicillin pretreated	Anterior hypothalamus	Ventromedial hypothalamus	Posterior hypothalamus	Mamillary bodies	Hippocampus	Fornix	Amygdaloid complex	Frontal cortex
Production of agglutinins	Normal	Increased[a]	Decreased[b]	Decreased[b]	Increased[b]	Increased[b]	Increased[b]	No change[c]	Increased[b]	No change[c]
Blastogenic response	Normal	Increased	Decreased	Decreased	Increased	Increased	Increased	No change	Increased	No change
Passive gutaneous anaphylaxis	Normal	Increased	Decreased	Decreased	Increased	Increased	Increased	No change	Increased	No change
Delayed-type hypersensitivity	Normal	Increased	Decreased	Decreased	Increased	Increased	Increased	No change	Increased	No change
Lymphocytic cAMP	Normal	No change	Increased	Increased	Decreased	Decreased	Increased	No change	Increased	No change
Lymphocytic cGMP	Normal	No change	Decreased	Decreased	Increased	Increased	Decreased	No change	Decreased	No change
Lymphocytic beta-adrenoceptor density	Normal	No change	Increased	Increased	Decreased	Decreased	Increased	No change	Increased	No change

[a] Statistically significant change relative to values obtained in sham-lesioned animals injected with heat-killed bacteria with no in vitro pretreatment with ampicillin.
[b] Statistically significant change relative to values obtained in sham-lesioned animals injected with heat-killed bacteria pretreated in vitro with ampicillin.
[c] No statistically significant change relative to values obtained in sham-lesioned animals injected with heat-killed bacteria pretreated in vitro with ampicillin.

treated groups showed a reversed pattern of change involving decreased production of anti-*E. coli* agglutinins, blastogenic response, passive cutaneous anaphylaxis, and delayed hypersensitivity. Furthermore, relative to the sham-lesioned ampicillin-pretreated control group there was an increase in the concentration of lymphocytic cyclic AMP and β-adrenoceptor densities together with the decreased level of cyclic GMP. With respect to the electrolytic lesions placed in the posterior hypothalamus there was a complete reversal of the pattern of responses found in the anterior and ventromedial hypothalamus and the same appears to be the case with electrolytic lesions placed in the mamillary bodies and hippocampus except in the behavior of cyclic nucleotide and β-adrenoceptor concentration. Lesions of the fornix and frontal cortex showed normal responses relative to the sham-lesioned heat-killed bacteria-injected group with no in vitro pretreatment with ampicillin. Lesioning of the amygdaloid complex produced immune parameters identical to those seen in the hippocampus group.

Discussion

The historically developed concept of antibiotic action is essentially the perception of antibiotics as substances having only selective toxicity. In this view the ideal antibiotic is one that has no adverse effects on the host, but is selectively destructive to the bacteria. Historically, therefore, penicillin G became the model antibiotic, and the acknowledgment of an antimicrobial agent as an antibiotic became patterned after penicillin G, resulting in research on antibiotic action essentially directed toward the bacterial cell [2, 8]. Patterned after this model antibiotic, certain interdependent criteria have been developed to identify other potential antibiotics, but also to prevent some overly enthusiastic investigators from using this term to cover new candidates for antibiosis before sufficient data were available to assure their antibiotic status. While such caution in any scientific inquiry is an elementary consideration, the set of criteria requiring fulfillment for assignment of antibiotic status would provide a perfect fit only for penicillin G in the nonallergic patient [28].

These circumstances became considerable handicaps in the evolution of our understanding of antibiosis, and they explain why the bacterium remained the almost singular focus in the exploration of the effects of these agents in the mammalian host. Another historical handicap in the development of our understanding of antibiotic action has been the fact that most investigations of antibiotic effects on bacteria have been carried out at antibiotic concentrations equal to or greater than the minimum inhibitory concentration (MICs) or the minimum bactericidal concentrations (MBCs). At concentrations lower than the MIC, antibiotics produce effects which are not milder than those seen with the MIC but which are qualitatively different. At these levels of concentration, the antibiotic actions are not considered to be on the multiplication mechanisms but rather on the modification of bacterial morphology and ultrastructure and their ultimate influence upon the host's anti-infectious mechanisms including immunogenic determinants [28].

The studies herein reported corroborate the findings of the recent literature on the actions of subinhibitory concentrations of antibiotics on the immunomodulatory effects of some antibiotic-induced changes in bacterial and host determinants. They also indicate, furthermore, that some regions in the mammalian brain exert profound influences on the immunomodulatory consequences of bacterial-antibiotic interactions. Nevertheless, at the time of this writing we do not know the nature of the cellular and molecular mechanisms involved in the operation of these immune-neuroendocrine circuits and extensive further investigations are needed to clarify their role in modulating bacterial-antibiotic interactions.

Summary

Hypothalamic structures play a critical role in the regulation of immune response; this was first described in 1952–1958 and was further confirmed by the identification of immune neuroendocrine circuits. In guinea pigs, the effects were examined of bilateral electrolytic lesions of hypothalamic and other brain areas on immunogenicity of *E. coli* pretreated with subinhibitory concentrations of ampicillin and tested by a variety of immune parameters. In sham-lesioned animals, pretreated bacteria increased the humoral and cellular immune responses whereas lymphocytic concentrations of cAMP and cGMP and β-adrenoceptor density remained unchanged. In contrast, lesions in the anterior as well as in the ventromedial hypothalamus resulted, under otherwise identical conditions, in decreased immune reactions together with increased lymphocytic cAMP and decreased cGMP levels and increased β-adrenoceptor density. Lesions in the posterior hypothalamus and the mamillary bodies showed completely opposite effects. Except the cyclic nucleotide level and β-adrenoceptor density, similar results were obtained by lesions in the hippocampus and the amygdaloid complex. Lesioning of the fornix and the frontal cortex had no effect in comparison with the sham-lesioned group injected with non-pretreated bacteria. These results show that some brain regions exert specific influences on immune response modulation of bacterial-antibiotic interactions.

References

1. Abramsky O, Wertman E, Reches A, Brenner T, Ovadia H (1987) Effect of hypothalamic lesions on experimental autoimmune diseases in rats. In: Jankovic BD, Markovic BM, Spector NH (eds) Neuroimmune interactions: proceedings of the second international workshop on neuroimmunomodulation. The New York Academy of Sciences, New York, pp 360–365
2. Adam D, Hahn H, Opferkuch W (eds) (1985) The influence of antibiotics on the host-parasite relationship II. Springer, Berlin Heidelberg New York
3. Ader R (ed) (1980) Psychoneuroimmunology. Academic, New York
4. Bishopric NH, Cohen HJ, Lefkowitz RJ (1980) Beta adrenergic receptors in lymphocyte subpopulation. J Allergy Clin Immunol 65:29
5. Boyum A (1968) Isolation of mononuclear cells and granulocytes from human blood. Scand J Clin Lab Invest 21 [Suppl 97]:77
6. Cross RJ, Brooks WH, Roszman TL, Markesbery WR (1982) Hypothalamic-immune interactions. Effect of hypophysectomy on neuroimmunomodulation. J Neurol Sci 53:557

7. Cross RJ, Markesbery WR, Brooks WH, Roszman TL (1984) Hypothalamic-immune interactions: neuromodulation of natural killer activity by lesioning of the anterior hypothalamus. Immunology 51:399
8. Eickenberg H-U, Hahn H, Opferkuch W (eds) (1982) The influence of antibiotics on the host-parasite relationship. Springer Berlin Heidelberg New York
9. Filipp G, Szentivanyi A (1958) Anaphylaxis and the nervous system, part III. Ann Allergy 16:306
10. Filipp G, Szentivanyi A (1957) Die Wirkung von Hypothalamuslasionen auf den anaphylaktischen Schock des Meerschweinchens. Allergie Asthma 1:23
11. Filipp G, Szentivanyi A (1956) Experimentelle Data zur regulativen Rolle des Neuroendokrinimus in experimenteller Anaphylaxie. I. Relazioni e Communicazioni 229. Il Pansiero Scientifico, Rome
12. Filipp G, Szentivanyi A, Mess B (1952) Anaphylaxis and nervous system. Acta Med Hung III 2:163
13. Frederickson RCA, Hendrie HC, Hingtgen JN, Aprison MH (eds) (1986) Neuroregulation of autonomic, endocrine and immune systems. Martinus Nijhoff, Boston
14. Hancock AA, DeLean AL, Lefkowitz RJ (1979) Quantitative resolution of beta-adrenergic receptor subtypes by selective ligand binding: application of a computerized model fitting technique, Mol Pharmacol 16:1
15. Harper JF, Brooker G (1975) Femtomole sensitive radioimmunoassay for cyclic AMP and cyclic GMP after 2'0 acetylation by acetic anhydride in aqueous solution. J Cyclic Nucleotide Res 1:207
16. Jankovic BD, Markovic BM, Spector NH (eds) (1987) Neuroimmune interactions: proceedings of the second international workshop on neuroimmunomodulation. The New York Academy of Sciences, New York
17. Kadlecova O, Masek K, Seifert J, Petrovicky P (1987) The involvement of some brain structures in the effect of immunomodulators. In: Jankovic BD, Markovic BM, Spector NH (eds) Neuroimmune interctions: proceedings of the second international workshop on neuroimmunomodulation. The New York Academy of Sciences, New York, pp 394–398
18. Katayama M, Kobayashi S, Kuramoto N, Yokoyama MM (1987) Effects ofl hypothalamic lesions on lymphocyte subsets in mice. In: Jankovic BD, Markovic BM, Spector NH (eds) Neuroimmune interactions: proceedings of the second international workshop on neuroimmunomodulation. The New York Academy of Sciences, New York, pp 366–376
19. Locke S, Ader R, Besedovsky H, Hall N, Solomon G, Strom T (eds) (1985) Foundations of psychoneuroimmunology. Aldine New York
20. Macris NT, Schiavi RC, Camerino MS, Stein M (1970) Effect of hypothalamic lesions on immune processes in the guinea pig. Am J Physiol 219:1205
21. Macris NT, Schiavi RC, Camerino MS, Stein M (1972) Effect of hypothalamic lesions on passive anaphylaxis in the guinea pig. Am J Physiol 222:1054
22. Quirico-Santos T, Valdimarsson H (1987) Modulation of systemic antibody response and tolerance by brain injury. In: Jankovic BD, Markovic BM, Spector NH (eds) Neuroimmune interactions: proceedings of the second international workshop on neuroimmunomodulation. The New York Academy of Sciences, New York, pp 384–387
23. Roszman TL, Cross RJ, Brooks WH, Markesbery WR (1982) Hypothalamic-immune interactions. II. The effect of hypothalamic lesions on the ability of adherent spleen cells to limit lymphocyte blastogenesis. Immunology 45:737
24. Steiner AL, Parker CW, Kipnis DM (1972) Radioimmunoassay for cyclic nucleotides. I. Preparation of antibodies and iodinated cyclic nucleotides. J Biol Chem 247:1106
25. Szentivanyi A (1961) Hypothalamic influences on antibody formation and on bronchial responses to histamine. Proceedings of the fourth Aspen conference on research in emphysema and asthma, p 48
26. Szentivanyi A, Filipp G (1958) Anaphylaxis and the nervous system, part II. Ann Allergy 16:143
27. Szentivany A, Filipp G (1956) Experimentelle Data zur regulativen Rolle des Neuroendokriniums in experimenteller Anaphylaxie. II. Relazioni e Communicazioni 237. Il Pansiero Scientifico, Rome
28. Szentivanyi A, Friedman H, Gillissen G (eds) (1987a) Antibiosis and host immunity. Plenum, New York

29. Szentivanyi A, Friedman H, Gillissen G, Szentivanyi J (1987b) Immunomodulatory effects of some antibiotic-induced changes in bacterial and host determinants. In: Szentivanyi A, Friedman H, Gillissen G (eds) Antibiosis and host immunity. Plenum New York, pp 3–11
30. Szentivanyi A, Szekely J (1958) Anaphylaxis and the nervous system, part IV. Ann Allergy 16:389
31. Szentivanyi A, Szekely J (1956) Effect of injury to and electrical stimulation of hypothalamic areas on the anaphylactic and histamine shock of the guinea pig. Ann Allergy 14:259
32. Szentivanyi A, Szekely J (1957d) Über den Effekt der Schädigung und der elektrischen Reizung der hypothalamischen Gegenden auf den anaphylaktischen und Histamin-Schock des Meerschweinchens. Allergie Asthmaforschung Bd 1:28
33. Szentivanyi A, Szekely J (1957b) Wirkung der konstanten Reizung hypothalamischer Strukturen durch Tiefenelektroden auf den histaminbedingten und anaphylaktischen Schock des Meerschweinchens. Acta Physiol Hung [Suppl V] Tomus XI:41
34. Van Oosterhout AJM, Nijkamp FP (1986) Anterior hypothalamic lesions decrease anaphylactic contractions in guinea pig trachea in vitro by reducing histamine and LTC_4 reactivity. Int J Immunopharmacol 8(8):975
35. Van Oosterhout AJM, Nijkamp FP (1984) Anterior hypothalamic lesions prevent the endotoxin-induced reduction of beta-adrenoceptor number in guinea pig lung. Brain Res 302–277
36. Williams LT, Snyderman R, Lefkowitz RJ (1976) Identification of beta-adrenergic receptors in human lymphocytes by (−)[^{3}H]alprenolol binding. J Clin Invest 57:149

In Vitro Effect of Different Antimicrobial Agents on Il-2 Production and Il-2 Receptor Expression of Human Lymphocytes

S. Pusztai-Markos and K. Hauss

Introduction

Among the first events of lymphocyte activation are the synthesis and surface expression of a receptor for interleukin-2 (Il-2R). The action of Il-2 results from binding to its specific receptors inducing the proliferation of activated T cells. Resting lymphocytes do not express their growth factor receptors on their surface, only as a consequence of antigenic or mitogenic stimulation [1]. Il-2 production and Il-2 receptor expression seem to be important in the development and termination of the T-cell immune response. Il-2R is also present on some activated B cells, and interaction of Il-2 with these receptors may play a role in B-cell growth and differentiation [2].

In this study, we investigated the influence of several antimicrobial agents on Il-2 production and Il-2R expression after mitogenic stimulation with a whole peripheral blood mononuclear cell (PBMC) population, with monocyte-depleted PBMCs, and with isolated T-lymphocytes. With antibiotics markedly modulating the above parameters, the T-cell-dependent in vitro immunoglobulin synthesis was also studied.

Material and Methods

Reagents. Ampicillin (Grünenthal), cefotaxim (Hoechst), tetracycline (Sigma), ofloxacin (Hoechst), ciprofloxacin (Bayer), and rifampicin sodium (Ciba Geigy) were used. All drugs were resolved in tissue culture medium immediately prior to use. Phytohemagglutinin (PHA-P, Difco) and concanavalin A (con A) (Sigma) were used for the Il-2 induction at a concentration of 5 μg/ml and pokeweed mitogen (PWM) (Gibco) at an optimal concentration of 1 μg/ml for induction of immunoglobulin synthesis. Highly purified interleukin-2 (200 U/ml) was purchased from Boehringer Mannheim and anti-Il-2 receptor (CD25) and fluoresceinated goat anti-mouse-Ig from Becton Dickinson.

Lymphocyte Preparation. Fresh peripheral blood mononuclear cells were isolated from healthy human volunteers by Ficoll-Hypaque density gradient centrifugation. Enriched populations of T cells were then isolated either after or without

Department of Medical Microbiology, Medical Faculty, Pauwelsstraße, 5100 Aachen, Federal Republic of Germany

The Influence of Antibiotics on the Host-Parasite Relationship III
Edited by G. Gillissen, W. Opferkuch, G. Peters, and G. Pulverer

monocyte depletion by the method of rosette formation with neuraminidase-treated sheep erythrocytes and density gradient centrifugation. Monocytes were depleted by adherence on plastic petri dishes for 1 h at 37 °C and this process was repeated.

Il-2 Induction. Lymphocytes suspended at 4×10^6 cells/ml in RPMI 1640 medium (Flow Labs.) supplemented with 10% AB serum, 2 m*M* L-glutamin, 100 U/ml penicillin, and 100 µg/ml streptomycin were incubated in microtiter plates at 37 °C in 5% CO_2 in a humidified incubator for 24 h in the presence or absence of mitogen and with or without the drugs at varying concentrations. At the end of the culture the supernatants were harvested, centrifuged, dialyzed at 4 °C overnight against medium to remove antibiotics, and stored at −70 °C until the assay.

Il-2 Receptor Detection. Lymphocytes similarly cultivated as for Il-2 induction for variable periods were washed three times at the end of the culture and subsequently incubated with the monoclonal antibody (5 µl/10^6 cells) and then washed and further incubated with the fluorescence-conjugated goat anti-mouse-Ig as described [3]. The percentage of fluorescein-labeled cells was established by counting on a Leitz Orthoplan microscope (Leitz, Wetzlar, FRG).

Assay for Il-2 Activity in Supernatants. Peripheral blood mononuclear cells from healthy volunteers were cultured in the presence of 5 µg/ml PHA in medium (see above) for 5 days. Thereafter, the cells were washed and resuspended in the same medium without PHA containing 20 U Il-2/ml. This splitting and feeding procedure was repeated five times every 4 days. After the last culture, cells were harvested and frozen in a programmed liquid nitrogen freezer. The procedure is described in detail elsewhere [4]. For the assay, the cells were thawed, adjusted to 4×10^5/ml with a serial dilution of culture supernatant and with 5% inactivated AB serum. The plates were incubated for 48 h at 37 °C in a humidified CO_2 incubator and then each well was pulsed with 0.5 µCi [^{3}H]thymidine (Amersham), and after a further 16 h of incubation cells were harvested with a cell harvester and washed, and radioactivity was determined by counting in a liquid scintillation counter. Serial dilutions of Il-2 with and without mitogen PHA and Con A were prepared as standards.

In Vitro Immunoglobulin Synthesis. For Ig synthesis 1×10^6/ml lymphocytes were incubated in medium supplemented with 10% fetal calf serum with and without PWM and different concentrations of drugs. At the end of the culture supernatants were harvested, centrifuged, and stored at −70 °C until assay for Ig secretion. Ig concentrations were determined with a Beckmann nephelometer using a modification of rate nephelometry [5].

Results

Dose-dependent Modulation by Drugs of Il-2 Production and Il-2R Expression of PBMCs. Ampicillin, tetracycline, rifampicin, or ciprofloxacin induced a dose-de-

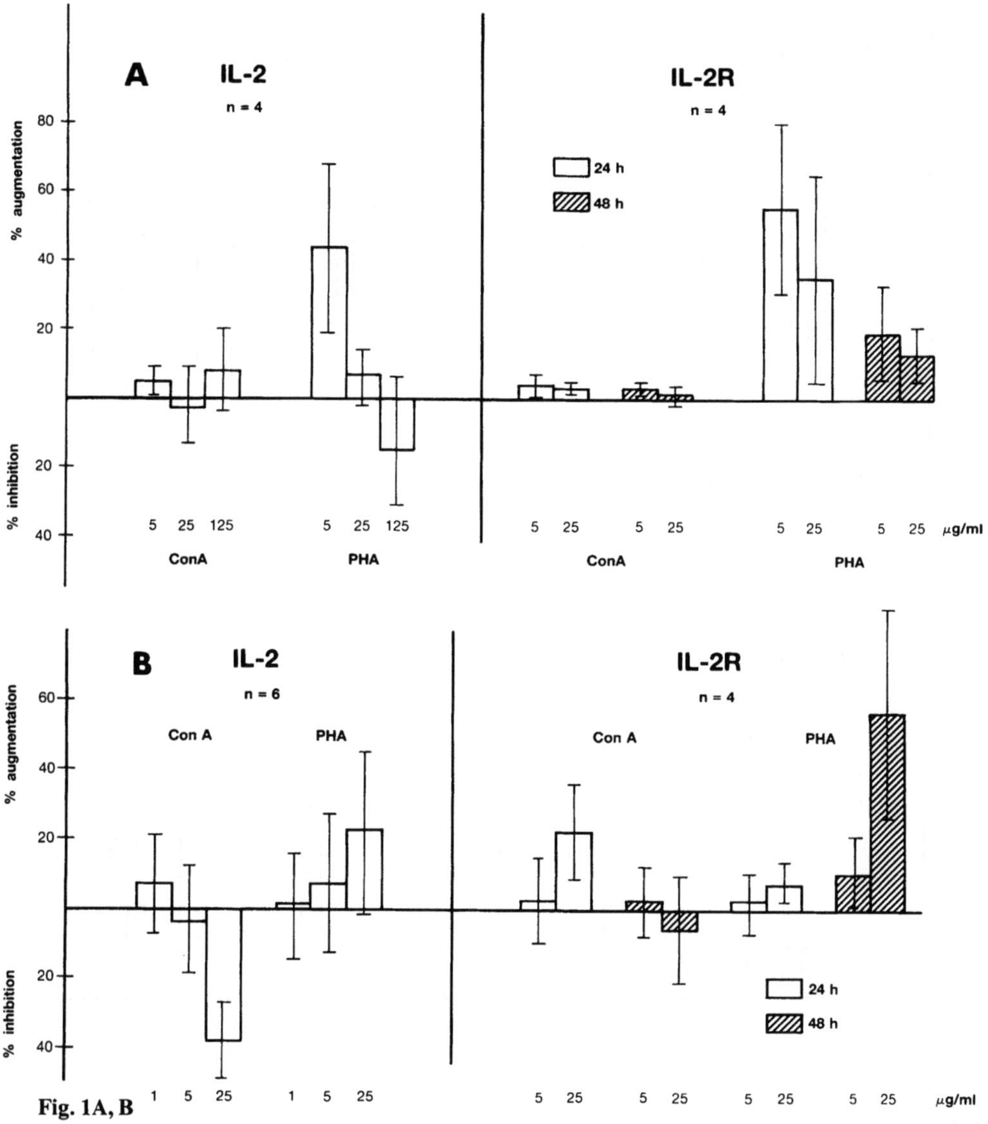

Fig. 1A, B

pendent modulation of Il-2 production and Il-2R expression of PBMCs when stimulated with optimal doses of con A or PHA (Fig. 1). With ampicillin a significant enhancement of Il-2 activity was detected a 5 μg/ml of the drug but only in the presence of PHA ($P<0.01$). Higher concentrations had no effect on Il-2 release, although a significant enhancement of Il-2R expression was registered at a dose of 25 μg/ml after 24 h ($P<0.01$). Tetracycline was found to suppress the con A-stimulated Il-2 production at a concentration of 25 μg/ml ($P<0.01$). The same concentration quite differently influenced the PHA-induced Il-2 release of cells of different donors but enhanced in each case the Il-2R expression after 48 h incubation ($P<0.001$). An overall inhibition was observed with rifampicin and

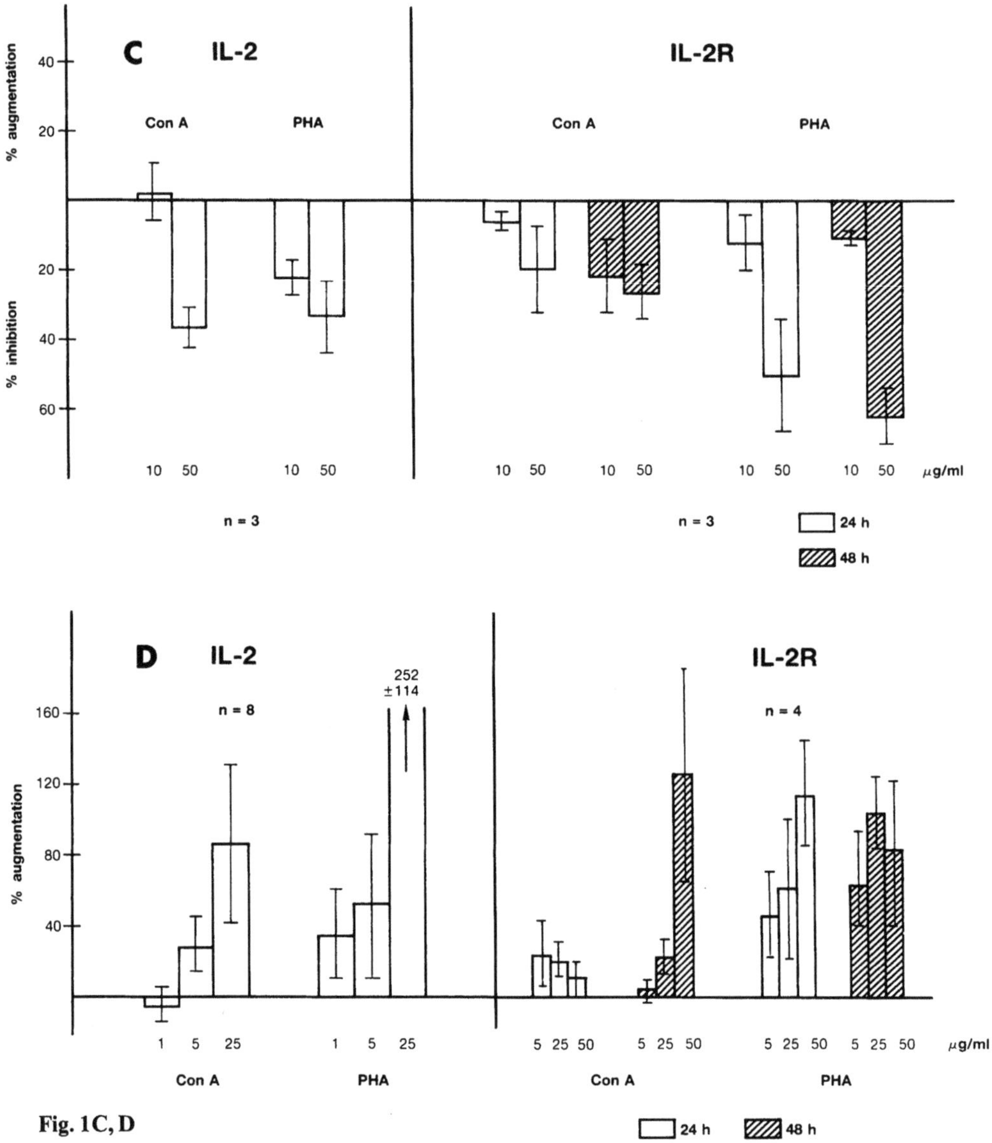

Fig. 1C, D

Figs. 1 A–D. Influence of ampicillin **A**, tetracycline **B**, rifampicin **C**, and ciprofloxacin **D** on mitogen-stimulated Il-2 production and Il-2R expression. Cells were incubated with 5 μg/ml con A or PHA with or without different amounts of the drugs. Il-2 activity was assayed after 24 h and Il-2R expression after 24 and 48 h. Inhibition was calculated:

$$100 \times \frac{\text{U/ml Il-2 or \% Il-2R-positive cells without drug} - \text{U/ml Il-2 or \% Il-2R-positive cells with drug}}{\text{U/ml Il-2 or \% Il-2R-positive cells without drug}}$$

Augmentation was calculated:

$$100 \times \frac{\text{U/ml Il-2 or \% Il-2R-positive cells with drug} - \text{U/ml Il-2 or \% Il-2R-positive cells without drug}}{\text{U/ml Il-2 or \% Il-2R-positive cells without drug}}$$

Results are means of experiments ± SD

this suppression was more pronounced when stimulated with PHA. In contrast to rifampicin, ciprofloxacin increased Il-2 activity in the supernatants significantly at concentrations of 5 ($P<0.05$) and 25 µg/ml ($P<0.01$). A similar augmenting effect was observed particularly on Il-2R expression after 48 h.

Effect of Drugs on Il-2 Production and Il-2R Expression of Mitogen-Stimulated PBMCs, Monocyte-Depleted PBMCs, and Enriched T Cells. To investigate which cell populations are mainly involved in the augmenting or inhibiting effect of the drugs, we examined with highly effective doses their influence on Il-2 production and Il-2R expression of PBMC, monocyte-depleted (MD), and T cells (Fig. 2). Tetracycline suppressed the Il-2 production of PBMC and MD cells but enhanced the Il-2R expression ($P<0.05$) of PBMCs in PHA-stimulated cultures, corresponding to the results shown in Fig. 1. In contrast, T cells showed an increase of Il-2 production ($P<0.01$) without an influence on the receptor expression after mitogenic stimulus with PHA, indicating the role of accessory cells in the tetracycline-mediated suppression. The inhibiting effect of rifampicin seems to be independent of accessory cells because Il-2 release of MD cells and T cells was likewise suppressed ($P<0.01$). The Il-2 release and Il-2R expression-enhancing effect of ciprofloxacin apparently depend on the presence of adherent cells as monocytes or B cells, because MD cells and T cells – the latter only in PHA-stimulated cultures – produced significantly less Il-2 than PBMCs, although still in a signifi-

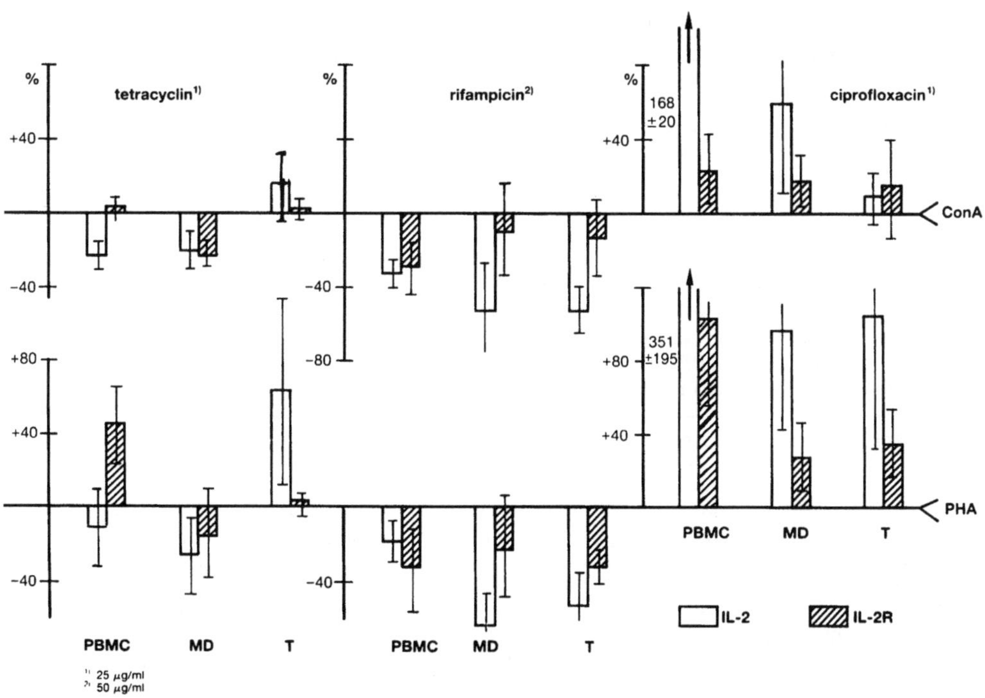

Fig. 2. Il-2 production and Il-2R expression of PBMCs and MD and isolated T cells. Cells were incubated with 5 µg/ml con A or PHA with or without 25 µg/ml tetracycline or ciprofloxacin and 50 µg/ml rifampicin. Il-2 activity and Il-2R receptor expression were assayed after 24 h. For calculation see Fig. 1

cantly raised quantity ($P < 0.01$). Ciprofloxacin had no influence on con A-stimulated T cells.

Influence of Drugs on Immunoglobulin Production. Interaction between Il-2 and its receptor provides not only a signal for T-cell proliferation, but also a differentiation-inducing mediator for immunoglobulin-producing B cells. Therefore, we

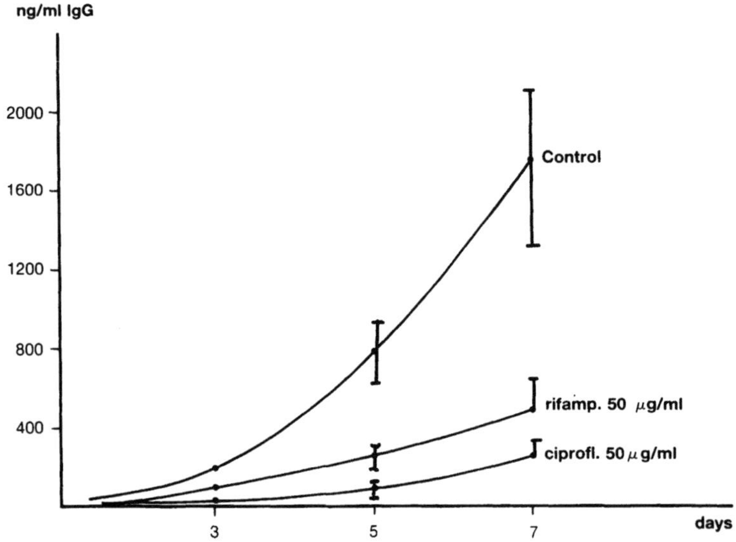

Fig. 3. Influence of rifampicin and ciprofloxacin on PWM-stimulated in vitro immunoglobulin production. Cells were incubated with 1 μg/ml PWM with or without 50 μg/ml rifampicin or ciprofloxacin. Supernatants were harvested on day 3, 5, and 7 and assayed for Ig concentration

Table 1. Influence of short-term and long-term treatment with ciprofloxacin on the PWM-stimulated immunoglobulin production of human lymphocytes. PBMCs were incubated without and with 1 μg/ml PWM. PWM-stimulated cultures were incubated with or without 25 μg/ml ciprofloxacin. One part of culture was washed out after 6 h and complemented either with medium containing 1 μg/ml PWM or with medium containing 1 μg/ml PWM and 25 μg/ml drug. Supernatants were harvested for assaying immunoglobulin concentration at day 7

Treatment	Exp. 1				Exp. 2			
	IgG		IgM		IgG		IgM	
	ng/ml	±%	ng/ml	±%	ng/ml	±%	ng/ml	±%
No stimulus	152	–	120	–	96	–	80	–
PWM	1630	100	1720	100	2150	100	1760	100
PWM + ciprofloxacin[a]	490	− 70	365	− 79	430	− 80	285	− 84
PWM + ciprofloxacin[a] 6 h → PWM	2120	+ 30	2370	+ 38	2910	+ 35	2320	+ 32
PWM + ciprofloxacin[a] 6 h → PWM + cipro[a]	770	− 53	458	− 72	690	− 68	480	− 73

[a] 25 μg/ml.

compared the influence of rifampicin – a substance which inhibits Il-2 production and Il-2R expression – and of ciprofloxacin – which has a quite opposite effect – on the in vitro immunoglobulin production (Fig. 3). Surprisingly both substances significantly suppressed the secretion of immunoglobulins in culture supernatants of PWM-stimulated cells over the whole culture period. In further experiments we investigated the influence of short-term and long-term treatment with ciprofloxacin on the PWM-stimulated immunoglobulin production (Table 1). When lymphocytes were stimulated with PWM and ciprofloxacin only for 6 h, which is sufficient time to induce enhanced Il-2 production, a rather increased concentration of immunoglobulins was found in comparison to the controls in the culture supernatants on day 7. If the washed cells were complemented not only with PWM but again with ciprofloxacin, immunoglobulin production was approximately inhibited to the same extent as in the cultures with PWM and ciprofloxacin without washing out after 6 h.

Discussion

In recent years the positive or negative immunomodulatory activities of antimicrobial agents have been investigated with growing interest. As most side effects of these substances are related to their direct interactions with mammalian cells, the influence on the proliferative response of lymphocytes after antigenic or mitogenic stimulation was also studied in in vitro experiments. In the lymphocyte activation process a sequence of very complicated events led from the activation signal to the DNA synthesis and cell division. It is, therefore, difficult to define the target site of exogenous substances when modifying effects are observed. Augmenting or suppressing effects on intermediate steps will not necessarily reflect a corresponding enhanced or suppressed proliferative capacity of cells.

In the present study we found differently modulating effects of antimicrobial agents on Il-2 production and Il-2R expression. Il-2 synthesis begins very early (4–8 h) after stimulation concurrently with Il-2R expression, with peak values between 24 and 72 h. Il-2 will be consumed by binding to its receptor followed by a progressive disappearance of the latter, probably due to different mechanisms such as discontinuation of synthesis, internalization, and/or release from the cell membrane. The mechanism for Il-2 production and Il-2R expression may also differ [6, 7]. Therefore, increased Il-2 production is not conclusive for an increased Il-2R expression. Nevertheless, Il-2 and each cell surface receptor have been shown to be essential components in the growth and proliferation of T- and most likely B-lymphocytes [1].

In general, significant suppression was not found on investigating human lymphocyte transformation by beta-lactam antibiotics only only at high concentrations [8]. We found that ampicillin stimulated Il-2 production parallel with enhanced Il-2R expression at low doses, whereas high doses (125 μg/ml) suppressed Il-2 production. Cefotaxime significantly inhibited Il-2 secretion at concentrations of 25 and 125 μg/ml (data not shown). Tetracycline, a mitochondriotropic antibiotic, seemed to influence Il-2 synthesis only at high doses without a corresponding suppressive effect on Il-2R expression. The significantly enhanced Il-2R positive cells after 48 h are most likely due to diminished consumption. The presence of elevated levels of such cells suggests that the cell function to express the membrane receptor is not impaired. Rifampicin has been shown to perturb immune reactions in vitro, although results of studies on a suppression of lymphocyte transformation are not unequivocal [8]. We demonstrated a clear-cut decrease of Il-2 production and Il-2R expression in particular at high doses. Suppression was only observed if rifampicin was added together with the mitogen. Ciprofloxacin exhibited a quite opposite effect. A significant enhancement of Il-2 production and receptor expression could be shown not only at high but also at low doses of the drug. The stimulation was more pronounced in PHA-stimulated cultures than in con A ones. It has been reported that high lectin concentrations favor Il-2 production, which is already initiated by con A concentrations as low as 1 µg/ml and by PHA concentration of 0.05 µg/ml respectively [9]. Therefore, 5 µg/ml PHA represents a more intense activating signal than the same dose of con A. Our data suggest that the higher the activation of the cells the more potent could be the modulating effect of the drugs.

Investigating the modifying effect of tetracycline, rifampicin, and ciprofloxacin on PBMCs and MD and T cells, we found that in the case of tetracycline the suppression was more pronounced in the presence of monocytes and other non-T cells. In contrast, isolated T cells produced significantly higher concentrations of Il-2 than the controls, probably due to a selective stimulating effect of tetracycline on T cells and to the abolition of the concomitant cellmediated inhibition. It should be noted that both Il-2 production and receptor expression were significantly less when isolated T cells were investigated (Il-2 concentration in supernatants of PBMCs: 14.7 ± 6.2 U/ml versus T cells: 4.2 ± 3.8 U/ml). The stimulation by ciprofloxacin was abrogated completely by using isolated T cells after stimulation with con A but not PHA. This again suggests the role of accessory cells in the drug-induced alteration; however, it could be caused by a suboptimal mitogen concentration. Rifampicin seems to exhibit a direct adverse effect on T cells at least under in vitro conditions.

The exceptionally pronounced augmenting effect of ciprofloxacin is even more interesting in view of the fact that Forsgren et al. [10, 11] described significantly increased thymidine incorporation by quinolones into lymphocytes without true stimulation of the cell proliferation. The authors demonstrated an inhibition of immunoglobulin production similar to that found in the present study. Furthermore, they observed that the inhibitory effect of ciprofloxacin on growth of HeLa cells was reversible when cells were exposed for only 24 h to the drug. We found that the short exposure to 25 µg/ml ciprofloxacin for 6 h did not influence the immunoglobulin synthesis but still augmented Il-2 production. These data suggest that ciprofloxacin may have a biphasic effect on activated cells. It probably interferes in the early state of mitogen-induced activation of lymphocytes stimulating the synthesis of macromolecules and metabolism, but inhibits other events in the later state of activation by which DNA replication and mitosis are blocked.

In conclusion, this study demonstrates that mitogen-activated lymphocytes but not resting cells may be modulated in Il-2 production and Il-2R expression in the presence of antimicrobial agents. The modifying activity seems to be mediated, at least in part, by monocytes and other non-T cells, suggesting a direct effect on the accessory cell population rather than on T cells. Furthermore, it should be emphasized that increased production of Il-2 does not necessarily reflect increased cell proliferation as in the case of ciprolfoxacin. Therefore, these early parameters of lymphocyte activation would need to be investigated together with other cell functions such as proliferative or immunoglobulin-producing capacity to provide a sensitive and helpful method for elucidation of the interactions between drugs and cells of the immune system.

Summary

The in vitro effect of antimicrobial agents with different modes of action was investigated on the Il-2 production and Il-2R expression of mitogen-activated lymphocytes. At low doses ampicillin enhanced Il-2 release and at high doses receptor expression. Tetracycline suppressed Il-2 activity only at high doses, whereas the percentage of Il-2R-positive cells was somewhat increased, suggesting a diminished consumption by Il-2. A pronounced decrease in Il-2 production and Il-2R expression was observed in the presence of rifampicin. In contrast, ciprofloxacin induced a highly significant stimulation. The results of experiments with isolated cell populations indicated the participation of accessory cells in the modulating effect of tetracycline and ciprofloxacin but not of rifampicin. Surprisingly, rifampicin and ciprofloxacin likewise inhibited the PWM-induced immunoglobulin syntheses independently of their opposite effect on Il-2 production and receptor expression. A biphasic effect of ciprofloxacin on the lymphocyte activation process was postulated because a short-term exposure of cells to the drug still induced an elevated level of Il-2 concentration without suppressing immunoglobulin synthesis.

References

1. Isakov N, Altman A (1986) Interleukin 2, an immunoregulatory hormone: biology and clinical implications. Clinical Immunology Newsletter Elsevier SC Pub Co 7:1–4
2. Zubler RH et al. (1984) Activated B cells express receptors for, and proliferate in response to, pure interleukin 2. J Exp Med 160:1170–1183
3. Pusztai-Markos ZS, Ebenfeld R, Scheiwe MW (1984) Fc receptors and human T lymphocytes in frozen-thawed peripheral blood cells. Cryobiology 21:427–434
4. Scheiwe MW, Pusztai-Markos ZS, Essers U, Seelis R, Rau G, Körber C, Stürner KH, Jung H, Liedtke B (1981) Cryopreservation of human lymphocytes and stem cells (CFU-c) in large units for cancer therapy – a report based on the data of more than 400 frozen units. Cryobiology 18:344–356
5. Geiersberger U, Pusztai-Markos ZS (1986) A modified method of rate nephelometry suitable to determine in vitro produced immunoglobulins: evidence of decreased synthesis by atopic subjects with perennial symptoms. Arbeitstagung der Deutschen Gesellschaft für Hygiene und Mikrobiologie (DGHM), Sektion II, III
6. Linch DC, Wallace DL, O'Flynn K (1987) Signal transduction in human T lymphocytes. Immunol Rev 95:137–159
7. Greene WC, Depper JM, Krönke M, Leonard WJ (1986) The human interleukin-2 receptor: analysis of structure and function. Immunol Rev 92:29–48

8. Hauser WE Jr, Remington JS (1984) Effect of antimicrobial agents on the immune response. In: Ristuccia AM, Cunha BA (eds) Antimicrobial therapy. Raven, New York, pp 55–79
9. Roosnek EE, Brouwer MC, Aarden LA (1985) T cell triggering by lectins I. Requirements for interleukin 2 production; lectin concentration determines the accessory cell dependency. Eur J Immunol 15:652–656
10. Forsgren A, Schlossman SF, Tedder TF (1987) 4-Quinolone drugs affect cell cycle progression and function of human lymphocytes in vitro. Antimicrob Agents Chemother 31:768–773
11. Forsgren A, Bredberg A, Pardee AB, Schlossman SF, Tedder TF (1987) Effects of ciprofloxacin on eucaryotic pyrimidine nucleotide biosynthesis and cell growth. Antimicrob Agents Chemother 31:774–779

Effect of 4-Quinolone Antibiotics on Cell Function, Cell Growth, and Pyrimidine Nucleotide Biosynthesis in Human Lymphocytes In Vitro

A. FORSGREN

Introduction

The new 4-quinolones such as ciprofloxacin, norfloxacin, and ofloxacin are strongly bactericidal, with activities approaching 1000 times that of nalidixic acid [12]. They are effective against a wider range of bacteria, including *Pseudomonas aeruginosa* and gram-positive cocci, which are considered resistant to nalidixic acid [6]. The activity of this family of drugs may be due to inhibition of bacterial DNA synthesis [5, 12]. Due to the great potential for the clinical use of these drugs it is important to investigate any possible positive or negative side effects on the host defense system.

In a previous study with human granulocytes no direct effects of the new quinolone derivatives were found, on granulocyte chemotaxis, chemiluminescence, phagocytosis, or bacterial killing [7].

This report summarizes work on the function of human lymphocytes cultured in the presence of 4-quinolone antibiotics.

Material and Methods

Antibiotics. Fresh solutions of the following preservative-free antibiotics were used: amifloxacin, ciprofloxacin, enoxacin, flumequine, pefloxacin, pipemidic acid (Bayer), norfloxacin (Astra), ofloxacin (Hoechst), A56619, A56620 (Abbot), cinoxacin (Lilly), and nalidixic acid (Sterling).

Lymphocytes. Heparinized blood from healthy donors was used in most experiments. Mononuclear cells were harvested by centrifugation on Ficoll-Paque [2]. B-lymphocytes were isolated by depletion of monocytes in plastic culture plates for 1 h at 37 °C and removal of T-lymphocytes from the nonadherent cells by rosette formation with sheep erythrocytes treated with 2-aminoethylisothiouronium bromide with subsequent density gradient centrifugation [13]. The Epstein-Barr virus-transformed cell lines Raji, Laz 388, and Laz 509, the human thymic tumor-derived cell line Rex and Hela cells were also used in some experiments.

Mitogens. T-lymphocytes were activated using phytohemagglutinin (PHA) at a final concentration of 1 μg/ml or concanavalin A (con A) (25 μg/ml). Pokeweed

Department of Medical Microbiology, University of Lund, Malmö General Hospital, 21401 Malmö, Sweden

The Influence of Antibiotics on the Host-Parasite Relationship III
Edited by G. Gillissen, W. Opferkuch, G. Peters, and G. Pulverer

mitogen (PWM) in a final dilution of 1:200 or Epstein-Barr virus (EBV) were used to stimulate Ig secretion. B-lymphocytes were activated using formalin-fixed *Staphylococcus aureus* Cowan strain 1 (SAC) or EBV.

Lymphocyte Culture Conditions. Triplicate samples were cultured in 96 well microtiter plates containing 1×10^5 lymphocytes per culture in 200 µl RPMI 1640 medium supplemented with 10% AB serum or 15% fetal calf serum, 2 m*M* glutamine, and 12 or 50 µg/ml gentamicin. The effect of quinolone antibiotics on human lymphocytes was identical in gentamicin-free medium. The proliferation of lymphocytes in the presence of ciprofloxacin was determined with an automatic cell counter (Coulter, Hialeah, Florida).

Radioactive Incorportion. A quantity of 0.5 or 1 µCi [^{3}H]thymidine (NET-072, specific activity 78 Ci/mmol), [6-^{3}H]deoxyuridine (NET-164, NEN Research Products, Boston, MA, specific activity 21.4 Ci/mmol), [^{3}H]uridine (NET 367, specific activity 40 Ci/mmol), [5-^{3}H] orotic acid (NET-134, specific activity 10–20 Ci/mmol), [8-^{14}C]hypoxanthine (NEC-149, specific activity 40–60 mCi/mmol), or [^{14}C]leucine (NEC-279, specific activity 337 mCi/mmol) was added to cell cultures 6–24 h before harvesting. Cultures were usually harvested in distilled water by an automatic harvesting machine onto fiberglass filters or by precipitation with 10% trichloroacetic acid (TCA). The radioactivity was measured in a Packard Tri-Carb liquid scintillation counter and data were calculated from the means of triplicate cultures.

Cell Cycle Analysis by Flow Cytometry. DNA content of individual cells stained with propidium iodide was analyzed by flow cytometry using a Coulter Epics C [3, 4, 10].

Radioimmunoassay for Immunoglobulin Secretion. Solid phase radioimmunoassays (RIAs) for IgG and IgM were performed in disposable flexible polyvinyl microtiter plates (Dynatech, Alexandria, VA) [1, 9]. Plates were coated with either 100 µl rabbit anti-human IgG or anti-human IgM (Dakopatts A/S, Denmark) overnight at room temperature.

Statistics. Wilcoxon's matched pair test was used to check the statistical significance of the results.

Results

Effects on [^{3}H]Thymidine Incorporation. Initial experiments (Fig. 1) demonstrated that the incorporation of [^{3}H]thymidine into DNA was increased in human lymphocytes stimulated with PHA and incubated with ciprofloxacin in clinically achievable concentrations for 3 days. In contrast, very high concentrations of the same drug inhibited the incorporation. The inhibitory effect was more pronounced when the lymphocytes were incubated with 4-quinolones for 5 days. The effect of 12 different 4-quinolones on [^{3}H]thymidine incorporation in human lym-

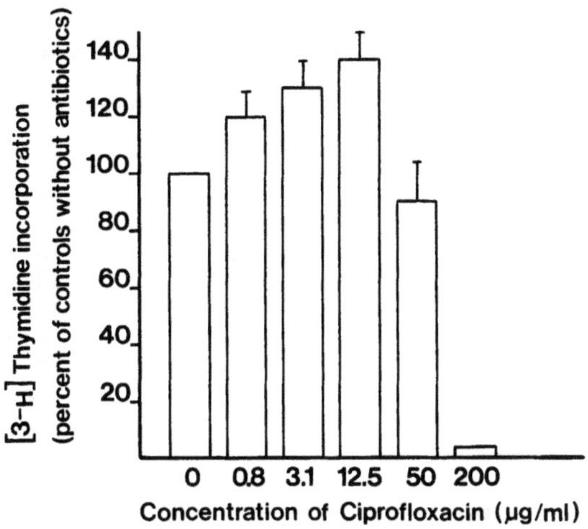

Fig. 1. Response ([^{3}H]thymidine incorporation) of PHA-stimulated human lymphocytes in the presence of ciprofloxacin during 3 days. The results (mean $\pm$ standard deviation), which are given as percentages of incorporation in controls without antibiotics, represent experiments with lymphocytes from seven volunteers. The increase in concentrations (0.8–12.5 μg/ml) is statistically significant ($P < 0.01$)

phocytes was examined (Table 1). Eight of the 4-quinolones at concentrations of 1.56–6.25 μg/ml significantly increased [^{3}H]thymidine uptake of stimulated lymphocytes. The effect was even more pronounced at 25 μg/ml of the drugs. Flumequine and pipemidic acid only had a significant effect at 25 μg/ml. Nalidixic acid and cinoxacin did not have any effect in the concentration range of 1.56–25 μg/ml.

It was determined whether ciprofloxacin also influenced thymidine incorporation of lymphocytes after stimulation with mitogens other than PHA. Con A, PWM, and SAC were added to human lymphocyte cultures containing 5–20 μg/ml ciprofloxacin. During the peak of incorporation, which varied for the different mitogens, there was an enhanced uptake of [^{3}H]thymidine in a similar fashion to that in PHA-stimulated lymphocytes.

Incorporation of Radioactive DNA, RNA, and Protein Precursors in the Presence of Ciprofloxacin. To determine whether increased incorporation of other nucleotides or amino acids occurs, the incorporation of radiolabeled thymidine, deoxyuridine, uridine, orotic acid, and leucine was studied in parallel cultures of PHA-stimulated human lymphocytes during 1- to 6-day cultures. From day 3 to day 5 of incubation, the incorporation of radiolabeled thymidine, deoxyuridine, uridine, and orotic acid was enhanced by the presence of ciprofloxacin. At a ciprofloxacin concentration of 80 μg/ml, incorporation was strongly inhibited.

The incorporation of [^{14}C]leucine was not significantly changed from control cultures at ciprofloxacin concentrations up to 20 μg/ml, while at 40 and 80 μg/ml leucine incorporation was inhibited. Similar results were obtained when the cell material was precipitated and washed with TCA, demonstrating radioactive precursor incorporation into nucleic acids and protein.

Table 1. [^{3}H]Thymidine incorporation of PHA-stimulated human lymphocytes cultured for 5 days with different quinolone derivatives[c]

Antibiotic	% of control ± SEM at a drug concentration (μg/ml) of		
	25	6.25	1.56
Ciprofloxacin	331 ± 39[a]	237 ± 20[a]	152 ± 7[a]
Norfloxacin	294 ± 31[a]	162 ± 16[a]	111 ± 4[b]
Ofloxacin	296 ± 25[a]	182 ± 10[a]	132 ± 6[a]
A 56619	233 ± 30[a]	177 ± 18[a]	119 ± 8[b]
A 56620	263 ± 34[a]	143 ± 8[a]	106 ± 4
Amifloxacin	240 ± 20[a]	146 ± 7[a]	114 ± 4[b]
Enoxacin	218 ± 38[a]	214 ± 16[a]	130 ± 4[a]
Pefloxacin	298 ± 26[a]	183 ± 11[a]	136 ± 6[a]
Flumequine	177 ± 11[a]	121 ± 9	107 ± 8
Pipemidic acid	163 ± 12[a]	111 ± 6	103 ± 5

[a] There was a significant increase ($P < 0.01$) in [^{3}H]thymidine incorporation.
[b] $P < 0.05$.
[c] Lymphocytes (1×10^5/well) from eight different healthy donors were incubated with all antibiotics and the results were statistically compared with control cultures without the drugs. The cells were incubated with [^{3}H]thymidine during the last 18 h of culture. The [^{3}H]thymidine uptake in control cultures without drugs was 100000–140000 cpm.

Table 2. Ciprofloxacin influences the total incorporation of nucleosides but not leucine during 6 days of culture

Radiactive nucleoside/ amino acid	% of control ± SD at a drug concentration (μg/ml) of[a]		
	20	5	1.25
[^{3}H]Thymidine	145 ± 15	142 ± 6	110 ± 4
[^{3}H]Deoxyuridine	142 ± 21	139 ± 5	102 ± 2
[^{3}H]Uridine	127 ± 11	119 ± 9	110 ± 3
[^{14}C]Leucine	82 ± 14	96 ± 7	92 ± 3

[a] Human lymphocytes were stimulated with PHA and incubated with ciprofloxacin. The cultures were pulsed with radioactive nucleosides or amino acid before harvesting at 24-h intervals on days 1–6. Incorporation (cpm) for each day was totaled and the results were calculated as percentage of control cultures not containing ciprofloxacin and are the mean ± SD obtained in three different experiments.

When the total radioactivity incorporated over a 6-day period was determined by daily pulsing and harvesting, it was found that at 20 μg/ml ciprofloxacin [^{3}H]thymidine and [^{3}H]deoxyuridine incorporation was increased by 42%–45%, [^{3}H]uridine uptake was increased by 27%, while leucine incorporation was decreased by 18% (Table 2). At 5 μg/ml, a similar effect was observed.

Thymidine, deoxyuridine, uridine, and orotic acid are incorporated through salvage pathways into steps of de novo pyrimidine nucleotide biosynthesis. Hypoxanthine is a precursor of purines in DNA synthesis. In contrast the incorpora-

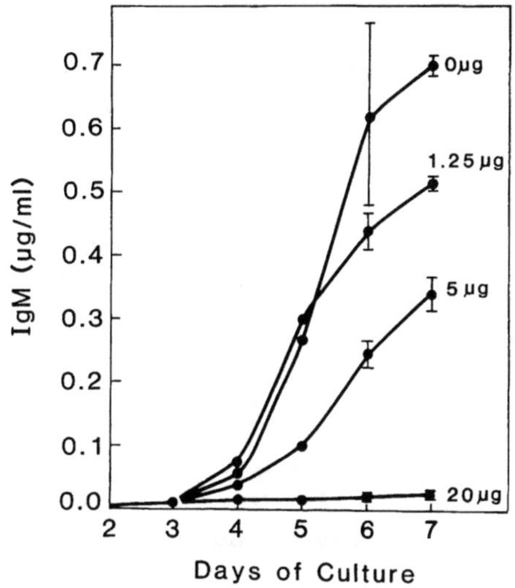

Fig. 2. Immunoglobulin secretion (IgG and IgM) by PWM-stimulated lymphocytes in the presence of ciprofloxacin. Lymphocytes were cultured in microtiter plates and supernatants harvested daily. The immunoglobulin content in the supernatants was determined with an RIA. These results were obtained in five experiments

tion of radiolabeled hypoxanthine was not increased by ciprofloxacin. The effect thus appears to affect pyrimidine and not purine pathways.

In hypoxanthine-aminopterin-thymidine (HAT) culture medium, nucleic acid metabolism is dependent on the uptake of thymidine and hypoxanthine through salvage pathways, since de novo thymidine and purine nucleotide biosynthesis is blocked by aminopterin. There was no increase in thymidine incorporation by cells cultured in HAT medium in the presence of 5 µg ciprofloxacin/ml, which indicates that ciprofloxacin affects de novo pyrimidine biosynthesis, resulting in increased uptake of radiolabeled thymidine through salvage pathways.

Immunoglobulin secretion. Lymphocytes (B + T cells) were stimulated with PWM and immunoglobulin secretion into the culture medium assessed (Fig. 2). Secretion of IgG and IgM was dramatically inhibited by 20 µg/ml ciprofloxacin, decreased to approximately half at 5 µg/ml, while 1.25 µg ciprofloxacin had a limited influence on immunoglobulin production. In addition, when isolated human B-lymphocytes were stimulated with EB virus, IgG and IgM production was inhibited to the same degree.

Cell Growth and Cell Cycle Progression. Phytohemagglutin-stimulated human lymphocytes were cultured in the presence of different ciprofloxacin concentrations and cell multiplication was determined with a cell counter. The lymphocytes were shown to grow slower, in approximately 50%, in the presence of 20 µg ciprofloxacin/ml than in the control cultures. Growth of lymphoblastoid cell lines was inhibited to the same degree. Growth of HeLa cells was also significantly inhibited ($P < 0.01$) at 20 µg ciprofloxacin/ml and there was no growth at all at

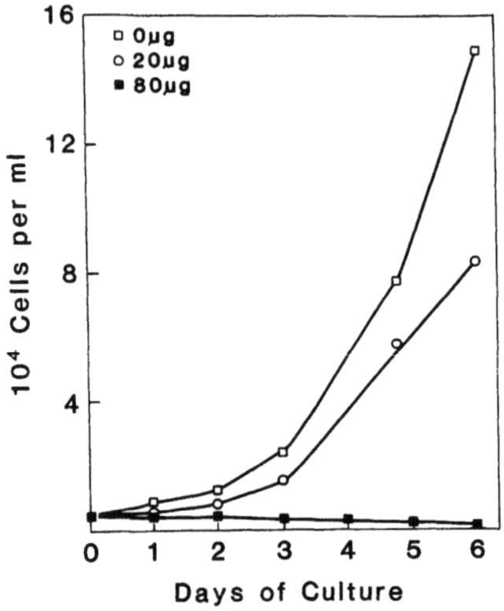

Fig. 3. Growth of HeLa cells in the presence of 0 (□), 20 (○), and 80 µg/ml (■) ciprofloxacin

80 µg drug/ml (Fig. 3). However, the inhibitory effect of ciprofloxacin on HeLa cell growth was reversible.

Although [^{3}H]thymidine incorporation is an estimate of DNA synthesis, it does not indicate the percentage of cells entering the cell cycle. By using a flow cytometry technique to quantitate the amount of DNA in individual cells, it was shown that ciprofloxacin at the highest concentration (20 µg/ml) inhibited the percentage of lymphocytes entering the $S+G_2/M$ phases during the first 3 days of incubation.

Discussion

The finding of a pronounced increase in incorporation of tritiated thymidine in the presence of 4-quinolones was remarkable [8–10]. The results are even more interesting in view of the fact that, with some of the new quinolones, the effect is even apparent at clinically achievable concentrations (Table 1).

The increased thymidine incorporation by quinolones into lymphocytes suggests a true stimulation of DNA synthesis. However, lymphocyte growth was inhibited at 20 µg/ml ciprofloxacin, and cell cycle analysis indicated a decrease in DNA synthesis and an inhibited progression through the cell cycle at 5 and 20 µg/ml. Thus, the increased [^{3}H]thymidine incorporated does not reflect increased DNA replication and cell growth. In addition, B-cell immunoglobulin secretion in T-cell-dependent and -independent assays was inhibited, suggesting that lymphocyte function in vitro is altered by the presence of ciprofloxacin.

There is a discrepancy between our results, which show an increased [^{3}H]thymidine uptake, and those of Gollapudi et al. [11], which do not demonstrate any effect in human lymphocyte cultures stimulated with PHA or con A for 3 days. In our kinetic experiments there was no increase in [^{3}H]thymidine uptake at day

2 in drug-treated cultures compared with control cultures. However, an increased [^{3}H]thymidine uptake by the drug-treated cells was significant at day 3 and even more pronounced on subsequent days. If the cells cultured by Gollapudi et al. grew slightly slower or were harvested somewhat earlier than our 3-day cultures, the effect of quinolones on [^{3}H]thymidine incorporation would not have been detected.

Exogenous thymidine, deoxyuridine, uridine, and orotic acid are precursors of pyrimidine nucleotides in different salvage pathways. Each of these precursors was incorporated at higher levels by cells cultured in the presence of ciprofloxacin. However, in HAT medium, where de novo pyrimidine synthesis is blocked, no increase in [^{3}H]thymidine uptake due to ciprofloxacin was detected. Incorporation of the purine, hypoxanthine, or the amino acid leucine were not increased in the presence of ciprofloxacin. These data suggest that ciprofloxacin inhibits de novo pyrimidine synthesis at a step before orotate synthesis. Such an inhibition could result in the increased uptake of pyrimidine nucleotide precursors. This was supported by results from experiments using (N-(phosphonacetyl)-2-aspartate (PALA), a well-defined transition state analog inhibitor of aspartate transcarbamylase [14].

The altered pyrimidine biosynthesis in the presence of 4-quinolones may represent a specific inhibition of one of the enzymes involved in the biosynthesis. However, a less-specific or another toxic effect of 4-quinolones which indirectly alters pools of pyrimidine nucleotides, particularly since the effect seen occurs after considerable delay, is also possible.

Summary

Several of the new 4-quinolones significantly increase the incorporation of [^{3}H]thymidine into the DNA of mitogen-stimulated human lymphocytes.

In spite of the apparent increase in DNA synthesis, lymphocyte growth of lymphocytes and several cell lines was inhibited by 20 μg/ml ciprofloxacin, and cell cycle analysis showed that ciprofloxacin inhibited progression through the cell cycle. In addition, immunoglobulin secretion by human lymphocytes stimulated by pokeweed mitogen (PWM) or Epstein-Barr virus (EBV) was inhibited by approximately 50% at 5 μg/ml ciprofloxacin.

This study suggests the ciprofloxacin inhibits de novo pyrimidine biosynthesis, thereby resulting in a compensatory increase in the uptake of pyrimidine precursors through salvage pathways.

References

1. Bensussan A, Meurer SC, Schlossman SF, Reinherz EL (1984) Delineation of an immunoregulatory amplifier population recognizing autologous Ia molecules. J Exp Med 159:559–576
2. Boyum A (1968) Separation of leukocytes from blood and bone marrow. Scand J Clin Lab Invest [Suppl]97:77

3. Crissman HA, Steinkamp JA (1973) Rapid simultaneous measurement of DNA, protein, and cell volume in single cells from large mammalian cell populations. J Cell Biol 59:766–771
4. Darzynkiewicz Z, Crissman H, Traganos F, Steinkamp J (1982) Cell heterogeneity during the cell cycle. J Cell Physiol 113:465–474
5. Drlica K (1984) Biology of bacterial dexyribonucleic acid topoisomerases. Microbiol Rev 48:273–289
6. Forsgren A (1985) Comparative in vitro activity of three new quinolone antibiotics against recent clinical isolates. Scand J Infect Dis 17:91–94
7. Forsgren A, Bergkvist PI (1985) Effect of ciprofloxacin on phagocytosis. Eur J Clin Microbiol 4:575–578
8. Forsgren A, Bergh AK, Brandt M, Hansson G (1986) Quinolones affect thymidine incorporation into the DNA of human lymphocytes. Antimicrob Agents Chemother 29:506–508
9. Forsgren A, Bredberg A, Pardee AB, Schlossman SF, Tedder TF (1987) Effects of ciprofloxacin on encaryotic pyrimidine nucleotide biosynthesis and cell growth. Antimicrob Agents Chemother 31:774–779
10. Forsgren A, Schlossman SF, Tedder TFT (1987) 4-Quinolone drugs affect cell cycle progression and function of human lymphocytes in vitro. Antimicrob Agents Chemother 31:768–773
11. Gollapudi SVS, Prabhala RH, Thadepalli H (1986) Effect of ciprofloxacin on mitogen-stimulated lymphocyte proliferation. Antimicrob Agents Chemother 29:337–338
12. Smith JT (1984) Awakening the slumbering potential of the 4-quinolone antibacterials. Pharm J 15:209–305
13. Tedder TF, Boyd AW, Freedman AS, Nadler LM, Schlossman SF (1985) The B cell surface molecule B1 is functionally linked with B cell activation and differentiation. J Immunol 135:973–979
14. Swyryd EA, Seaver SS, Stark GR (1974) *N*-(Phosphoracetyl)-L-aspartate, a potent transition state analog inhibitor of aspartate transcarbamylase, blocks proliferation of mammalian cells in culture. J Biol Chem 249:6945–6950

Enhancement by Ampicillin or Cyclacillin Pretreatment of *E.coli* of Phagocytosis, Blastogenesis, and Production of Lymphokines, Interferons, and Tumor Necrosis Factor

H. FRIEDMAN [1], A. SZENTIVANYI [2], T. W. KLEIN [1], and G. WARREN [3]

In recent years, the emergence of antibiotic-resistant bacteria has prompted a reevaluation of the nature of the host immune defense system as a primary reistance mechanism to infectious diseases, even in the presence of antibiotics [3, 26, 28]. Studies from a number of laboratories, including this one, have focused attention on the influence of antibiotics on host immune mechanisms and alteration of susceptibility of a microorganism to the immune response system [4, 5, 15, 18, 22, 33]. For example, previous studies in this laboratory have shown that the semisynthetic penicillins, cyclacillin and ampicillin, may cause a susceptible bacterium such as *Escherichia coli* to develop increased vulnerability to antibody-mediated complement-dependent bacteriolysis as well as increased susceptibility to phagocytosis by macrophages [6, 7, 9, 10, 12].

Antibiotic-pretreated bacteria also evinced increased activity as an immunogen, stimulating heightened specific antibody responses to the bacteria [8]. In this context, it is noted that macrophage-phagocytized antibiotic-pretreated bacteria may increase the immunogenic moieties of the bacteria as shown by subsequent injection of cell-free extracts of macrophages into recipient animals. Thus, it seemed likely that the immunogenic components of bacteria may increase in either concentration or potency by prior exposure to antibiotics.

In the present study, the immunogenicity of antibiotic-pretreated bacteria was examined in further detail. The effect of antibiotic pretreatment, on blastogenic responsiveness of normal lymphoid cells, as well as on the induction of these cells to produce cytokines important in immunoregulation, was studied. Among the cytokines examined were interleukin 1 considered a lymphocyte-activating factor produced by antigen or mitogen-stimulated macrophages, as well as interferons and tumor-necrotizing factor, a potent immunoregulatory substance [26, 28–32].

Experimental Design and Procedures

Phagocytosis was performed with adherent spleen cells or thioglycollate-induced peritoneal exudate cells using standard methods [6, 12]. The cells were counted

[1] Departments of Medical Microbiology and Immunology, and
[2] Pharmacology and Therapeutics, University of South Florida College of Medicine, 12901 N 30th Street, Tampa, FL, 3361–24742 USA
[3] Department of Microbiology, Thomas Jefferson University School of Medicine, Philadelphia, PA, USA

The Influence of Antibiotics on the Host-Parasite Relationship III
Edited by G. Gillissen, W. Opferkuch, G. Peters, and G. Pulverer

microscopically and trypan blue stain procedure was used for viability testing. Over 85% of the cells were morphologically similar to macrophages and readily phagocytized latex particles within 15 min at 37 °C. For the phagocytic assay, suspensions of 10^8 peritoneal cells in 0.5 ml medium were added to individual wells of 20 well Linbro plates. To each well was added 0.1 ml of a fresh suspension of *E. coli,* either untreated or previously treated with antibiotic. The cultures were incubated in an atmosphere of 95% air and 5% CO_2 for up to 4 h. Samples of each culture were placed on microscope slides which were then stained with Giemsa and examined microscopically [8]. At least 100 macrophages were examined per sample. The number of *E. coli* present per macrophage was scored and the percentage of macrophages with two or more ingested bacteria was determined.

In order to assess the immunogenicity of *E. coli* antigens in the macrophage after phagocytosis, freeze thaw lysates were prepared from 10^6 cells and injected in 0.5-ml quantities intraperitoneally into three to four BALB/c mice [8]. Blood was obtained from each animal by retroorbital venus plexus puncture at varying times thereafter, usually 5 or 10 days, and anti-*E. coli* agglutinin titers determined in the resulting serum by standard agglutination test in microtiter plates. The ability of the macrophages which had phagocytized *E. coli* to induce normal mouse spleen cells to produce anti-*E. coli* plaque-forming cells (PFCs) was determined by the standard plaque assay with viable *E. coli* in agar plates exactly as described previously [4, 8]. The number of individual PFCs to *E. coli* was determined for 10^6 whole mouse spleen cell suspensions. The numbers of PFCs were averaged for three or more spleens. In all cases the antibody response was determined for the spleen of mice injected with lysates of macrophages exposed to *E. coli* which had been previously treated with antibiotics as compared with lysates of macrophages which had phagocytized untreated *E. coli.*

The ability of the antibiotic-pretreated *E. coli* to stimulate normal spleen cell blastogenic responses was also studied. In brief, 10^6 or 10^8 washed *E. coli,* either untreated or at various times after exposure to graded amounts of antibiotics, followed by washing and resuspension in saline, were assessed for stimulation activity by the standard spleen cell blastogenic procedure. The heat-killed bacteria (80 °C for 30 min) were added to cultures of 10^6 spleen cells from normal BALB/c mice in 0.5 ml medium in 20 well Linbro plates. The plates were incubated for 48 h at 37 °C in an atmosphere of 5% CO_2, 95% air, and then pulsed with 0.5 Ci [^{3}H]thymidine. After 18 h of additional incubation, the amount of radioactivity taken up into the cultures was determined by standard scintillation counting and the stimulation index (SI) calculated as cpm for stimulated cultures −cpm for control cultures divided by cpm for control cultures $\times 100$.

In further experiments cell-free culture supernatants from 10^6 normal adherent spleen cells stimulated in vitro with bacteria, either untreated as a control or pretreated with graded amounts of antibiotics, were assessed for the presence of cytokines by the standard assays for IL-1 ([^{3}H]thymidine proliferation assay with thymus cells from C_3H/HeJ indicator mice), for interferons [protection of Vero cell cultures from infection with 4000 PFUs (plaque-forming units) vascular stomatitis virus], or for tumor necrosit factor (TNF) by protection of WIHI cells using procedures exactly as described previously [1, 2, 16, 23, 24].

Experimental Results

As seen in Table 1, pretreatment of *E. coli* with graded amounts of ampicillin or cyclacillin, but not penicillin G to which they were resistant, resulted in a time-dependent alteration in the susceptibility of the bacteria to be phagocytized by normal mouse peritoneal exsudate (PE) cells. Several hours of incubation of the bacteria with the antibiotic resulted in more bacteria being phagocytized by nor-

Table 1. Effect of antibiotic pretreatment on phagocytosis of *E. coli* by normal mouse peritoneal exudate cells

Antibiotic treatment[a]		Phagocytosis after incubation at 37 °C[b]		
		1 h	2 h	4 h
None (control)		2.6±8	7,8±8.2	11.2±2.1
Ampicillin	1.0 µg	–	18.5±2.1	29.1±6.1
	5.0	8.1±1.16	29.2±4.6	30.9±4.6
	10.0	9.4±2.2	28.4±3.6	26.5±1.9
Cyclacillin	1.0	–	23.7±3.4	–
	5.0	15.0±3.4	31.2±5.2	33.6±2.4
	10.0	11.3±2.1	28.0±2.9	30.5±4.6
Penicillin G	50 U	3.9±0.8	8.1±1.2	10.4±1.2
	200	21.2±1.1	9.8±0.9	12.3±1.8

[a] *Escherichia coli* (10^8) incubated with indicated concentration of antibiotics for 2 h before washing and incubation with 10^6 PE cells for indicated length of time before assay for phagocytosis.
[b] Average percentage of PE cells ± ASD with two or more *E. coli* after incubation in vitro.

Table 2. Effect of antibiotic pretreatment of *E. coli* on the immunogenicity of phagocytized *E. coli* in recipient mice injected with macrophage extracts

Antibiotic pretreatment[a]		Antibody response[b]		
		Agglutination titer	Anti E. coli PFCs/ 10^6 splenocytes	Percentage of control
None (control)		1:480	383±22	100
Ampicillin	1.0 µg	1:1250	495±32	130
	5.0	1:1280	450±48	170
Cyclacillin	1.0	1:960	542±30	142
	5.0	1:1280	586±42	153
Penicillin G	50 U	1:480	310±60	81

[a] *Escherichia coli* (10^8) pretreated for 2 h with indicated antibiotic before phagocytosis for 1 h by 10^6 normal mouse PE cells.
[b] Average antibody response for three to four normal recipient mice/group injected 7–10 days earlier with 1.0 ml cell-free homogenate of PE cells which phagocytized *E. coli*; control mice injected with homogenate from 10^6 normal PE cells which had not phagocytized *E. coli* had agglutination titer of 1:20 or less and fewer than 50 PFCs/10^6 spleen cells.

mal macrophages, as compared with phagocytosis of untreated *E. coli*. A greater percentage of macrophages phagocytized the antibiotic-pretreated bacteria and there were also more *E. coli* per positive macrophage (data not shown).

Extracts of the macrophages which had phagocytized the antibiotic-pretreated bacteria were also more immunogenic in terms of inducing specific antibody to *E. coli* in normal mice as compared with similar extracts of macrophages which had ingested the same number of nontreated *E. coli* or penicillin G-treated *E. coli* (Table 2). The increased numbers of specific PFCs to the *E. coli* in the spleen of indicator mice injected with lysates of macrophages incubated with the antibiotic-treated bacteria showed that there was a greater amount of immunogenic *E. coli* material in the macrophages exposed to the antibiotic-pretreated bacteria compared with those exposed to untreated bacteria.

Direct examination of the antibiotic-pretreated bacteria for immunogenic potential in normal mice injected with bacteria which were treated for 2 h in vitro with subinhibitory doses of either ampicillin or cyclacillin, as compared with untreated bacteria incubated for the same length of time in medium alone without antibiotic, revealed greater immunogenicity. As is evident in Table 3, 10 days after injection of the pretreated bacteria into normal mice there was a marked enhancement of the number of antibody PFCs to *E. coli* as compared with the number in the spleen of mice injected with untreated bacteria.

Since *E. coli* is a B-cell mitogen (3, 14, 17, 25, 27, 29], it is noted that this organism also induced potent stimulation of normal lymphocyte blastogenesis, as shown in Table 4. Ampicillin- or cyclacillin-pretreated *E. coli* were stronger stimulators of blastogenesis of normal spleen cells than were normal untreated *E. coli* or *E. coli* pretreated with penicillin G. Ampicillin- or cyclacillin-pretreated bacteria resulted in a greater SI as compared with that induced by untreated bacteria.

The antibiotic pretreatment also increased markedly the stimulatory activity of the bacteria in terms of soluble mediator production. These pharmacologically active effector molecules are immunoregulatory agents produced by antigen- or mitogen-stimulated lymphoid cells [25, 29, 31, 32]. Interleukin 1 was described over a decade ago as being produced when adherent spleen cell populations or

Table 3. Immunogenicity of antibiotic-pretreated *E. coli* injected into normal mice

Antibiotic pretreatment[a]		Anti *E. coli* PFCs on day[b]			
		+3	+6	+10	+15
None (control)		121±15	865± 32	652± 42	210±16
Ampicillin	1.0 μg	210±32	1750±138	1230±130	428±60
	5.0	265±40	1830±246	1445± 62	325±40
Cyclacillin	1.0	152±10	1410±193	1140± 16	570±48
	5.0	242±18	1563±120	1336±141	652±48

[a] *Escherichia coli* (10^8) treated with indicated antibiotic for 2 h before washing and injection into mice.
[b] Average number of anti-*E. coli* PFCs ± SD per spleen for three to four mice/group on indicated day after injection of bacteria.

Table 4. Effect of antibiotic treatment on blastogenic-stimulating activity of *E. coli*

Antibiotic pretreatment[a]	Dose of bacteria	Blastogenic response[b]	
		cpm ± SD	SI
None (control)	10^6	12345 ± 1940	7.9
	10^8	24658 ± 2870	15.9
Ampicillin (5.0 μg)	10^6	17340 ± 2456	11.1
	10^8	39760 ± 4866	25.5
Cyclacillin (5.0 μg)	10^6	22450 ± 3978	14.4
	10^8	37286 ± 4535	23.9
Penicillin G (50 U)	10^6	14310 ± 2390	9.2
	10^8	22768 ± 4310	14.6

[a] *Escherichia coli*, either 10^6 or 10^8, incubated with indicated antibiotic for 2 h before washing, heat killing, and stimulation of blastogenesis of 10^6 normal mouse spleen cells.
[b] Average blastogenic responses ± SD for three to four cultures/group after 72 h stimulation with antibiotic-pretreated *E. coli;* cpm for control cultures not stimulated with bacteria = 1560 ± 240.

Table 5. Effect of antibiotic pretreatment of *E. coli* on stimulation of IL-1 production by normal adherent murine spleen cells as assessed by the C_3H/HeJ thymocyte proliferation assay

Antibiotic pretreatment[a]		Thymocyte proliferation[b]	
		cpm ± SD	Percentage of control
None (control)		3978 ± 976	100
Ampicillin	1.0 μg	5230 ± 940	132
	5.0	9765 ± 1631	246
	10.0	8346 ± 1450	210
Cyclacillin	1.0	6300 ± 1200	159
	5.0	10741 ± 3316	270
	10.0	7398 ± 1186	186
Penicillin G	50 U	4136 ± 681	104

[a] Indicated antibiotic added in indicated concentration to 10^8 *E. coli* for 2 h at 37 °C before washing and use as stimulator of IL-1 production by cultures of 10^6 normal mouse spleen cells.
[b] Average stimulatory activity of three to four cell-free culture supernatants of normal mouse spleen cells incubated for 24 h with 10^8 antibiotic-treated *E. coli* as cpm ± SD for three to four cultures of indicator C_3H/HeJ thymocytes after 24 h incubation with [^{3}H] thymidine.

Table 6. Effect of pretreatment length of time of *E. coli* with antibiotics on stimulatory activity for IL-1 production by normal adherent mouse spleen cells

Antibiotic pretreatment[a]	Pretreatment length of time (h)	cpm ± SD[b]
None (control)	4	4736 ± 965
Ampicillin (5.0 μg)	1	5440 ± 1100
	2	11765 + 2316
	4	10326 ± 1970
Cyclacillin (5.0 μg)	1	5238 ± 736
	2	9836 ± 1210
	4	11720 ± 2160
Penicillin G (50 U)	2	4210 ± 732
	4	4896 ± 688

[a] Indicated antibiotic preincubated with 10^8 *E. coli* for indicated length of time before washing bacteria and stimulation of 10^6 normal mouse spleen cells for 24 h.
[b] Average cpm ± SD for three to four cultures/group after 24 h incubation with 1.0 ml cell-free culture supernatants from *E. coli*-stimulated mouse spleen cells.

Table 7. Stimulatory activity of antibiotic-pretreated *E. coli* for interferon and TNF production by adherent spleen cells

Antibiotic pretreatment[a]		Interferon[b]	TNF[c]
None (control)		100 (40)	24
Ampicillin	1.0 μg	200 (40)	48
	5.0	200 (40)	64
Cyclacillin	1.0	150 (20)	48
	5.0	200 (20)	48
Penicillin G	50 U	100 (20)	16

[a] Indicated concentration of indicated antibiotic used to pretreat 10^8 *E. coli* for 2 h at 37 °C before washing and stimulation of 10^6 normal mouse spleen cells.
[b] Average activity (U/ml) of IFN in 24-h culture supernatants from three to four adherent spleen cell cultures; ( ), activify after neutralization with anti-alpha/beta IFN.
[c] Average TNF activity (U/ml) in 24-h culture supernatant from three to four adherent spleen cell cultures stimulated for 24 h with antibiotic-pretreated *E. coli.*

peritoneal cells rich in macrophages are activated by endotoxin [27], resulting in a soluble lymphocyte-activating factor which enhanced T-cell immune function [31]. As is evident in Table 5, antibiotic pretreatment of *E. coli* increased their ability to stimulate mouse-adherent spleen cell populations to produce IL-1 in comparison to untreated *E. coli* or *E. coli* previously treated with penicillin G.

Table 8. Effect of injection of antibiotic-pretreated *E. coli* on production of cytokines by normal mouse spleen cells in culture

Escherichia coli injection[a]	Spleen cell supernatant acticity[b]		
	IL-1	IFN	TNF
Untreated (control)	100	100	100
Antibiotic pretreated			
Ampicillin (5.0 μg)	210	150	100
Cyclacillin (5.0 μg)	170	150	120
Penicillin G (50 U)	100	100	100

[a] *Escherichia coli* (10^8) pretreated with indicated antibiotic for 2 h, washed, heat killed, and then injected i.v. into groups of mice.
[b] Response as average percentage of indicated cytokine activity as compared with control cell-free supernatants of 10^6 adherent spleen cells from three to four untreated or treated mice. 3–6 h after injection, and 24 h after culture.

Treatment of the *E. coli* with ampicillin or cyclacillin for as little as 2 h was sufficient to increase their stimulatory activity in terms of IL-1 production by adherent spleen cell cultures in comparison to stimulation by the same numer of bacteria incubated for 4 h in medium alone or after treatment with penicillin G for 2–4 h (Table 6).

Pretreatment of *E. coli* with subinhibitory doses of ampicillin or cyclacillin but not penicillin G increased the ability of the bacteria to stimulate normal mouse spleen cells to produce interferon or TNF (Table 7). The resulting interferon was neutralized by monoclonal anti-alpha/beta-interferon, indicating that, except for about 20%–40% of the interferon activity, mostly alpha/beta-interferon was produced. More TNF activity was also stimulated by antibiotic-pretreated bacteria as compared with control nontreated bacteria. Similar results were obtained when pretreated bacteria were injected directly into intact mice as seen in Table 8. Antibiotic-pretreated bacteria injected into normal mice enhanced the subsequent formation of IL-1, IFN, and TNF by murine splenocytes.

Discussion

Much evidence exists that antibiotic-pretreated bacteria become more susceptible to host defense mechanisms, either cellular or humoral, as compared with untreated organisms [11, 13, 15, 18, 20, 21]. Thus, a number of studies from various laboratories, including this one, have shown that antibiotic treatment of susceptible bacteria with subinhibitory doses of certain antibiotics results in increased susceptibility to phagocytosis by macrophages both in vivo and in vitro. For example, our laboratory has shown that adherent peritoneal cells derived from either normal or adjuvant-stimulated mice show a strong ability to phagocytize and kill bacteria such as *E. coli* after pretreatment of the microbe with subinhibitory doses of an effective semisynthetic antibiotic such as ampicillin or cyclacillin [7,

10, 11]. In addition, the studies described herein showed that susceptibility to phagocytosis correlates with increased susceptibility of the bacteria to antibody-mediated, complement-dependent bacteriolysis. The greater enhancement of phagocytosis by macrophages from adjuvant-stimulated donor mice appears to be due to a synergism between the effects of the antibiotic on the bacteria and increased activation of macrophages after adjuvant stimulation. No increased phagocytosis occurred when bacteria were first killed by heating before treatment with the antibiotic. In this regard, it is noted that previous studies showed that soluble mediators derived from adjuvant-activated macrophages had the ability to enhance phagocytic activity by normal macrophages exposed to antibiotic-pretreated bacteria [12].

In harmony with these considerations are the findings of our present study indicating that culture supernatants from adherent spleen cells as well as peritoneal exudate cells stimulated with antibiotic-pretreated bacteria also released increased amounts of soluble mediators of immunity. The latter include interleukin-1, tumor necrosis factor, and interferons. Of these, the alpha/beta interferons, among others, are considered a product of antigen- or mitogen-stimulated T-lymphocytes, and the tumor necrosis factor has been recently recognized as an important immunoregulator involved not only in antitumor reactivities but also in responses to microorganisms such as bacteria, viruses, and fungi [31, 32].

Pretreatment of the bacteria with the antibiotics followed directly by injection into indicator mice also resulted in increased antibody formation. In accord with this was also the finding that pretreatment of these bacteria enhanced their ability to stimulate lymphocyte blastogenic responsiveness of normal murine spleen cells together with the already-mentioned enhanced production of immunoregulatory molecules. Similar observations were made on the enhanced production of tumor necrosis factor in normal spleen cell cultures by antibiotic-pretreated bacteria. The latter, furthermore, when injected into normal mice, also increased the production of immunoregulatory soluble effectors. It is apparent, therefore, that pretreatment of *E. coli* even with subinhibitory concentrations of the appropriate antibiotics not only alters their immunogenicity but also their ability to stimulate proliferation of normal spleen cells and production of cytokines considered important in immunoregulation [26, 28, 30–32].

Of course, the ultimate question raised by these pretreated bacterial effects is the nature of the mechanisms responsible for their development. At the time of this writing, we know very little about the developmental mechanisms possibly involved in these effects but it is felt by many investigators that they may be due to altered cell surface components of the bacteria following exposure to an antibiotic even in subinhibitory concentrations [26, 28, 35]. For example, filamentous forms of gram-negative bacteria often develop after exposure of the organism to subinhibitory concentrations of antibiotics to which they are susceptible. Such doses of antibiotics do not appear to interfere with the viability of the bacteria in vitro and similar numbers of colony-forming units are generally observed with such pretreated bacteria as compared with untreated ones [28]. It is possible that viable bacteria become more susceptible to increased phagocytosis because of altered surface components which become more readily available to opsonizing serum proteins. Macrophages may be able to degrade more effectively bacterial antigens and the potent immunogens when these organisms are first pretreated with an appropriate antibiotic [26, 28]. This may be reflected by the finding that incubating macrophages with ampicillin- or cyclacillin-pretreated *E. coli* resulted in increased numbers of specific anti-*E. coli* antibody when lysates of the macrophages were injected into test mice [5]. In any case it would certainly appear warranted to investigate in more depth the interaction of antibiotics with microbes which become more potent stimulators of immune responses in vitro as well as in vivo.

Summary

The influence of subinhibitory concentrations of antibiotics on *E. coli* was examined with regard to a modulation of immunogenicity and the ability to stimulate spleen cell proliferation and cytokine production. The experiments showed that both ampicillin – and cyclacyllin – but not penicillin-pretreated bacteria were more easily phagocytosed by peritoneal exudate cells than non-pretreated ones. They caused increased immunogenicity, as demonstrated by the induction of increased numbers of antibody-forming spleen cells. Lysates of macrophages which had ingested pretreated bacteria were also more immunogenic in terms of agglutination titer and *E. coli*-specific plaque-forming cell response than those which had phagocytosed equal numbers of normal or penicillin-pretreated bacteria. Ampicillin- and cyclacillin-pretreated *E. coli* revealed increased stimulation activity on normal lymphocyte blastogenesis compared with untreated or penicillin-pretreated bacteria. Similarly, pretreated bacteria increased interleukin-1 (Il-1) production by normal adherent spleen cells as well as the production of interferon (IFN), mostly alpha/beta IFN, and tumor necrosis factor (TNF). Pretreatment of bacteria with subinhibitory concentrations of antibiotics may, therefore, not only alter their immunogenicity but also their capacity to stimulate blastogenesis and the production of cytokines.

Acknowledgment. We thank Ms. Catherine Newton and Dr. Kay Blanchard as well as Mrs. Christine Abarca, for their excellent assistance in the cytokine assays, and the editorial development of the manuscript, respectively.

References

1. Blanchard DK, Djeu JY, Klein TW, Friedman H, Stewart II WE (1986) Dependence of interferon gamma induction by lipopolysaccharide. Involvement of interleukin 2 and macrophages. J Immunol 136:963
2. Blanchard DK, Djeu JY, Klein TW, Friedman H, Stewart II WE (1987) Induction of tumor necrosis factor by *Legionella pneumophila*. Infect Immun 55:433
3. Friedman H, Klein TW, Szentivanyi A (eds) (1981) Immunomodulation by bacteria and their products. Plenum, New York
4. Friedman H, Warren GH (1976) Antibody-mediated bacteriolysis: enhanced killing of cyclacillin-treated bacteria. Proc Soc Exp Biol Med 153:301
5. Friedman H, Warren GH (1977) Cyclacillin-induced potentiation of *Escherichia coli* immunogenicity in vivo and in vitro. Chemotherapy 23:324

6. Friedman H, Warren GH (1974) Enhanced susceptibility of penicillin-resistant staphylococci to phagocytosis after in vitro incubation with low doses of nafcillin. Proc Soc Exp Biol Med 146:207
7. Friedman H, Warren GH (1982) Increased phagocytosis of *Escherichia coli* pretreated with subinhibitory concentrations of cyclacillin or ampicillin. Proc Soc Exp Biol Med 169:301
8. Friedman H, Warren GH (1983) Increased susceptiblity of bacteria treated with subinhibitory concentrations of antibiotics to phagocytosis and killing. ICAAC 23:178
9. Friedman H, Warren GH (1984) Antibacterial activity of cyclacillin in vivo and in vitro: effects on gram negative organisms. Prog Chemother 2:119
10. Friedman H (1985) Synergism between the host defense mechanism and antibiotic treatment of bacteria. In: Pulverer G, Jeljaszewicz J (eds) Chemotherapy and immunity [Suppl 13] Gustav Fischer, Stuttgart, pp 105–113
11. Friedman H (1985) Synergism between the host defense mechanism and antibiotic treatment of bacteria. Zbl Bakt Hyg [A] Suppl 13:104
12. Friedman H, Warren GH (1984) Muramyl dipeptida-induced enhancement of phagocytosis of antibiotic pretreated *Escherichia coli* by macrophages. Proc Soc Exp Biol Med 176:765
13. Gillissen G (1980) Antibiotics and immune response, concomitant effect of chemotherapy, Immun 8:79
14. Hadden JW, Szentivanyi A (eds) [1985) The pharmacology of the reticuloendothelial system. Plenum, New York
15. Hahn H, Mielke M (1985) Influence of antibiotics on interactions between *Listeria*-specific T cells and antigen in vitro. In: Pulverer G, Jeljaszewicz J (eds) Chemotherapy and immunity. [Suppl 13] Gustav Fischer, Stuttgart, pp 143–154
16. Kaido TJ, Stewart II WE (1987) A plaque assay for detection and quantitation of TNF. International Conf on TNF, Heidelberg, pp 14–18
17. Klein TW, Specter S, Friedman H, Szentivanyi A (eds) (1983) Biological response modifiers in human oncology and immunology. Plenum, New York
18. McDonald PJ, Wetherall BL, Druel H (1981) Post-antibiotic leukocyte enhancement. Increased susceptibility of bacteria pretreated with antibiotics to activity of leukocytes. Rev Infect Dis 3:38
19. Munster AM, Loodholdt CB, Leary AG, Barnes MA (1977) Effect of antibiotics on cell-mediated immunity. Surgery 81:692
20. Opferkuch W, Buscher K-H, Karch H, Leying H, Pawelzik M, Schuman U, Wiemer C (1985) The effect of sublethal concentrations of antibiotics on the host-parasite relationship. In: Pulverer G, Jeljaszewicz J (eds) Chemotherapy and immunity. [Suppl 13] Gustav Fischer, Stuttgart, pp 165–177
21. Root RK, Istunz R, Molavi A, Metcalf JA, Malech HL (1981) Interaction between antibiotics and human neutrophils in the killing of staphylococci. Studies with normal and cytochalasin B treated cells. J Clin Invest 67:247
22. Roszkowski W, Ko HL, Roszkowski K, Jeljaszewicz J, Pulverer G (1985) Effect of selected antibiotics on the cellular and humoral immune response in mice. In: Pulverer G, Jeljaszewicz J (eds) Chemotherapy and immunity. [Suppl 13] Gustav Fischer, Stuttgart, pp 59–72
23. Scala G, Djeu JY, Allaveva P, Kasahara T, Ortaldo JR, Herberman RB, Oppenheim JJ (1984) Human natural killer (NK) cells are high producers of interleukin-1. Nature 309:56
24. Stewart II WE (1981) Interferon assays: CFE-reading methods. In: Stewart WM (ed) The interferon system, Springer, Vienna, pp 15–21
25. Szentivanyi A (1971) Effect of bacterial products and adrenergic blocking agents on allergic reactions. In: Samter M et al. (eds) Textbook of immunological diseases. Little, Brown, Boston, pp 356–374
26. Szentivanyi A, Friedman H, Gillissen G, Szentivanyi J (1987) Immunomodulatory effects of some antibiotic-induced changes in bacterial and host determinants. In: Szentivanyi A, Gillissen G, Friedman H (eds) Antibiosis and host immunity. Plenum, New York, pp 3–11
27. Szentivanyi A, Friedman H, Nowotny A (eds) (1986) The immunobiology and immunopharmacology of bacterial endotoxins. Basic and clinical aspects. Plenum, New York
28. Szentivanyi A, Gillissen G, Friedman H (eds) (1987) Antibiosis and host immunity. Plenum, New York

29. Szentivanyi A, Middleton E, Williams JF, Friedman H (1983) Effect of microbial agents on the immune network and associated pharmacologic reactivities. In: Middleton E, Reed CE, Ellis EF (eds) Allergy: principles and practice, 2nd edn. CV Mosby, St Louis, MO, pp 211–236
30. Szentivanyi A, Szentivanyi J (1985) Cellular and molecular foundations of immunity, immunologic inflammation and hypersensitivity. Component parts and their relation to neurohumoral control mechanisms. In. Sodeman WA, Sodeman TM (eds) Sodeman's pathologic physiology – mechanisms of disease, 7th edn. WB Saunders, Philadelphia, pp 113–150
31. Szentivanyi A, Szentivanyi J, Williams JF, Middleton E Jr, Friedman H (1988) The pharmacology of microbial modulation in the induction and expression of immune reactivities. I. The pharmacologically active effector molecules of immunologic inflammation, immunity, and hypersensitivity. Immunopharmacol Ref (in press)
32. Szentivanyi J, Szentivanyi A, Krzanowski JJ, Polson JB, Friedman H (1988 b) The pharmacology of microbial modulation in the induction and expression of immune reactivities. II. Effector mechanisms in the afferent and efferent limbs of the immune response. Immunopharmacol Rev (in press)
33. Taylor PW, Gaunt H, Unger FM (1981) Effect of subinhibitory concentrations of mecillinam on the serum susceptibility of *E. coli* strains. Antimicrob Agents Chemother 19:786
34. Verhoef J, Milatovic D (1985) Influence of antibiotics on opsonization of staphylocci. In: Pulverer G, Jeljaszewicz J (eds) Chemotherapy and immunity. [Suppl 13] Gustav Fischer, Stuttgart, pp 115–122
35. Vosbeck H, Handschin A, Menge B, Zak G [1979) Effects of subinhibitory concentrations of antibiotics on adhesiveness of *Escherichia coli* in vitro. Rev Infect Dis 1:845

Effect of Beta-Lactam Antibiotics on Eukaryotic DNA Replication: Possible Impact on the Host-Parasite Relationship

K. A. Neftel [1], U. D. Huynh [2], and U. Hübscher [2]

Introduction

According to Waksman, antibiotics are substances produced by microorganisms which exhibit either an inhibitory or destructive effect on other microorganisms. That therapeutically effective concentrations of such products can be tolerated by humans and animals relates primarily to their highly specific interaction with well-defined target structures or functions of the microorganisms attacked which the human or animal cell lack. A prominent example of this is the functioning of the β-lactam antibiotics (BLAs). They specifically bind to and inhibit a number of enzymes involved in bacterial cell wall synthesis, the penicillin-binding proteins, thereby initiating the deleterious effects on growing bacteria [29].

In eukaryotes analogous target structures for BLAs are unknown. Some years ago, however, we began to observe the effects of BLAs and, in particular, of some of their degradation products on proliferating eukaryotic cells from various sources [9, 16, 18, 20, 21]. BLAs and even more so some of their degradation products dose dependently inhibited cell growth and modified various biosynthetic activities relating to proliferation. Analogies in the structure-effect relationship for inhibition of different cell typus suggested a common mechanism underlying the antiproliferative effects. Eukaryotic DNA replication was then identified as one, if not the only, primary target function mediating these unexpected BLA effects [3, 8] and DNA polymerase α was found to be a specific target structure for BLAs and especially some degradation products thereof [8, 10].

These BLA effects are likely to explain some adverse reactions to prolonged high-dose BLA treatment [20, 22]. In addition, there are reasons to believe that they have clinical impact in other, distinct fields [22]. Here, we summarize some results from in vitro and animal studies indicating that high-dose BLA treatment might influence the host-parasite relationship by affecting proliferating cell populations at different levels.

Effects of BLAs on Proliferating Eukaryotic Cells

A broad array of effects on cells involved in host defense mechanisms has been ascribed to antibiotics of all classes [4, 7, 15, 23, 25]. Since 1973 selected BLAs,

[1] Medical Clinic, University Hospital, Rämistr. 100, 8091 Zürich, Switzerland
[2] Institute of Pharmacology and Biochemistry University Zürich-Irchel, Winterthurer Str. 190, 8057 Zürich, Switzerland

The Influence of Antibiotics on the Host-Parasite Relationship III
Edited by G. Gillissen, W. Opferkuch, G. Peters, and G. Pulverer

particularly cephalosporins, have repeatedly been found to inhibit growth of cultured lymphocytes in a concentration-dependent fashion [1, 2, 11, 12, 26]. Although the underlying mechanism remained unknown, such findings were thought possibly to reflect immunosuppressive potencies of BLAs in vivo. Comparable antiproliferative effects of high penicillin-G concentrations have been found further in cells not belonging to the immune system, namely in culture of rat liver cells [27, 30] and of human fibroblasts [5].

Some years ago we analyzed 50 cases of BLA-induced neutropenia from various hospitals and 140 well-documented literature cases [20]. The data suggested a direct toxic effect of BLAs on granulopoietic precursor cells rather than an immune mechanism underlying this side effect of BLAs. The strongest argument was the clear dependence of neutropenia upon duration and total dose of BLA treatment even in cases that have been reexposed to BLAs after an initial episode of neutropenia.

Later, we indeed found that more than 50 BLAs and related compounds dose dependently inhibit human in vitro granulopoiesis in a semisolid agar system [18, 20]. Others have confirmed the toxicity of BLAs for human in vitro granulopoiesis [13, 14] and have found an analogous suppression of megakaryocyte-colony formation [14]. Altogether, BLA effects can explain the clinical findings in BLA-induced neutropenia without contradiction although not being a formal proof for a toxic pathogenesis.

Subsequently a variety of cells from other sources – malignant and nonmalignant – were found to be susceptible to BLAs when brought to proliferate under appropriate conditions in vitro (see Table 1). Resting cells, on the other hand, were unsusceptible even to very high BLA concentrations. As an example, viability and proliferative capacity of human bone marrow cells is maintained during preincubation periods of up to 24 h, provided cells are carefully washed before being cultured [18].

Table 1. Cells found to be susceptible to the antiproliferative effect of BLAs in vitro

Cell Type	References
Nonmalignant	
Human granulocyte-macrophage progenitors	[13, 14, 16, 18, 20]
Human megakaryocyte progenitors	[14]
Human and animal lymphoid cells	[1, 2, 9, 11, 12, 26]
Human fibroblasts	[5]
Rat liver cells	[27, 30]
Chick embryo liver cells	[21]
Malignant	
HL-60 (human promyelocytic leukemia)	[31]
K-562 (human erythroleukemia)	[3]
EL-4 (murine T-cell lymphoma)	[9]
YAC-1 (murine T-cell lymphoma)	[9]
BCL-1 (murine B-cell lymphoma)	(Unpublished data)
NS-1 (murine myeloma)	[6]

The main argument for believing that there is a common mechanism underlying the antiproliferative effects of BLAs came from attempts to elucidate the structure-activity relationship for inhibition of cells from very different sources [9, 17, 21]. In all cell culture systems used a similar hierarchy of activity was reproduced. Considering BLA concentrations in culture media, cephalosporins as a group were 3 to over 25 times more active than penicillins, while monobactams were practically inactive. The activity of compounds that were active at all was invariably and strongly enhanced if they were allowed spontaneously to degrade for up to 96 h in aqueous solution under cell culture conditions. A similar increase of activity was seen immediately after pretreatment with β-lactamase. On the other hand, further spontaneous degradation of β-lactamase-treated BLAs in some instances finally led only to very weak products. Hence, unidentified intermediates of BLA degradation – probably having an opened β-lactam ring still fused to a second six-membered ring structure – might be the most active compounds.

Effects of BLAs on Eukaryotic DNA Replication

Data from flow cytometrically monitored liquid cultures of K-562 cells indicated that (1) BLAs might act primarily on DNA synthesis and (2) their effects are cell cycle dependent [4]. Accordingly, K-562 cells that were arrested at the Gl-S boundary were almost completely protected from BLA effects, whereas cells in the S-phase were much more susceptible than unsynchronized cell populations. These findings suggested that DNA replication might be the biological function primarily affected by BLAs.

Indeed, recent experiments using an in vitro DNA replication system have suggested that one intracellular target of BLAs and in particular of some of their degradation products is the DNA-polymerase α [8, 10]. BLAs dose dependently inhibited crude and highly purified DNA-polymerase α from various eukaryotic sources including human, while DNA-polymerases β and γ involved in DNA repair and mitochondrial DNA replication, respectively, were insensitive. Not unexpectedly, BLA degradation products were again more active. The difference in inhibitory activity between fresh and aged compounds was even more pronounced and in some instances increased more than 200-fold following degradation [10].

Although these data seem to reflect BLA toxicity in living cells, the link between BLA effects on cultured cells and on cell-free DNA replication has not yet been formally established. One major obstacle is the lack of information about cellular uptake of BLAs and their degradation products.

Can BLAs Affect the Host-Parasite Relationship Through Their Influence on Proliferating Cells?

Beta-lactam antibiotic effects on eukaryotic cells, possibly being correlates of an in vivo influence on host defense mechanisms, have been studied in many respects. In most studies nondividing cells were used. Based on the above results, it is easily conceivable that BLAs might also influence the functioning of cells involved in host defense mechanisms by means of their antiproliferative effects. In the following, we summarize some results suggesting that this might happen at different levels.

Lymphoid Cells

According to the studies mentioned above, we first found that BLAs inhibit growth of normal lymphocytes and continuously growing T-cell lymphomas (EL-4 and YAC-1) from animal sources [9].

Later, we looked at possible effects of BLAs on the generation of immunological effector T-cells. Generation of virus-specific cytotoxic T-cells and proliferation of lymphocytes were studied in a secondary in vitro antiviral immune response (for methods see [9]). Spleen lymphocytes of vaccinia virus-primed mice were restimulated in a secondary culture in vitro. Syngeneic peritoneal macrophages that had been infected with UV-inactivated vaccinia viruses were used as stimulator cells. BLAs at various concentrations were added to the cultures at the outset. The cytotoxic activity of the cultures as assessed on day 5 was dose dependently suppressed by BLAs of different classes. The reduction of cytotoxic activity by five selected β-lactam compounds at 1 mM concentration is exemplified in Fig. 1.

Regarding the structure-activity relationship, BLAs tested in this system behaved exactly as previously found in various other cell culture systems. In addition, an identical rank of toxicity was found when measuring [^{3}H]thymidine incorporation on day 3 of an alloreactive mixed lymphocyte culture in the presence of BLAs.

We have, so far, no data documenting a similar effect of BLAs on generation of cytotoxic T-cells in vivo. In another type of experiment, however, BLAs were likely directly to affect growth of a distinct population of lymphoid cells in vivo, which, however, do not directly take part in host-defense functioning. Using a B-

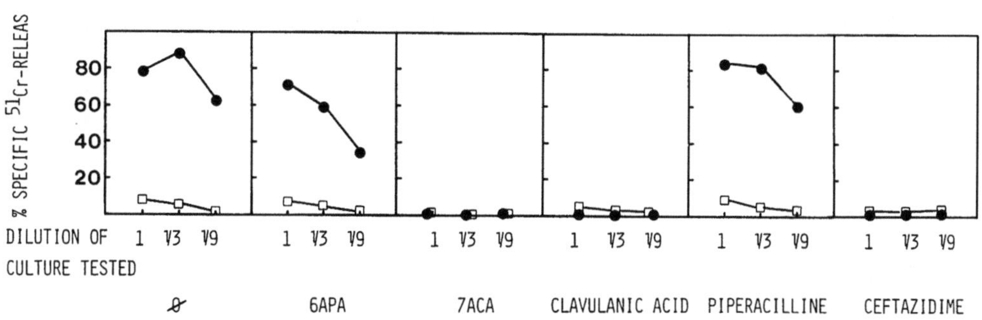

Fig. 1. Effects of various beta-lactams (1 m*M*) on in vitro generation of cytotoxic T-cells (see text). ——□——, uninfected target cells; ——●——, vaccinia-infected target cells; *6APA*, 6-aminopenicillianic acid; *7ACA*, 7-amino-cephalosporanic acid (from [9] with permission)

cell-lymphoma model in the mouse, namely BCL-1 [28], we have seen that subcutaneous adminstration of high-dose cephalosporins but not penicillins and monobactams significantly prolonged duration of cytosinearabinoside-induced remission and survival (Guldenschuh et al., unpublished). Cultured in vitro, this particular cell type proved to be similarly sensitive to BLAs as the various lymphoid cells with T-cell characteristics studied previously.

Granulopoiesis

Clinical data of cases with BLA-induced neutropenia and the well-documented toxicity of BLAs for in vitro granulopoiesis raise the possibility that high-dose BLA treatment could prolong duration of granulocytopenia after cytostatic treatment. Analysis of historical cases with acute myelogenous leukemia gave first support to this hypothesis, in that the early beginning of BLA therapy, independently from other factors, predicted a longer duration of granulocytopenia [19]. Accordingly, total doses of BLAs given were disproportionally higher with a longer duration of granulocytopenia. Later, Osterwalder et al. found similar results in 115 patients after bone marrow transplantation [24], while Kibbler et al., comparing a single BLA/aminoglycoside regimen with a double BLA regimen (also in 115 patients but with various diseases), detected no significant differences between the two groups (personal communication). On the other hand, in another study a double BLA combination was associated with more patients having persistent granulocytopenia ($\leqq 100$ granulocytes/mm^3) than a BLA/aminoglycoside combination [32]. In mice no evidence was found that BLA delayed recovery from cytosine arabinoside-induced bone marrow damage, one problem in this species being the very short serum half-life of BLA as compared with humans [31]. In sum, a definite answer to the question awaits further data.

Effect of Beta-Lactam Antibiotics on Polymerases from Microorganisms

In addition to DNA-polymerase α from various eukaryotic sources, BLAs inhibited the two DNA-polymerases from herpes simplex and vaccinia viruses [10]. Furthermore, from experiments comparing BLA effects in mycoplasma-contaminated versus mycoplasma-free cultures of K-562 cells, we have indirect evidence that BLAs also affect mycoplasmal DNA-polymerase even at concentrations lower than those leading to visible growth inhibition of K-562 cells [6]. It is unclear, however, whether this can also happen in a biologically relevant fashion in the infected host.

Concluding Remarks

Besides specifically interacting with bacterial targets, BLAs can apparently affect proliferating eukaryotes. Data suggest that interaction of some as yet undefined BLA-degradation products with DNA-polymerase α is a key event. Furthermore,

DNA polymerases from some viruses and from mycoplasmas also appear to be sensitive to BLAs.

Whether BLAs can thereby really influence the host-parasite relationship remains speculative. The preliminary studies summarized here lead us to believe that the question must be further clarified. The main prerequisite for this will consist in the identification of the relevant BLA-derived compounds and the capability of detecting them in biological fluids.

Summary

Beta-lactam antibiotics (BLAs) and in particular some of their degradation products have been found dose dependently to inhibit growth of various eukaryotic cells in vitro. According to experiments using in vitro DNA-replication systems, this proliferation inhibition appears to be mediated by interaction of BLA derivatives with the key enzyme of DNA replication, namely DNA-polymerase α. In addition, DNA polymerases from other than eukaryotic sources have been found also to be susceptible to BLAs.

Based on preliminary experiments, it is speculated here that high-dose BLA treatment could influence the host-parasite relationship by affecting (1) generation of cytotoxic T-cells, (2) proliferative activity of granulopoietic precursor cells, or (3) directly acting on DNA polymerases from various microorganisms.

References

1. Banck G, Forsgren A (1979) Antibiotics and suppression of lymphocyte function in vitro. Antimicrob Agents Chemother 16:554–560
2. Chaperon EA, Sanders WE (1978) Suppression of lymphocyte responses by cephalosporins. Infekt Immun 19:378–384
3. Cottagnoud P, Neftel KA (1986) Beta-lactams act on DNA-synthesis in K-562 cells. Cell Biol Toxicol 2:523–529
4. Daschner FD (1985) Antibiotics and host defence with special reference to phagocytosis by human polymorphonuclear leukocytes. J Antimicrob Chemother 16:135–141
5. Götz IE, Moklebust R, Warren CJ (1979) Effects of some antibiotics on the growth of human diploid skin fibroblasts in cell culture. In Vitro (Rockville) 15:114–119
6. Guldenschuh I, Cottagnoud P, Neftel KA (1987) Betalactam antibiotics affect mycoplasmal DNA-synthesis in vitro. Annu Meet Swiss Soc Microbiol Berne (abstr)
7. Hauser WE, Remington JS (1982) Effect of antibiotics on the immune response. Am J Med 72:711–716
8. Hübscher U, Huynh UD, Hässig M, Neftel KA (1986) Effects of beta-lactams on DNA replication. Cell Biol Toxicol 2:541–548
9. Hügin AW, Cerny A, Zinkernagel RM, Neftel KA (1986) Suppressive effects of beta-lactam-antibiotics on in vitro generation of cytotoxic T-cells. Int J Immunopharmacol 8:723–729
10. Huynh UD, Neftel KA, Spadari S, Hübscher U (1987) Betalactam-antibiotics interfere with eukaryotic DNA-replication by inhibiting DNA polymerase α. Res 15:10495–10506
11. Larson ST, DaMert GJ, Collins-Lech C, Sohnle PG (1980) Direct stimulation of lymphokine production by cephalotin. J Infect Dis 142:265–272
12. Manzella JP, Clark JK (1973) Effects of moxalactam and cefuroxime on mitogen-stimulated human mononuclear leukocytes. Antimicrob Agents Chemother 23:360–363

13. Marie JP, Thevenin D, Zittoun R (1986) Inhibition de la granulopoièse in vitro par les betalactamines (comparaison entre piperacilline, mezlocilline, cefriaxond et ceftazidime). Presse Mèd 15:2358–2361
14. Maruyama T, Uchida K, Hara H (1987) Suppressive effect of antibiotics on colony formation from human megakaroycyte progenitors (CFU-M) and granulocyte-macrophage progenitors (CFU-GM) Jpn J Pharmacol 43:423–428
15. Milatovic D (1983) Antibiotics and phagocytosis. Eur J Clin Microbiol 2:414–425
16. Müller MR, Neftel KA, Wälti M, Hauser SP, Erni J (1983) Inhibition of in vitro granulopoiesis by betalactam antibiotics. Exp Hematol 11 [Suppl 14]:181
17. Müller M, Erni J, Neftel KA (1985) The myelotoxicity of betalactam-antibiotics: is there a structure-effect relationship? Exp Hematol 13:359
18. Neftel KA, Müller MR, Wälti M, Erni J, Gugler M, Arrenbrecht S (1983) Penicillin-G degradation products inhibit in vitro granulopoiesis. Br J Haematol 54:255–260
19. Neftel KA, Spirig M, Berchtold W, Notter H, Grob P, Calandra T, Hauser S, Glauser M (1984) Is the myelotoxic effect of betalactam antibiotics (BLA) relevant for the treatment of the granulocytopenic patient 24th Interscience Conference on Antimicrob Agents Chemother (abstr 388)
20. Neftel KA, Hauser SP, Müller MR (1985) Inhibition of granulopoiesis in vivo and in vitro by betalactam antibiotics. J Infect Dis 52 1:90–98
21. Neftel KA, Müller MR, Widmer U, Hügin AW (1986) Beta-lactam antibiotics inhibit human in vitro granulopoiesis and proliferation of some other cell types. Cell Biol Toxicol 2:513–521
22. Neftel KA, Hübscher U (1987) Effects of betalactam-antibiotics on proliferating eukaryotic cells. Antimicrob Agents Chemother 31:1657–1661
23. Oleske JM (1984) Effects of antimicrobials on host defence mechanism. J Antimicrob Chemother 13:413–415
24. Osterwalder B, Haberthuer C, Gratwohl A, Speck B (1986) Können Betalactam-Antibiotika die Myelopoiese in vivo hemmen? Eine Studie bei 115 Patienten mit allogener Knochenmarkstransplantation. Schweiz Med Wochenschr 116 [Suppl 20]:26
25. Peterson PK (1982) How antibiotics augment host defence. Eur J Clin Microbiol 1:335–337
26. Schneider CH, de Weck AL (1981) Allergy towards beta-lactam antibiotics. In: Mitsuhashi CS (ed) Beta-lactam antibiotics. ISSP Springer, Tokyo, pp 299–316
27. Schwarze PE, Seglen PO (1981) Effects of antibiotics on protein synthesis and degradation in primary cultures of rat hepatocytes. In Vitro (Rockville) 17:71–76
28. Slavin S, Strober S (1978) Spontaneous murine B-cell leukemia. Nature 272:624–626
29. Spratt BG (1983) Penicillin-binding protein and the future of beta-lactam antibiotics. J Gen Microbiol 129:1247–1260
30. Vonen B, Morland J (1982) Penicillin toxicity in isolated rat hepatocytes revealed by decreased incorporation of valine into proteins. Acta Pharmacol Toxicol 51:81–86
31. Weston BJ, Spackmann VM, Dewdney JM (1986) Effects of beta-lactam antibiotics on a human myeloid cell line: investigation of potential in vivo correlates in the mouse. Cell Biol Toxicol 2:549–557
32. Winston DJ, Barnes RC, Ho WG, Young LS, Champlin RE, Gall RP (1984) Moxalactam plus piperacillin versus moxalactam plus aminkacin in febrile granulocytopenic patients. Am J Med 77:442–450

Interaction Between the DNA-Gyrase Inhibitor Coumermycin and the Membrane of Human Neutrophils

P. Van der Auwera [1], M. Husson [1], J. M. Ruysschaert [2], and R. Brasseur [2]

Introduction

We have previously shown that coumermycin, a DNA-gyrase inhibitor, was a potent inhibitor of superoxide generation stimulated by PMA (PMA = phorbol-12-myristate-13-acetate), chemotaxis induced by fMLP (FMLP = n-formyl-methionyl-leucyl-phenylalanine), or opsonized zymosan, phagocytosis, and other membrane-related functions of human polymorphonuclear leukocytes (PMNs) [1–4]. In order better to characterize the interaction between coumermycin and the membrane of PMNs, we studied the inhibition of adenyl cyclase activity. In addition, the conformational analysis of the interaction was studied by computer model.

Materials and Methods

Neutrophils

Neutrophils were obtained from the peripheral blood of healthy volunteers. Blood was collected on ACD (Acetate, Citric acid, Dextrose; Gibco, Ghent, Belgium). Sedimentation in dextran for 1 h was allowed, followed by separation of the leukocyte-rich supernatant on Ficoll-Hypaque (Pharmacia). After lysis of the residual erythrocytes by hypotonic shock, the cells were resuspended in Hank's balanced salt solution (HBSS) (Gibco) and stored on ice until used. Counting and viability tests were done before each experiment. Viability was >97% by the trypan blue exclusion method. Purity of the preparation was >97% as assessed by May-Grünwald-Giemsa stain or by flow cytometry. PMNs were preincubated with variable concentrations of coumermycin for 30 min at 37 °C.

Adenyl Cyclase Activity

A quantity of 10 PMNs/ml was centrifuged at 800 g for 10 min then resuspended in cold distilled water, homogenized (Potter), frozen in liquid nitrogen, then tha-

[1] Service de Médecine Interne et Laboratoire d'Investigation, Clinique H. J. Tagnon, Institut Jules Bordet, Centre des Tumeurs de l'Université Libre de Bruxelles, rue Héger-Bordet 1, 1000 Brussels, Belgium

[2] Laboratoire des Macromolécules aux Interfaces, CP 206-2, Université Libre de Bruxelles, Campus de la Plaine, 1050 Brussels, Belgium

The Influence of Antibiotics on the Host-Parasite Relationship III
Edited by G. Gillissen, W. Opferkuch, G. Peters, and G. Pulverer

wed, rehomogenized, and adjusted to 15–30 μg protein for the test. Adenyl cyclase activity was measured according to the method of Salomon et al. [5], modified by Waelbroek et al. [6] using alpha[^{32}P]ATP. The following agonists were used: GppNHp (10^{-4} *M*), NaF (10^{-2} *M*), and forskolin (10^{-5} *M*).

Conformational Analysis

The theoretical conformational analysis (molecular structure) analysis of coumermycin is based on a semiempirical procedure [7–9]. In this approach the total conformational energy was calculated as the sum of all the contributions due to Van der Waal's interactions, torsional potentials, and the electrostatic interactions [10]. The conformational energy was calculated for a large number of conformations in a systematic analysis structure tree [11–13]. The conformers which yield the highest probability were then submitted to the energy function minimization procedure [14] with a precision of 10 ° on each torsional angle. The values used for the valence angles, boundary lengths, atomic charges, torsional potentials, and energy values for Van der Waal's interactions were those currently used in conformation analysis [9, 15–17]. The systematic and minimization procedures were carried out in a medium of intermediate dielectric constant representative of the membrane-water interface [18, 19].

The interaction energies between coumermycin and DL-alpha-dipalmitoyl-phosphatidyl-choline (DPPC) were calculated as described previously [7]. Calculations were performed on an Olivetti M28 computer equipped with the 80287 arithmetic coprocessor using the PC-MSA program (molecular structure analysis) and the PC-TAMMO procedure (theoretical analysis of molecular membrane organization); graphs were drawn with the PC-MGM program (molecular graphics manipulation) (Datavision, Brussels).

Results

Inhibition of Adenyl Cyclase

Table 1 shows the results of the study of adenyl cyclase activity in PMNs preincubated for 30 min with coumermycin. For the three agonists studied, the concentration of coumermycin inhibiting 50% of the control activity was 1–2 mg/liter.

Conformational Analysis

Coumermycin has 22 rotational angles and if these angles were affected by systematic 60° changes, more than 10^{10} conformers could be designed. To avoid these large numbers of conformations, a systematic anaylsis was carried out in a stepwise manner on different parts of the molecules to give a structure tree. Figure 1 a shows the structural formula and the torsional angles of coumermycin. Following application of the energy minimization procedure at the lipid interface, one most

Table 1. Inhibition of adenyl cyclase of human polymorphonuclear leukocytes by coumermycin. Preincubation for 30 min at 37 °C. Viability >97%

Coumermycin concentration (μg/ml)	Adenyl cyclase activity as a percentage of control agonists		
	GppNHp 10^{-4} *M*	NaF 10 m*M*	Forskolin 10^{-5} *M*
0.1	97.0	87.0	86.0
0.5	100.0	93.0	100.0
1.0	60.6	73.8	65.0
2.0	25.6	24.9	–
5.0	3.0	5.0	3.0
10.0	3.0	4.2	5.4

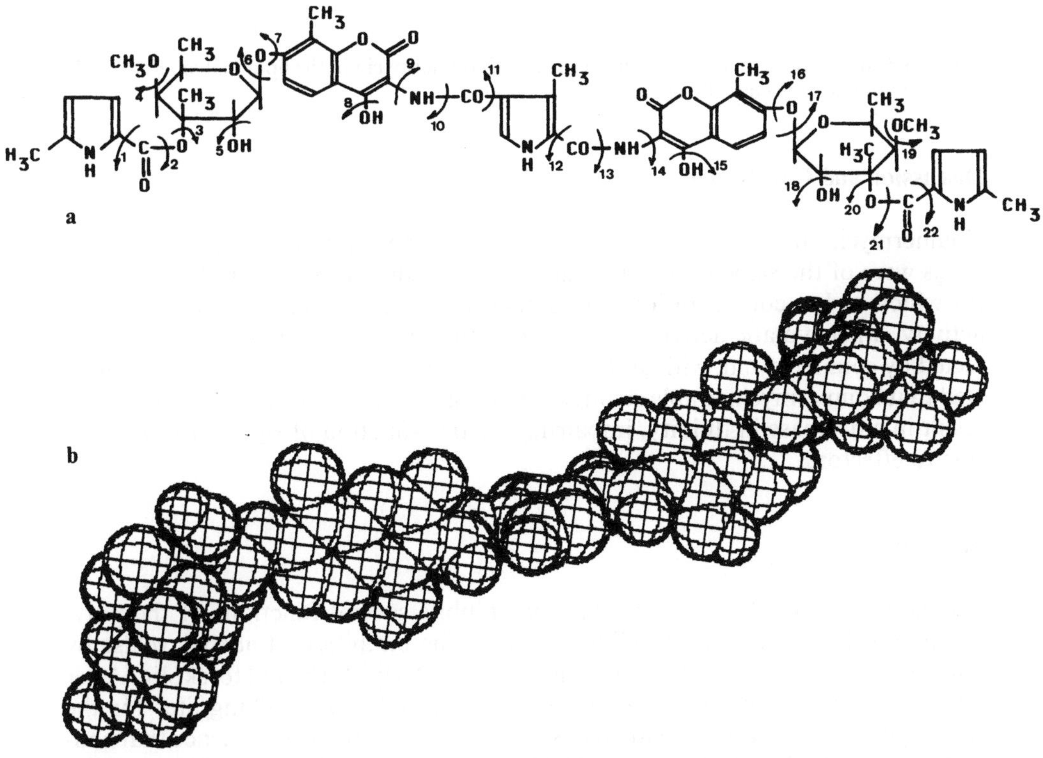

Fig. 1. a Structural formula of coumermycin with numbering of torsional angles. **b** Space-filling cross-hatching representation of the most probable conformers obtained after structure tree analysis and minimization procedure at the lipid-water interface

probable conformer was obtained (Fig. 1 b). This conformer was inserted into a DPPC monolayer. Figure 2 shows a stereoview of the mode of insertion of coumermycin in the lipid matrix. Five lipid molecules surround one coumermycin molecule and the mean energy of interaction between coumermycin and lipids is −13.43 kcal/mol. The mean energy of interaction between DPPC molecules in a monolayer is −13.0 kcal/mol.

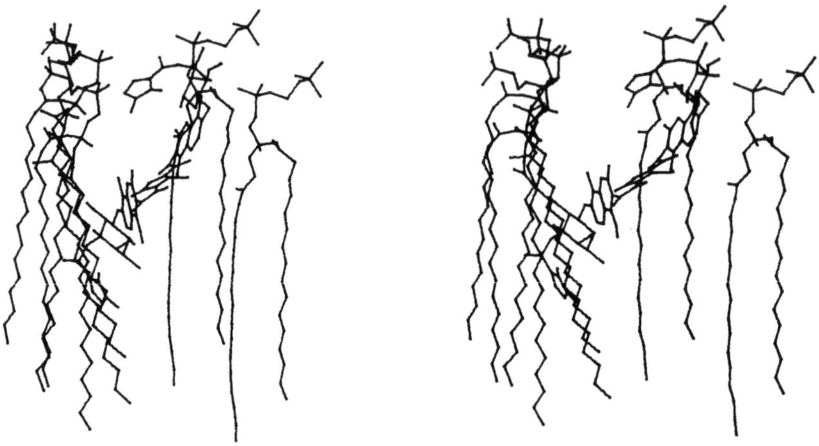

Fig. 2. Skeleton stereoscopic view of the insertion of coumermycin in the lipid matrix. Five lipids interact with one molecule of coumermycin

Discussion and Conclusion

Coumermycin inhibits several functions of the PMNs in vitro [1–4]. Most of the IC_{50}s were of the same order of magnitude, with the exception of phagocytosis, for which higher concentrations of coumermycin were required. Adenyl cyclase activity, an enzymatic activity associated with the membrane, was markedly affected by coumermycin, with an IC_{50} of 1–2 mg/liter. Computer modeling suggested that coumermycin is able strongly to interact with the membrane. This might result in a decrease in fluidity, impairing the transduction of signals from receptors to effectors.

Summary

Coumermycin, a DNA-gyrase inhibitor, inhibits several functions of the polymorphonuclear leukocytes (PMNs) in vitro. The inhibition of adenylcyclase by coumermycin was studied using the agonists GppNHp, NaF, and forskolin. After 30 min of preincubation with coumermycin, the IC_{50} was 1–2 mg/liter for the three agonists. Conformational analysis by computer provided evidence that coumermycin strongly interacted with PMN membranes, probably resulting in a decreased fluidity.

Acknowledgements. We are grateful to Dr. P. Robberecht, Laboratoire de Chimie Biologique et de la Nutrition, Université Libre de Bruxelles, who performed the adenyl cyclase assays.

References

1. Van der Auwera P, Petrikkos G, Husson M, Klastersky J (1986) Influence of various antibiotics on superoxide generation by normal human neutrophils. Arch Int Physiol Biochim 86:S23–S28
2. Van der Auwera P, Husson M, Frühling J (1987) Influence of various antibiotics on phagocytosis of *Staphylococcus aureus* by human polymorphonuclear leukocytes. J Antimicrob Chemother 20:399–404
3. Van der Auwera P, Matsumoto T, Husson M (1988) Intraphagocytic penetration of antibiotics. J Antimicrob Chemother 22:185–192
4. Petrikkos G, Van der Auwera P, Husson M, Klastersky J (1987) Influence of the DNA-gyrase inhibitor coumermycin on the functions of human neutrophils. Annual meeting of the American Society of Clinical Microbiology, March 1987. Atlanta, p 94 (abstract D 135)
5. Salomon Y, Londos C, Rodbell MA (1974) A highly sensitive adenylate cyclase assay. Anal Biochem 58:541–544
6. Waelbroeck M, Robberecht P, Coy DH, Camus JC, de Neef P, Christophe J (1985) Interaction of growth hormone-releasing factor (GRF) and 14 GRF analogs with Vasoactive Intestinal Peptide (VIP) receptors of rat pancreas. Discovery of (N-Ac-Typ^1, D-Phe^2)-GRf (1–2g)-NH_2 as a VIP antagonist. Endocrinology 116:2643–2649
7. Brasseur R, Goormaghtigh E, Ruysschaert JM (1981) Theoretical conformational analysis of phospholipids bilayers. Biochem Biophys Res Commun 103:301–310
8. Brasseur R, Deleers M, Malaisse WJ, Ruysschaert JM (1982) Conformational analysis of the calcium-A23187 complex at a lipid-water interface. Proc Natl Acad Sci USA 78:2835–2897
9. Brasseur R, Hurwitz HD (1983) A conformational analysis of propylene carbonate molecule absorbed at the mercury electrode. J Electro Chem 148:249–270
10. Brasseur R (1986) Theoretical analysis of membrane molecular organization. J Molec Graphics 1:117–120
11. Brasseur R, Deleers M (1984) Conformational analysis of 6-cis- and 6-trans-leukotriene B_4-calcium complexes. Proc Natl Acad Sci USA 81:3370–3379
12. Brasseur R, Deleers M (1983) Theoretical study of conformation-related activity of hypoglycemic sulfonylurease. Pharmacol Res Commun 15:901–907
13. Brasseur R, Ruysschaert JM (1984) Evidence of a thromboxane A2$-$CA2$+$ complex: a conformational approach. Res Commun Chem Pathol Pharmacol 46:175–185
14. Nelder JA, Mead R (1965) A simplex method for function minimization. Computer J 7:308–313
15. Hopfinger AJ (1973) Conformational properties of macromolecules. Academic, New York
16. Tanford C (1973) The hydrophobic effects: formation of micelles and biologic membranes. Wiley, New York
17. Ralston E, DeCoen JL (1973) Folding of polypetide chains induced by the amino-acid side chains. J Mol Biol 83:65–92
18. Brasseur R, Ruysschaert JM (1986) Conformation and mode of organization of amphiphilic membrane components: a conformational analysis. Biochem J 238:1–11
19. Brasseur R, Deleers M, Ruysschaert JM (1986) Mode of organization of amphiphilic molecules at the lipid-water interface: a conformational analysis. J Colloid Interface Sci 114:277–281

Concluding Remarks

J. S. REMINGTON

This symposium has contributed new and substantive data and concepts on the subject of the influence of antibiotics on the host-parasite relationship. The breadth of disciplines covered by the speakers and the broadly based expertise represented by the participants, as evidenced by the eclectic nature of the open discussions, resulted in a well-rounded symposium which was both enlightening and enjoyable. Its scientific content was interesting, instructive, and important and the concerted attempt to stimulate discussion was highly successful and edifying for us all.

The narrow view that antibiotics act solely by themselves to effect killing of microorganisms is no longer tenable. As highlighted by the papers delivered at this symposium, they are able in vitro to modify both cellular and humoral immune responses of the host and to alter pathogens in such a way as to increase their susceptibility to inhibition or killing by effector mechanisms of host resistance. The speakers were careful to point out that further work will be required to clarify the importance and clinical relevance of these in vitro observations to the in vivo situation in humans.

It is apparent from the presentations and discussions that substantial progress has been made in the technological development of newer methods to evaluate host-cell–parasite interactions. Advances have also been made in the biochemical, physicochemical, and molecular biological manipulation of the parasites to allow for closer and more objective scrutiny of their relationships with the cellular and humoral mechanisms of host resistance.

We were informed that a number of different antibiotics, representative of most of the classes of antimicrobial agents, and even some new ones, can themselves have a profound influence in vitro on functions of both the afferent and efferent limbs of host resistance. This effect may be on the host's phagocytes or lymphocytes per se, on the ability of the organisms to interact with these cells, or both.

In the studies on phagocytosis of bacteria, it became obvious that there is a vital need for standardization of both materials and methods. This is essential if unifying concepts are to be drawn from results obtained by different investigators. Examples are: the importance of differences in reactivity of cells and antibodies of different species and even between different individuals within the same species; the constituents of the bacterial growth medium; the phase in the growth

Research Institute, Palo Alto Medical Foundation, 860 Bryant Street, Palo Alto, CA 94301, USA

The Influence of Antibiotics on the Host-Parasite Relationship III
Edited by G. Gillissen, W. Opferkuch, G. Peters, and G. Pulverer

cycle that an organism is in which is being used in an assay; the presence or absence on an organism of pili, K1 polysaccharide, or protein A, the length of time that organisms are allowed to produce slime; and the duration of antimicrobial treatment on the susceptibility of organisms to phagocytosis and intracellular killing. Since the participants in this symposium made up the vast majority of scientists working in this field of investigation, it became obvious that it is their obligation, and indeed their charge, to accomplish this task of standardization. In addition, whenever feasible, it was agreed that an attempt should be made to determine whether there is an in vivo correlate for the in vitro observation.

The preeminence of the staphylococcus and of *Escherichia coli* in the presentations was obvious. Their use was not so much by conviction or concept as it was by necessity. The dominance of these organisms in studies of the effect of antibiotics on the host-parasite relationship is understandable when one places into perspective the available techniques to study host effector cell function and our knowledge of the mechanisms of action of available antimicrobial agents.

A number of investigators focused our attention on the often dual nature of an antibiotic in relation to host resistance – the antibiotic may act as a double-edged sword – at least in vitro – one edge cutting the organism and the other incapacitating a major means of host defense, the oxidative burst which occurs during phagocytosis of microorganisms. This was exemplified by the studies with certain of the macrolide antibiotics and clindamycin.

The elucidation of the nature of the neutrophil receptor for clindamycin and of the necessity of an active transport system for entry of this antibiotic into the host cell should serve as an impetus to search for similar requirements for other antibiotics which attain higher intracellular than extracellular levels. The subcellular compartments where these drugs are concentrated and the reasons for the lack of intracellular microbicidal activity by some of them remain to be defined.

The area of investigation of lectins and their receptors is rapidly evolving and its importance to pathogenicity of bacteria and other infectious organisms is clear. Its value to the disciplines addressed by this symposium was equally obvious. The effect of antimicrobials, particularly on expression of these lectins by pathogens, and thereby their capacity to influence the ability of an organism to colonize or invade the host or paraphernalia such as indwelling catheters, was discussed and has become a critical area for investigation – the host cell receptor can now be identified and the antibiotic activity manipulated to alter expression of a specific lectin and thereby its organ specificity. One of the problems discussed in the work on adherence was the differences in adherence due to variability in response of different bacterial strains (e.g., strains of *Staphylococcus aureus*) to a given antibiotic. Hopefully, this will not prove to be a significant deterrent to solving certain of the complexities of the effects of antibiotics on adherence.

An important aspect of future studies will be the use of in vivo models in laboratory animals and humans to study the influence of antibiotics on the host-parasite relationship in the mileau where "it counts." The worthwhile data that have emanated from the models in mice and humans presented at this symposium, and the clear demonstration of the lack of concordance between in vitro and in vivo results, such as in the rat endocarditis model, emphasizes that one cannot necessarily extrapolate directly from results obtained in vitro to what might occur in vivo.

Despite the fact that the effect of each antibiotic will be greater on the parasite than on the host, there is a need for additional information on the effect of these drugs on monocytes, macrophages from different anatomical sites, NK cells, LAK cells, T-cell subsets, and B cells and the receptors on these cells (e.g., complement, Fc, major histocompatibility complex). In addition, there is need to define further the effects of antibiotics on production and secretion of the various cytokines including interleukin 1 and interleukin 2, the various colony growth factors, and tumor necrosis factor, and on the expression of their receptors. Surely there will be important complementary interactions of these cytokines and antibiotics on pathogenic organisms, host cells, and host resistance against a variety of pathogens.

Subject Index

MIX
Papier aus verantwortungsvollen Quellen
Paper from responsible sources
FSC® C105338

If you have any concerns about our products,
you can contact us on
ProductSafety@springernature.com

In case Publisher is established outside the EU,
the EU authorized representative is:
Springer Nature Customer Service Center GmbH
Europaplatz 3, 69115 Heidelberg, Germany

Printed by Libri Plureos GmbH
in Hamburg, Germany